Primary Nursing
in Perspective

Edited by

Steven Ersser

BSc (Hons), RGN
Clinical Lecturer in Nursing, Institute of Nursing (Oxford)

and

Elizabeth Tutton

MSc, BSc (Hons), RGN, PGCEA
Principal Lecturer in Nursing, Buckinghamshire College

SCUTARI PRESS

© Scutari Press 1991

A division of Scutari Projects, the publishing
company of the Royal College of Nursing

First published 1991
Reprinted 1992

British Library Cataloguing in Publication Data
  I. Ersser, Steven   II. Tutton, Elizabeth
  Primary nursing in perspective.
  1. Great Britain. Medicine. Nursing
  610.730941

  ISBN 1-871364-36-3

Typeset by MC Typeset Limited, Gillingham, Kent
Printed and bound in Great Britain by The Alden Press, Oxford, London and Northampton

Contents

Foreword vii

Preface ix

Acknowledgements x

Contributors xi

Part 1: Preparation for Primary Nursing 1

1 Primary Nursing – A Second Look 3
  Steven Ersser and Elizabeth Tutton

2 Introducing and Managing Change – The Move to Primary Nursing . . 31
  Christopher Johns

3 Educational Preparation for Primary Nursing 49
  Mary Fitzgerald

4 Accountability and Legal Issues in Primary Nursing 61
  Julie Goulding and John Hunt

Part 2: Primary Nursing in Practice in the United Kingdom 75

5 Primary Nursing in a Surgical Unit 77
  Chris Allsopp

6 A Change for the Better – Primary Nursing in a Medical Ward . . . 87
  Sue Chilton

7 Primary Nursing in a Unit for the Young Disabled 103
  Jan Dewing

8 Primary Nursing in a Continuing Care Unit 117
  Catherine Miller

9 Meeting the Needs of People with Acquired Immune
  Deficiency Syndrome 127
  Ann Taylor

10 Close Enough to Touch – Primary Nursing in a Psychiatric Unit . . . 141
   Chris Hart

11 Consensus – A Basis for Introducing Primary Nursing into an
   Acute Respirology Ward 153
   Angela Heslop and Shelagh Sparrow

Part 3: The Implications of Primary Nursing 165

12 Primary Nursing – Implications for the Patient 167
   Steven Ersser and Elizabeth Tutton

13 Primary Nursing – Implications for the Nurse 183
   Jan Dewing

14 Managerial Implications of Primary Nursing 197
   Heather Jane Sears and Shirley Williams

15 Power and Communication Issues in Primary Nursing 217
   Richard McMahon

16 Educational Implications of Primary Nursing 227
   Sarah Burns

Part 4: Conclusion 239

17 Primary Nursing in Perspective 241
   Steven Ersser and Elizabeth Tutton

Appendix I Primary Nursing Network Information 261

Appendix II Examples of Job Descriptions 263

Cumulative Bibliography 272

Index 287

Foreword

"To move forward requires flexibility and critical evaluation, and therefore we expect to continue to learn and modify this approach to care". Thus writes one of the authors of this text which combines a critical and authoritative review of primary nursing, with practical and detailed accounts of the introduction and practice of primary nursing in the United Kingdom, in a number of different settings. All the authors are nurses with experience of primary nursing and some, in addition, are teachers and researchers.

The result is a rich source of help to those who are just beginning the journey of introducing primary nursing, those who want to evaluate the results so far and to reflect on the benefits or otherwise of primary nursing to patients and nurses, and those who want to undertake research. A key chapter reviews the research on patient satisfaction and the quality of nursing care, and there is an extensive bibliography.

This is a book to dip into: it has different seams of gold for beginners and established practitioners of primary nursing, for those with responsibility for managing the big changes of introducing primary nursing and for the associated teaching and research.

Primary Nursing in Perspective offers the opportunity to stand back mentally and emotionally and think more critically about the development of primary nursing in the United Kingdom. This opportunity is an important contribution to nursing and one that I believe will be valued and widely used. I recommend this book to you.

Susan Pembrey OBE, RGN, FRCN, Ph.D
Director, Institute of Nursing, Oxford
& Clinical Practice Development Nurse, Oxfordshire Health Authority

Preface

This book grew out of our interest and experience as primary nurses on the Oxford Nursing Development Unit. As a method of organising nursing care, primary nursing raises many issues about nursing practice which go far beyond the question of how nursing is best organised. The shape of the book is the product of our discussions with many nurses, our reading and our work experience.

The theoretical underpinnings and practicalities of primary nursing within the British hospital system have, however, only recently begun to be explored. It is our purpose to continue this exploration of the relationship between theory and practice by presenting experiences of individuals practising primary nursing in a variety of nursing specialties. All the contributors to this book have been involved, to some degree, in the practice of primary nursing and were eager to share their trials and tribulations with other nurses. The intention is not to sell primary nursing but rather to consider the issues involved in changing the way nursing is organised. To consider a change in practice of this scale is quite a responsibility and so we have tried to present a realistic, and constructively critical picture of the practice of primary nursing.

To provide a clear structure for the reader the book has been divided into four sections:

- Part 1: Preparation for Primary Nursing
- Part 2: Primary Nursing in Practice in the United Kingdom
- Part 3: The Implications of Primary Nursing
- Part 4: Conclusion

Part 1 begins with an exploration of the underlying concepts of primary nursing. The historical context of primary nursing is also considered, and justification for its use is made by arguing that primary nursing has the potential to counterbalance the dehumanising effect of today's health care system. Primary nursing constitutes a change in practice for many nurses and any change in nursing has repercussions at many different levels of the organisation. A discussion of the effects of change and guidance on how to plan change are provided. Educational preparation for primary nursing is essential for the maintenance of the new norms and for the continued provision of high quality nursing care. Significant changes in accountability and certain legal issues are also given consideration.

The reality of practice described in part 2 constitutes the 'heart' of the book. It is our belief that, at the expense of a minimum of repetition, nurses will be able to learn from the description of different personal experiences of those engaged in the practice of primary nursing. Each setting is unique, proving a need for flexibility and individuality in the setting up and day-to-day running of primary nursing.

Part 3 describes many implications arising from primary nursing. For instance, how does primary nursing affect patients' experience of health care? What effect does primary nursing have on the welfare of patients and nurses? How does one manage primary nursing? Does the balance of power at ward level change in primary nursing. Does primary nursing foster or inhibit the clinical education of learners? As always there are many more questions than answers, and the chapters have only just begun to scratch the surface of these issues. Our intention is to provide a review of the literature so that nurses can make their own decisions about the development of their nursing practice.

Part 4 attempts to synthesise issues from the practice chapters and the literature by addressing some of the key issues in the practice of primary nursing in the UK today.

We hope this book will serve as a resource or ideas book for nurses that raises many issues but does not provide all the answers. The intention is that nurses will dip into individual chapters, depending on their areas of interest.

Our commitment to the development and exploration of primary nursing arises from our belief in the opportunities it can create for patients and primary nurses. Changes in practice will never be all things to all people, but we hope that you will discover some of the many opportunities that primary nursing can create.

For reasons of convention and not because of our beliefs about gender stereotyping we will refer to nurses as 'she' and patients as 'he'.

Acknowledgements

Many people have helped us with this project. Firstly we must give our thanks to all the contributors who have suffered our editorial badgering for the last year. We are also most grateful for the assistance and comments of Kate Robinson, Anne-Marie Rafferty, Marg Johnson and Alison Binnie. We cannot avoid mention of all those staff who worked on the Oxford Nursing Development Unit who created such a marvellous environment for developing clinical nursing. This stimulus had a great influence on our writing.

Special thanks also extend to Kate, Richard and long suffering Charles for their help and encouragement.

Contributors

Chris Allsopp, MSc, BSc(Hons), RGN, Lecturer-Practitioner, formerly Primary Nurse, John Radcliffe Hospital, Oxford

Sarah Burns, RGN, SCM, DN(Lond), DNEd(Lond), Lecturer-Practitioner, John Radcliffe Hospital, Oxford

Sue Chilton, BNurs, Macmillan Nurse, Bromsgrove and Reddich District Health Authority. Formerly Ward Sister, Alexander Hospital, Redditch

Jan Dewing, DN(Lond), RGN, Lecturer-Practitioner, Ritchie Russell House. Formerly Staff Support Nurse, Ritchie Russell House, Churchill Hospital, Oxford

Steven Ersser, BSc(Hons), RGN, Clinical Lecturer in Nursing, Institute of Nursing (Oxford). Department of Dermatology, Slade Hospital Oxford. Formerly Nurse Practitioner, Oxford Nursing Development Unit.

Mary Fitzgerald, MN, RGN, DN(Lond), CertEd(FE), Lecturer-Practitioner, John Radcliffe Hospital, Oxford

Julie Goulding, RGN, FETC, Resource Management Project Manager, Sandwell District General Hospital. Formerly Ward Sister, John Radcliffe Hospital, Oxford

Chris Hart, MA, RMN, RGN, Care Group Manager, Bloomsbury HA Mental Health Unit. Formerly Senior Charge Nurse, Maudsley Hospital, London

Angela Heslop, RGN, RCNT, DN(Lond), Joint Appointment Ward Sister/Respiratory Health Worker, Charing Cross Hospital, London

E. John Hunt, LLB, FHSM, MIPM, General Manager, Harefield Hospital, Middlesex

Christopher Johns, MN, RMN, RGN, Cert Ed, Head of Nursing Development Unit, Burford Community Hospital, Burford, Oxfordshire

Richard McMahon, MA, DN(Lond), RGN, Senior Nurse (Elderly Care), Horton General Hospital, Banbury, Oxfordshire. Formerly Nurse Practitioner, Oxford Nursing Development Unit

Catherine Miller, RGN, FETC, Senior Nurse, Royal Marsden Hospital, London

Heather Jane Sears, RGN, DMS, LHSM, MBIM, Regional Nurse, Oxford RHA; formerly Hospital Manager, Didcot Community Hospital, Oxfordshire

Shelagh Sparrow, MA, DN(Lond), RGN, Research Teacher Bloomsbury and Islington Health Authority. Formerly Joint Appointment Ward Sister Senior Nurse Research, Charing Cross Hospital, London

Ann Taylor, RGN, DN(Lond), Clinical Nurse Specialist, Mildmay Mission Hospital, London

Elizabeth Tutton, MSc, BSc(Hons), RGN, PGCEA, Principal Lecturer in Nursing, Buckinghamshire College; formerly Nurse Practitioner, Oxford Nursing Development Unit

Shirley Williams, RGN, RHV, Director of Nursing Services (Community Unit), Radcliffe Infirmary, Oxford. Formerly DNS (Acute Unit), Radcliffe Infirmary

PART 1

Preparation for Primary Nursing

1

Primary Nursing – A Second Look

Steven Ersser and Elizabeth Tutton

The intention of this chapter is to provide some background to primary nursing for the subsequent chapters. Its title reflects the need to take a deeper look at the issues that surround primary nursing and the complexities of its practice. The information is organised around three central themes. The first explores the nature of primary nursing, taking into account the major concepts surrounding this approach and comparing them with those within team nursing, patient allocation and task allocation. The following historical section establishes the place of primary nursing within the development of the organisation of nursing work documenting in particular issues and trends within the UK since the mid-nineteenth century. Finally the humanising hospital care theme covers various complex interrelated issues that are of current concern to nurses. In particular we look at the possible place of primary nursing in counteracting the dehumanising features of hospital care.

THE NATURE OF PRIMARY NURSING

Primary nursing, according to Manthey (1980), is a method of organising nursing care. However, like the nursing process, it is said to encompass also a philosophy of care (Hegyvary, 1982). It is therefore important to analyse the concepts reflected by the term to clarify its meaning. One important benefit of this approach is that it may help nurses to identify movement or progress towards particular aspects of nursing that are seen as desirable such as the degree of continuity of care or the level and pattern of accountability exercised by particular nurses on the ward.

The issue of whether or not a unit is practising primary nursing is not as significant as the need to identify movement towards conditions that are seen as desirable in the organisation of nursing. Alternatively, questions may be asked such as to what extent the nurse planning care is providing it, or, to what extent this nurse is engaged in direct communication with the patient, his family and the ward team.

To facilitate the process of clarification, the concepts within primary nursing will also be compared with those within three other methods of nurse assignment:

● Team nursing
● Patient allocation, also called day-to-day patient or case assignment
● Functional or task assignment

The labels given to the different organisational patterns suggest that there is a clear-cut division between assignment methods and that they are easily identified. Munson and Clinton (1979) suggest that nurse assignment patterns are not clear cut but maybe a mixture of one or more methods. They developed a tool to measure assignment patterns along a continuum. The continuum was based on Horn and Parker's (1975) four main attributes of quality care:

- Comprehensiveness of care
- Accountability for care
- Continuity
- Co-ordination of care

Primary nursing may be depicted as positioned at some point along a continuum for each of these attributes. Furthermore, those who describe their practice as 'primary nursing' may be able to distinguish their position along the various continua from those of other units also said to be practising primary nursing. To identify the key concepts inherent in primary nursing, four global definitions of primary nursing were considered (see figure 1.1). Analysis of these definitions suggests that the key concepts of primary nursing relate to:

Marram *et al.* (1976)

... the delivery of comprehensive, continuous co-ordinated and individualized patient care through the primary nurse who has autonomy, accountability and authority to act as a chief nurse for her patients.

Anderson and Choi (1980: 29)

Primary nursing is a system organised to maximise continuous and comprehensive delivery of nursing care to patients. Emphasis is on one nurse having professional/organisational autonomy in assuming responsibility and retaining accountability for planning and when possible personally administering total care to designated patients throughout their hospital-isation. Ideally, this responsibility is expanded to include such patients episodes as readmissions, home care clinic visits and other outpatient related activities.

Manthey (1980: 31)

1. Allocation and acceptance of individual responsibility for decision-making to one individual.
2. Assignment of daily care by case method.
3. Direct person-to-person communication.
4. One person operationally responsible for the quality of care administered to patients on a unit 24 hours a day, seven days a week.

Point 4 has since been updated to 'total responsibility for a patient while he receives nursing services from a particular department or agency' (Manthey 1988: 645).

Hegyvary (1982: 3)

1. *Accountability.* One nurse, the primary nurse, answerable for the nursing care of a patient 24 hours a day throughout the patient's hospitalization.
2. *Autonomy.* The primary nurse has and acts on the authority to make decisions about nursing care of her patients in the mode of professional self governance.
3. *Co-ordination.* Nursing care is continuous around the clock, with smooth, uninterrupted flow from shift to shift and with direct communication from care giver to care giver.
4. *Comprehensive.* Each care giver performs all required nursing care for a patient during a specific time period such as a shift.

Fig. 1.1 Definitions of primary nursing.

● Particular patterns of responsibility, authority, autonomy and accountability
● Continuity of care
● Care planner as care giver
● Direct communication

These concepts are closely aligned to Manthey's (1980) four design elements, which are:

● Responsibility for the quality of nursing care
● Daily assignment by the case method
● Direct channels of communication
● Care giver as care planner

The concepts derived from the definitions of primary nursing could be viewed on a continuum from a high degree to a low degree according to the particular organisational method, and also were specific to its practice in individual units (see figure 1.2). Depending on what is valued as desirable movement, along this continuum such an approach may be used as a crude indicator of development. Figure 1.3 (overleaf) seeks to demonstrate how each of the concepts in figure 1.2 may be viewed from within the four major methods of nurse assignment.

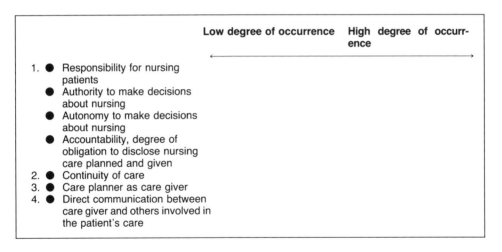

Fig. 1.2 The concepts of primary nursing depicted as a continuum.

For the purpose of discussion the four major methods of nurse assignment will be viewed as 'ideal types'. Abercrombie *et al.* (1980) see ideal types as hypothetical constructions that have explanatory value. These constructions will not have all the characteristics of a real situation, but real situations can be understood by comparison with an ideal type. If the four assignment methods described are seen as ideal types they may be positioned along the continua as demonstrated in figure 1.3.

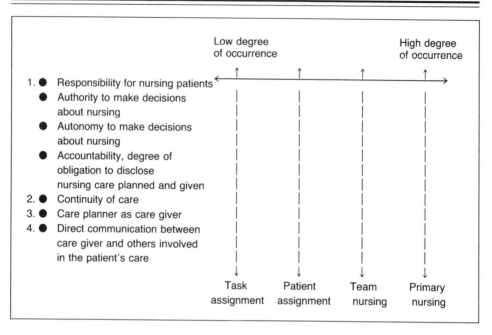

Fig. 1.3 The four assignment methods depicted on a continuum using the concepts derived from the definition of primary nursing.

Primary Nursing

Responsibility/Authority/Autonomy/Accountability

All the definitions of primary nursing consider one nurse to be answerable for decisions about nursing – in particular its overall direction – and also for a named group of patients on a continuous basis. The primary nurse is presented as being responsible for particular actions, or accountable for them, or both. The use of terms may vary between authors, and chapter 4 considers these terms in some depth. Lewis and Batey (1982) provide perhaps the clearest distinction between the terms, saying that responsibility is the charge, and accountability is 'to disclose about the charge'. Manthey (1980) proposes that nurses who opt to be primary nurses accept the responsibility accompanying the role, which implies that it cannot be imposed.

The assumption is also that the nurse is qualified and is legitimately able to accept this responsibility. A nurse therefore needs to accept this responsibility formally before taking on the role of primary nurse. The charge in primary nursing is both to plan and provide direct nursing care for a named group of patients. Disclosure concerning the nursing care provided for the patients may be demonstrated in written form in care planning or verbal form at handover sessions. Emphasis needs to be placed on proactive planning as opposed to reactive planning (Lewis and Batey, 1982). As such, patient goals and nursing intervention should be orientated towards forward planning instead of merely reacting to or describing present events.

Both Manthey (1980) and Hegyvary (1982) suggest that responsibility and accountability for nursing care extend over the 24 hour day. This implies that care planning by the primary nurse must be proactive so that a plan of care can be left for other nurses to follow. Hegyvary (1982: 4) does not consider 24-hour accountability to mean 'hands on care around the clock'. The primary nurse provides the overall direction of the nursing care but does not, of course, have to be present all the time. Some clinical areas operated an on-call system where primary nurses were called at home when changes in care were needed. This was very successful in the Oxford Nursing Development Unit but this system is not essential.

It is important that a unit adopts a protocol acceptable to all concerned, which sets out what should happen in the absence of the primary nurse when the patient's circumstances change and nursing decisions have to be made. Twenty-four hour accountability is embodied within the care plan, which enables the primary nurse's instructions to continue over this period. When the primary nurse is absent, associate nurses perform the nursing care in accordance with the set plan, but have to justify changes in care to the primary nurse on her return. The primary nurse retains the right to change the care plan on her return and as such retains accountability for the overall direction of nursing care. The associate nurse's role in decision making in the absence of a primary nurse may be considered on a continuum as displayed in figure 1.4.

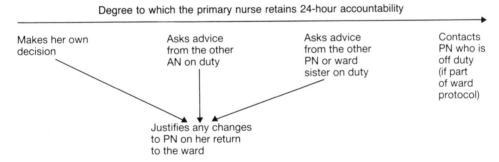

Fig. 1.4 The role of the associate nurse in decision making in the absence of the primary nurse: AN, associate nurse; PN, primary nurse.

The difference between the primary and associate nurse's levels of accountability may also be demonstrated on a continuum using a sample of an off-duty rota as in figure 1.5.

Authority (the power to act) and autonomy (freedom to act) (Lewis and Batey, 1982) are present in three of the definitions of primary nursing. This is not surprising, as the four concepts are all interrelated. In fact it is impossible to be accountable if authority and autonomy are not also present.

Traditionally authority and autonomy for decision making are invested in the role of ward sister. In primary nursing, authority and autonomy are devolved to the primary nurse. The primary nurse needs to have achieved a level of competence in which she can use her authority and autonomy to benefit the patient.

	Weekdays						
	Monday	Tuesday	Wednesday	Thursday	Friday	Saturday	Sunday
PN	Early	Early	Off	Off	Early	Early	Early
Degree of accountability							
AN 1	Late,	Late,	Early,	Early,	Off	Off,	Late,
Degree of accountability							
AN 2						Late,	Late,
Degree of accountability							

Fig. 1.5 Diagram to demonstrate the difference between primary and associate nurses' levels of accountability: PN, primary nurse; AN, associate nurse; Early, day duty; Late, evening duty; Off, off duty.

Continuity of Care

Continuous accountability by one nurse for a named group of patients is integral to all the definitions, although there is some variation in the duration of the continuity. Hegyvary (1982: 3) suggests that continuity is for the duration of hospitalisation whereas Anderson and Choi (1980: 29) expand this to include readmissions and clinic visits. From experience of working with nurses in Accident and Emergency and Outpatients departments, Manthey (1988: 645) also widened her definition to include continued outpatient attendance. Continuity of care may have implications for the formation of a nurse–patient relationship and its consequences.

Care Planner as Care Giver

In primary nursing the nurse who has responsibility for planning care for a patient also provides that care for her patients when on duty. However, Anderson and Choi (1980: 29) qualify this by stating 'when possible'. This raises the issue of how much care the primary nurse has to provide to maintain her position of accountability for a case load of patients.

Manthey (1988: 644) said that the primary nurse 'needs to give enough direct care to assess the patient's status and the effectiveness of the decisions currently in place'. How much direct care time a primary nurse has depends on the skill mix of the ward, the nature of patients' needs, and the roles adopted by the individuals within the team. Environmental factors such as the geographical position of the patient may also affect time available for direct care. The number of hours a nurse works may affect nurses' ability to become care planners and care givers. In acute areas, where patient changes are rapid primary nurses may need to be in full-time posts. In areas where changes in the patient's condition are at a slower rate this may not need to be the case (see chapter 14).

Direct Communication

The necessity for direct person-to-person communication within primary nursing is referred to by Manthey (1980) and Hegyvary (1982:3). This refers to the commitment that the primary nurse will be the key communicator with all the people concerned with the patient's welfare. The primary nurse as the care planner will use the information gained through opportunities to interact with the patient to make key decisions regarding the patient's care. Hegyvary (1982: 3) implies that the primary nurse communicates directly with the nurse who cares for the patients on the next shift to facilitate co-ordinated care. Manthey (1980: 37) extends this to responsibility for initiating communication directly with other members of the health team who either have information she needs or who need information she has. Emphasis is also placed on open and direct communication with the patient and his family. This concept also has implications for the role of the ward sister, who has traditionally held the position of key communicator within the nursing team.

Team Nursing

Responsibility/Authority/Autonomy/Accountability

Walters (1985) describes team nursing as a method of allocating a group of nurses to a group of patients; a definition wide enough to include a myriad of different practices. The number of nurses and patients and the duration of their allocation is not specified. Work assignment could be task-centred, patient-centred or a mixture of both. Team nursing may also be seen within a historical context (see the Historical overview below). Kron (1971), one of the early writers on team nursing, suggests that the key worker for particular patients is the team leader. The team leader is a registered nurse who accepts delegated responsibilities and duties from the ward sister. The exercise of responsibility, authority, autonomy and accountability for the quality of nursing care a patient receives may therefore be held by the team leader. The team leader is responsible for matching team members' skills to the needs of the patient and providing overall continuity of care (Kron, 1971). All the nurses in the team attempt to get to know all the patients cared for by that team and contribute to care planning so that all the patients benefit from the combined nursing skills of the team members.

Continuity of Care

Team nursing presents limitations in the extent to which the care planned is carried out by the same nurses and is proactive. The duration of continuity between the team of nurses and groups of patients is not specified. If the team is allocated to patients for only part of their stay in hospital, the overall responsibility for the quality of patient care will be fragmented. Responsibility for the quality of care a patient receives for the duration of his stay remains partly with the ward sister, who is often required to ensure continuity between team changeovers. Continuity of care may also be disrupted by changes within the nursing team unless there is a policy to maintain team stability. Manthey (1980) and Marram *et al.* (1974) criticise team nursing on the basis that the team holds group responsibility and hence no one person may be responsible for the overall quality of care received by patients. In comparison Walters (1985) argues that team nursing can provide continuity of care as the same group of nurses is able to work with the same group of patients over a period of time. Opportunities are also present for nurses to understand their patients' individual needs and to develop relationships.

Care Planner as Care Giver

In team nursing the team leader carries the responsibility for care planning but is not necessarily carrying out direct nursing care. The nursing work is shared among the team members on the basis of individual competence. Manthey (1980) and Marram *et al.* (1974) suggest that this may lead to disjointed care provision, with the most experienced nurse – the team leader – providing the least 'hands-on' care. However, there are some benefits. Walters (1985) sees the educational opportunities of student nurses working with registered nurses as advantageous. She suggests that team leaders are also more able to develop their managerial and leadership skills.

Direct Communication

Ward communication patterns are complex within team nursing (Manthey, 1980). With team nursing, all changes in the patient's condition are passed through the team leader, who will take appropriate action. If she is unable to do this the ward sister's advice is typically sought (Kron, 1971). Walters (1985) suggests that problems may occur if multidisciplinary team members are unsure of whom they should communicate with about patients' treatments. However, this may also occur within primary nursing. Manthey (1980) proposes that the team leader's position is untenable as she has to remember vast amounts of information and recall it at a moment's notice. (Presumably this is because of the anticipated larger patient group size than with primary nursing.) It has been suggested that the ward sister may feel that her role has been eroded as the team leaders have more information about the patients than she has (Walters, 1985). Kron (1971) proposes that the ward sister's role becomes one of a specialist nurse involved in co-ordinating nursing activities, supervising team leaders and providing education support.

Patient Assignment/Patient allocation

Responsibility/Authority/Autonomy/Accountability

Patient allocation is a form of nursing assignment which involves the allocation of one or more nurses to a group of patients (Berry and Metcalf, 1986). The duration of nurse assignment to patients may change on a day-to-day basis (Pearson, 1988), although there is potential for this period to be longer. Within this method of assignment the overall responsibility, authority, autonomy and accountability for the quality of care remains with the sister/nurse in charge. Care planning may be performed by the sister/nurse in charge (Chavasse, 1981) or she may choose to delegate this to the nurses who are providing direct care. The sister/nurse in charge, however, maintains overall control of this activity and hence retains authority over nursing actions. Individual nurses are responsible and accountable (within their level of competence) for the care they provide for a group of patients for the duration of the shift.

Continuity of Care

Continuity of care is provided for the duration of the shift or longer, depending on the duration of the allocation. Each nurse is accountable for the care she provides on each shift. However, accountability for the overall direction of care is fragmented as each nurse may plan care differently or may change the previous nurse's plan. Unless the sister/nurse in charge is able to keep a tight control over care planning, care may become fragmented, making evaluation difficult. Pearson (1988) said that lack of continuity may prevent nurses from developing a close nurse–patient relationship. Consequently this may reduce the nurses' abilities to plan care effectively as they may have a limited knowledge of the patients' interrelated needs.

Care Planner as Care Giver

Care planning may be performed by the sister/nurse in charge or may be jointly shared between the nurse providing the direct care and the sister. Matthews (1975) considers it to be beneficial for the care giver to be the care planner so that the nurse understands the patient's individual needs. However, even if this does occur, care planning for the duration of the patient's stay will be disjointed as the patient may have a different nurse planning his care on each shift. The extent to which the care planned is proactive is also limited as the nurse who planned the care may not be able to follow it through.

Direct Communication

The major channel of communiction is through the sister/nurse in charge. Changes in patients' care are channelled through the sister/nurse in charge to the multidisciplinary team and vice versa as necessary. Individual nurses communicate with the rest of the nursing team through the nursing notes and at handover between shifts (Matthews, 1975). Communication channels remain complex.

Task Assignment/Task Allocation

Responsibility/Authority/Autonomy/Accountability

Task assignment is an established bureaucratic working method where, for managerial convenience, nursing activities are broken down into small components (Berry and Metcalf, 1986; see Historical Overview below). It is said that the nurse within a task-oriented system 'operates within an explicit hierarchy' (Webb, 1981: 373). Thus small components or tasks are further ordered into a hierarchy of status based on the perceived hierarchy of skill necessary for its performance. Each nurse accepts responsibility for a single task or group of tasks relating to her abilities. For instance, a third-year student nurse may be allocated the aseptic dressings and a first-year student nurse the blood pressure recordings. Implicit in this hierarchy of status is the assumption that 'basic' or fundamental nursing care is simple (Hall, 1969). Overall accountability for the quality of care a patient receives for the duration of his stay and the accompanying authority and autonomy of decision making is held by the sister. Accountability and authority are held by the individual nurse mainly in respect of the assigned task.

Continuity of Care

Continuity of care is provided only in the sense that one nurse may perform several different tasks for the same patient. Otherwise, in contrast to primary nursing, task assignment represents a high level of fragmentation and discontinuity. The sister retains continuous overall accountability for the quality of care a patient receives.

Care Planner as Care Giver

The planning of nursing care within task assignment is performed by the sister/nurse in charge (Merchant, 1985). Care is then delegated to the nurse with the appropriate skills. The sister/nurse in charge may perform some traditionally high status tasks that require her expertise, such as administering medications. Care planning and providing direct nursing care are therefore separate activities. The patient is subject to a large number of carers, each concerned with providing a particular aspect of care. Typically those providing care are in a position of having to act without detailed information on any one patient or an awareness of the interrelated nature of his needs, because of the organisation of work. Manthey (1980) criticises this system on the basis that it fragments the patients' nursing care. Patients' own needs or requests may be seen to interrupt important work assignments. Webb (1981) suggests that it may force patients into a position of passivity where they are unable to control or take part in their care. This could be potentiated by the distance between the care planner and the care giver. It could, however, be argued that separating the care planner from the care giver is an efficient means of organising care. The care is planned by the qualified nurse and the subsequent work can be easily divided between student nurses and untrained staff depending on their level of competence. Melia (1987) suggests that this is a useful method of allocating work when dealing with a mobile workforce (see Historical Overview).

Direct Communication

'In a task-orientated system communications are hierarchically passed in a vertical direction' (Webb, 1981: 374). Nurse-to-nurse, shift-to-shift, and nurse-to-multidisciplinary team members' communications occur through this hierarchy of status. For instance, a junior nurse may convey a change in the patient's condition to a staff nurse, who then informs the sister, who in turn may inform the doctor. This is both a lengthy process and a complex channel for information which is subject to varying interpretation as it passes up the hierarchy.

HISTORICAL OVERVIEW OF THE ORGANISATION OF HOSPITAL WORK IN THE UK

In discussing the merits and shortcomings of the various ways of organising nursing work, it is easy to focus only on affairs at ward level and the local context within which nurse's work. A historical overview of the transitions involved in the way hospital nursing has been organised will be provided here. It is hoped that this may help to reveal something of the context in which particular practices develop or regress, and the factors shaping them. It will be seen that the natural history of such changes has not necessarily arisen from deliberate shifts in policy decisions taken by nurses, but rather by wider social influences, such as the need for economic regulation within the health service. Firstly, an examination will be made of the historical background to the emergence of primary nursing in the USA described by Marie Manthey (1970; 1980), the innovator of the approach.

To explore the changes in the organisation of nursing work in the UK it is argued here that it is inappropriate to translate the situation in the USA directly to the UK. Although some parallels will be evident, the transition from community to hospital care and from one method of organisation to another in the UK was a process of great complexity which does not follow a pattern of ordered sequential development. Some attempt has been made here to avoid the traditional interpretation of the history of nursing as unproblematic evolutionary progress, as described by Davis (1980).

A Return to the Case Method

Manthey (1980) describes the rapid expansion of hospital care from the 1920s in the USA. Before this time nursing was a predominantly community based private practice, with nursing being organised on the case method which refers to the assignment of nurses to particular patients. Attention is drawn to the similarities between the case method and public health nursing practice of the 1920s–1930s period. A central feature of Manthey's argument is that the transition of nursing into the hospital institution led to the case method being rapidly abandoned. The subsequent difficulties this created were said to account for the eventual transition from nursing organised on the basis of task (functional method) to a cyclic return, via team nursing, to the adoption of the case method in the form of primary nursing.

Expansion of Hospital Nursing in the UK

During the early nineteenth century most sick people were nursed in their homes rather than hospital (Baly, 1980) The prosperous classes of this period saw no need for hospital care since they could readily employ nurses in their own homes (Abel-Smith, 1964). They were anxious to avoid the stigma of being associated with charitable institutions serving the poor. Also, the perceived advantages of institutional care were few; the unreliability of treatments at this time would have made home nursing far more attractive to those who could afford it.

Despite the preference of the prosperous classes for home nursing rapid expansion of hospital care took place across the nineteenth century. A corresponding expansion in the in-patient population took place in the second half of the nineteenth century, a change related to the state of local economies (Abel-Smith, 1964). Maggs (1987) emphasised the constant concern administrators faced in maintaining the economic viability of their hospitals. The expansion of hospital care from the mid-nineteenth century coincided with a phase of economic stability with the rise of industrial capitalism (Baly, 1980). The majority of voluntary hospitals relied heavily on subscriptions and donations from local companies and wealthy individuals.

During this period the number of nurses working in hospitals and workhouses grew in response to the demand created by the extra beds (Abel-Smith, 1960: 50). The cost of both employing extra nurses and accommodating them was significant. Pinker (1966) provides an analysis of hospital statistics from the time of the 1861 Census to 1938. These figures reveal the difficulty and unreliability of the early data, which can only serve as a crude guide to the demand for hospital care. The statistics nonetheless reveal a doubling of in-patients in hospitals and related institutions for the physically ill from 1861 to 1891.

The development of hospital care was influenced by other areas of social change: the growth of medical science; the greater provision made for the prosperous class; the Boer War; and the increasing difficulty maintaining adequate asepsis in the home (Dingwall et al. 1988). In the 1880s the middle and upper classes began to make greater use of voluntary hospitals, which now had pay-beds, and the developing of private nursing homes (Abel-Smith, 1964).

The abandonment of the case method following the rise in the numbers of nurses practicing in hospital in the USA will now be compared with the organisation of hospital nursing in the UK at the turn of the century. An image of ward organisation at this time is drawn from the biographical studies of Maggs (1983: 108), who studied general hospital nursing of the period. He concludes that:

● . . . in most accounts of wardwork of the period it is possible to differentiate

between the tasks performed by the different grades of trainees; there was . . .
a hierarchy of tasks determined by the seniority of service and training.

Therefore, as in the USA, the organisation of nursing work in hospitals led to a
move away from the allocation of nurses on the basis of the patient to one in which
a number of nurses were assigned to complete a specific task for each patient. Baly
(1980: 227) said that practices such as 'task allocation' were deeply embedded in the
nineteenth century notion of work, that is, 'the nature of the task defines the status
of the worker'. However, reference to the existence of this notion is not made and
its relevance to nursing work is not explored. Maggs (1987) argues that such a
division of labour was based mainly on class and gender power relations and less on
skill.

Despite the rapid growth of hospital care approximately half of all nurses in the
UK continued to work in patients' homes at the turn of the century (Abel-Smith,
1960). Private nurses formed an important proportion of all nurses at this time
(Maggs, 1983). From 1891 to 1921, again, the number of hospital beds doubled;
however, during the interwar years, the prevailing economic crisis produced a
slower rate of increase (Pinker, 1966).

Post-war Organisation of Hospital Nursing

Following World War II and the birth of the National Health Service (NHS) in 1948
there was a need to tackle the nursing manpower shortage and to ensure efficiency
in the new nationalised nursing system, within manageable financial limits.

The RCN Nursing Reconstruction Committee produced a series of four reports
under Lord Horder from 1942 to 1949. The Horder Committee advocated the
industrial model of ward nursing, namely task allocation based on a firm belief that
a hierarchy of skill in nursing work legitimated an organisational approach based on
a hierarchy of tasks. Concern was expressed that boredom among SRNs might
cause them to leave the NHS. An increase in the proportion of unqualified staff
relative to qualified was proposed, with emphasis on an assistant nurse's role.
Horder also expressed anxiety about the poor supply of well educated women and
the expense of training. The Horder committee was wide ranging in the scope of its
enquiry. Despite reference to the fact that it attracted a remarkable lack of interest
in the nursing press (White, 1985: 18), such a response was not unusual at this time;
whether meritorious or not, nursing reports were not guaranteed take-up.

Continued anxiety about the adequacy of nurse training and recruitment for the
new NHS led to the establishment of the Wood Committee. The Wood Report
(1947) was a publication of the Ministry of Health and other government
departments. In contrast to the Horder enquiry the Wood report criticised the
ritualistic features of ward organisation arising from the hierarchy of tasks. It was
felt that the assistant nurse grade should not be perpetuated. Wood suggested that
the roll established in 1943 should lapse while retaining the single SRN grade
supported by student nurses and by a new nursing orderly grade. Despite these
suggestions by the Wood Committee to break the hierarchy of tasks by reducing the
stratification of nursing grades; the related Cohen (Minority) Report (1948)
following a year later advocated the continuation of the industrial model.

It is interesting that in North America at this time the practice of task or functional nursing was also seen as an acceptable method of organising nursing compatible with the demands created by an expansion of hospital care and rising financial pressures (Brown, 1966), a situation not unlike that in the UK. However, it remains unclear from Brown's paper to what extent this system became an inevitable consequence of such pressures or, rather, of other factors such as the bureaucratic organisation of hospitals or the socialisation of nurses.

By the 1950s there was growing evidence of dissatisfaction with task allocation and the advocacy of team nursing. The Nuffield Provincial Hospital Trust commissioned a study to undertake a job analysis of hospital nursing. This study, *The Work of Nurses in Hospital Wards* (Goddard Report), published in 1953, expressed its dissatisfaction with task allocation. Emphasis was placed on interpreting its proposal that nursing work be divided into three components, in rank order:

● Technical, performed by senior nurses
● Basic, performed by junior nurses
● 'Non-nursing', performed by the untrained

But White (1985) claims that the report was in fact misrepresented since it referred to the existence of such practice already and expressed concern about the difficulty of meeting specific patient needs in isolation and about the little time given to emotional care with task allocation. The Report expressed concern with the segregation of technical and basic nursing activities. Bedside care was thought to be best provided by SRNs within a group assignment system which assured that non-nursing activities were left to others (White, 1985: 197/202). It was reported that the RCN believed that the Nuffield team's objective to increase the number of qualified nurses would be neither numerically possible nor economically justifiable (Blair-Fish 1954).

The Goddard Report (1953) was referred to the Standing Nursing Advisory Committee by the Ministry of Health, who encouraged trials of case or patient assignment. Miss M. Powell, Matron of St George's Hospital, London, described a trial of 'group' or 'case' assignment which took the form of team nursing (*Nursing Times*, 1953). Powell described the trial as a successful 'educational experiment'; however, the main problems encountered were the provision of adequate supervision of juniors and ward geography (*Nursing Times*, 1953a). It was later described as an improvement on the existing arrangements for patients and staff (Jackson, 1958). Nevertheless, the Central Health Services Council (1958) Report on the success of these trials was inconclusive. Evaluation was said to be difficult because the conditions under which the trials were conducted did not ideally match this novel assignment method. However, despite these comments, the Report recommended that 'group assignment as a method of ward organisation should be introduced into hospitals as soon as practicable'. Support for group or team assignment also arose from anxiety about the significant demands placed on the ward sister's role, in particular those arising from medical developments (*Nursing Times*, 1958b).

Team nursing was said to be practised in few hospitals by the late 1950s (Watkin, 1958). White (1958: 207) speculates that difficulties with case assignment arose from organisational problems, such as maintaining cover by the team during off-duty periods, because of serious shortages of trained nurses. She also makes reference to the difficulty in identifying the cause of the problems owing to the inadequate documentation of these experiments.

The RCN (1956) policy statement, *Observations and Objectives*, stated its concern with the existing pattern of nursing organisation based on the allocation of tasks. The RCN proposed that there be both a vertical and a horizontal expansion of the nursing structure in order to meet patients' needs for total patient care. This would take the form of team nursing: a group assignment with the SRN as team leader. As such, this report was in sympathy with the Goddard Report (1953).

In contrast to the situation in the UK, team nursing was said to have swept the USA in the 1950s (Manthey, 1980: 16). However it would seem that the label 'team nursing' was often deceptive in conveying that the orientation of ward nursing had shifted from task to patient orientation. Brown (1966: 189–190) indicates that team nursing took the form of task assignment in practice, with the team leader delegating the perceived hierarchy of tasks.

During the 1950s interest was also growing in the concept of 'total patient care' (Brown, 1966). There are some indications to suggest that this notion became popular with nursing leaders in the USA to a point perhaps where it began to influence the organisation of hospital nursing. This rather nebulous concept expressed the need to give due consideration to meeting the patient's psychosocial needs. One centre that promoted this patient-centred concept of nursing was the Columbia University Teachers College (CUTC), which could be described as an important crucible for developing American nurses who were going to have a significant effect on nursing subsequently, both in the USA and, it would seem, in the UK. Meleis (1985) has described the influence that nurses such as Peplau, Henderson, Hall, Abdellah, King, Wiedenbach and Rogers had on the development of nursing theory from the 1950s. The Dean of CUTC, Francis Reiter, had a great interest in the understanding of the psychosocial determinants of behaviour: the importance of nurses enhancing their interaction skills and the importance of the distinctions between 'technical' and 'professional' nursing. Ciske (1980: 1) describes Reiter's (1966) influential writing on the 'nurse clinician' on the belief that there was a need to bring nurses of most experience and expertise to the bedside. In the light of such emphasis it was not surprising that the subsequently influential nurses educated at CUTC were to place great emphasis on patient-centred or individualised nursing.

From Brown's (1966) analysis of 1950s and 1960s in the USA it can be seen that nurses were facing problems that interfered with the organisation of hospital nursing. Severe staff shortages and the difficulty of finding a delivery system that would accommodate nursing auxiliaries, whose number proliferated in the 1940s, produced a reliance on the functional method. As the complexity of hospital care and pace of work in the USA grew, the role of the graduate nurse underwent transition, with an expansion of her technical-supervisory role. These nurses began to act as team leaders within a system of team nursing. However, problems continued with team and functional nursing.

These difficulties were compounded for those American nurses who attempted to develop a patient-centred approach to organising nursing. This is illustrated by the writing of Lydia Hall. Hall was one of the nurses from the CUTC who developed a conception of nursing in the late 1950s which she attempted to introduce in 1963, with the founding of the Loeb Centre for Nursing and Rehabilitation in New York (Meleis, 1985). Hall *et al* (1975: 2–3) had expressed concern about the current state of nursing organisation and attempts to improve on functional and team nursing. Particular reference was made to the difficulty in providing patients with continuity of care. There was said to be emphasis on both the frustration and discouragement of nurses in the USA and the fragmented, depersonalised care received by patients (Manthey, 1980: 18). Other evidence of the dissatisfaction of nurses with hospital nursing is given by Kramer's study in the 1960s (published in 1974).

In the UK not only had the NHS inherited a shortage of nurses in the post-war period, but also the service as a whole was dominated by the major problem of controlling its financial demands. Webster (1988) describes the concern to bring under greater control the costly elements of the service, such as the cost of hospital employees, of which nurses formed the largest group. Tighter control of establishments rather than remuneration was chosen as the most feasible strategy.

By the 1960s nurses working in hospitals were facing significant pressures. The rising number of in-patients in proportion to the number of hospital beds, the increasing number of consultants and the greater use of technology further exacerbated the strain of manpower shortages (Baly, 1980: 245–246).

In addition to these demands, dissatisfaction with task allocation in the UK was to continue into the 1970s. The Briggs Committee (1972) remarked on the frustration of nurses experienced with this method. They claimed that in almost two-thirds of acute hospitals the nursing work was allocated by tasks. Other evidence of its continuation throughout the decade exists (Pembrey, 1975; Bellaby and Oribabor, 1980).

There were various obstructions in the move towards patient-orientated practice which may account for the persistence of the task-orientated approach. Financial cuts and staff shortages were said to be important factors (Baly, 1980). This would support observations made in the USA (Brown, 1966). There was also the issue of whether such a change was desirable. The performance of basic care would have been considered a status threat by some nurses.

Another perspective on the tenacity of task-orientated nursing was provided by Menzies, (1960b) who conducted a case study of nursing in general hospitals. It was argued that the social organisation of nursing had unconsciously developed as a means of socially constructed defence against anxiety, which arose from the emotion aroused in the nurse when she had long or intense contact with patients (see chapter 13).

Study of the organisation of nursing work from the 1950s to the present in both the UK and the USA reveals that change has been piecemeal rather than sequential. Broadly speaking, there seemed to be a gradual shift in emphasis, if not in practice then certainly in theory from task-centred to patient-centred organisation. The RCN research reports of the 1970s (e.g. Lelean, 1973; Jones, 1975a) provided some indication that there were problems in providing patient-centred nursing.

Throughout the 1970s there was more evidence of interest in patient or case assignment methods (Matthews, 1975; Jones, 1977). It would seem that where patient-centred nursing was practised in the UK this often took the form of patient allocation. However, in the USA, team nursing appeared to be the focus of interest. These methods are described earlier in the first section of this chapter.

Attempts to introduce patient-centred approaches to nursing in the 1970s continued to face problems. Staff shortages were said to jeopardize patient allocation (Matthews, 1975). Ostensive reference to the notion of individualised nursing was seen with the growing interest in the nursing process (Crow, 1977a,b; Kratz, 1979a).

De la Cuesta (1983) examined the development of the nursing process from the 1950s in the USA to the UK in the 1970s. She argued that it emerged from the context of four main areas of discontent:

- Task-orientated nursing
- Lack of individualised care
- Low level of job satisfaction for nurses
- The superficial nature of the nurse–patient relationship

She highlights the mismatch between the theory of the nursing process and its practice and, in particular, the sacrifice of the individualised approach. This development was in part seen to be hampered by the ward organisational approach.

De la Cuesta (1983: 9369) explains that, although the nurse had patients allocated to her instead of tasks, her work was nevertheless still organised around task routine. This is consistent with Merchant's (1985: 69) observations that 'when patient allocation or team nursing are in use the nurses, if inadequately supervised, may use their discretion to institute a type of task allocation within their own group or team of nurses'. So it would seem that from the 1970s into the 1980s, far from emerging as discrete organisational approaches in hospital, nursing had constructed a range of hybrid forms. Furthermore, there is some indication across the literature that nurses may use terms to describe the various approaches to organising nursing in different ways. As such it is difficult to obtain any clear picture of the actual patterns of organisation. Whatever the form such approaches took, it would seem that nurses found it difficult in practice to provide nursing which was actually suited to the individual's needs. Chapman (1983) drew attention to the paradox within nursing that much patient care was not individualised despite frequent descriptions in the literature to the contrary.

Primary Nursing

Primary nursing is believed to have originated in the USA in the 1960s. It developed from nurses' concern with two main problem areas of nursing practice according to Manthey (1980: 18). She among other American nurses observed that team nursing was very problematic; patients were receiving fragmented, depersonalised and discontinuous care, and nurses were discouraged and frustrated with their job. Manthey (1970) said that they began to consider organisational approaches that would permit nurses to take increased responsibility for fewer patients and provide them with comprehensive care. Primary nursing was established at the University of Minnesota hospitals late in 1968.

Reference is often made to Manthey being the founder of primary nursing. Despite indications from the literature that primary nursing was being practised earlier by Lydia Hall at the Loeb Centre from 1963 (Hall, 1963: 805–806), this was not actually the case. Although acknowledging the influence of the Loeb centre on the development of primary nursing, Ciske (1980) says that the approach practised there was not primary nursing, but rather what she calls a system of 'total care' in which one nurse was responsible for the total nursing of a patient to whom she was allocated for a shift (what is generally described as patient allocation). The Loeb system was seen as advanced because all registered nurses were employed. Ciske also makes reference to the development of primary nursing at the university hospitals of Minnesota, Vanderbuilt and Michigan during the 1960s.

The few accounts referring to the development of primary nursing, such as McDonald (1988), tend to focus on changes in the USA. Both Lee (1979) and Kratz (1979b) made early reference in the UK to primary nursing in the *Nursing Times*. They described its development in the Sir Charles Gairdner Hospital in Australia after staff concern about the fragmentation of nursing arising from task assignment.

It is difficult to obtain any accurate picture of the early experiments with primary nursing in the UK: it is only possible to draw on claims made about practices in certain high profile units.

Castledine (1980) depicted the evolution of primary nursing at the Manchester Royal Infirmary. Implicit reference was made to what appears to be patient allocation as a starting point (Castledine, 1980: 14): 'on a daily basis, we allocated whoever was on duty to their patients'. However, the final pattern which emerged was that of a system involving case assignment and improved continuity of care, but from this account it is not explicit where the locus of accountability lay. In 1982 McFarlane and Castledine made a clear statement about the practice of primary nursing at the Infirmary. Later Walters (1985) described the successful practice of team nursing in the same unit. It is of note that little reference is made to team nursing in the UK literature thereafter.

In the early descriptions of primary nursing at both Manchester and Burford, Oxfordshire (Alderman, 1983) there is evidence of a close link between the need to extend individual care through the nursing process, such as ensuring greater continuity of nurse–patient contact following the initial assessment, and the need to rethink the ward level organisation of nursing.

Oxfordshire Health Authority has strategically supported a policy of each patient having a named nurse who is responsible and accountable for named patients. Work organisation that allows nurses to be responsible for individual patients over long periods of time, such as primary nursing, is said to be actively encouraged. (Pembrey, 1987). It was within this framework that nursing at Burford Community Hospital began to develop from the summer of 1982 (Punton, 1985). This development continued in some parts of Oxfordshire including a ward at the Radcliffe Infirmary (Tutton, 1986) and the John Radcliffe Hospital (Binnie, 1987).

The chapters in part 2 of this book are intended to capture a realistic picture of units trying to practise primary nursing today. 1988 could be said to have been a highly visible year for primary nursing. It would seem that the nursing media have an increasingly important influence on the promotion of ideas about nursing practice. This would certainly appear to be the case with primary nursing. Firstly, the *Nursing Times* Conference 'Challenge on the Ward' took place in June and was repeated several times thereafter. This was followed by a Scutari/RCN conference 'The Future Starts Here' in October 1988, which devoted a day to exploring primary nursing. Also, the 'Primary Nursing Network' organised from the King's Fund Centre for Health Service Development London, was launched at the Manchester conference. The Network aims to serve as a national forum for sharing information about primary nursing in the UK to help units wanting to try, develop and monitor its value for patients and staff. It has, up to November 1990, over 800 contact nurses representing units covering most health authorities in this country and also extending to Scotland and Jersey. The inaugural meeting was held on 6 January 1989 at the King's Fund with the launch of the newsletter *Primary Nursing News* (see Appendix 1.)

Many of the factors influencing the way nursing has been organised in the past are present in the late 1980s. Celia Davis (1976, 1977) has made a valuable analysis of the development of hospital nursing since the Nightingale era, which she argues has followed a remarkable continuity in occupational strategy. This strategy has involved a continuation of hierarchical nursing structure, routinisation, a focus on nursing tasks and a deference to doctors. Davis argues that two influential nursing reports, the Salmon Report (1966) and the Briggs Report (1972), reinforced this strategy. The weaknesses of this strategy were said to make it very susceptible to external pressures, of which nursing manpower shortages were of note. For example routine job activities were said to make it considerably easier to deal with staff shortages and rapid turnover of staff since new members are readily slotted in with a minimum of preparation.

It is interesting that during the 1980s there have been some major changes and proposals for the nursing service which may help break the enduring occupational strategy described by Davis (1976, 1977). These include radical changes such as the nursing process, the UKCC (1986) educational proposals 'Project 2000', and perhaps the rising popularity of primary nursing. However, the external pressures remain: an ever-increasing demand to provide a service within tight budgets; threat of an erosion of the nursing role due to changes largely in medical practice (Department of Health, 1989) and, in particular, the diminishing availability of skilled manpower (RCN 1985). Furthermore, there is some indication that features of the strategy described by Davis persist today (Melia, 1987). It remains to be seen whether radical educational reforms and practice reforms, such as primary nursing, will provide sufficiently strong alternative occupational strategy which can resist the external pressures, such as staff shortage, and help nurses to respond effectively to the demands facing the nursing service into the next century.

HUMANISING HOSPITAL CARE

This section is concerned with the issue of the dehumanisation of hospital care and the response that the nursing service could make to the alleviation of this problem. In particular, the potential impact of primary nursing will be explored.

Alienating Aspects of Hospital Care

● The central historical paradox in the delivery of health care . . . is, the practice of medicine is at once an intrinsically human concern and an increasingly dehumanised process.

Cobbs, 1975

Preserving the 'human' or personal quality of hospital care remains a significant continuing challenge for the health service today. Cobbs' viewpoint applies to both medicine and nursing alike. It could be said that nurses have a particular responsibility to provide this aspect of care because of the opportunity provided by their close and continuous proximity to the patient (Henderson, 1980). The term to 'dehumanise' could be described as 'to make impersonal'. This verb is often used interchangeably in the literature with the term 'to alienate'. For simplicity this practice will be continued here.

The nature and origins of alienation are complex and difficult to pinpoint clearly (Fein, 1975; Levanthal, 1975). Alienating features are often intrinsic to the hospital organisation itself and may also arise from the way nursing and medical care are practised. Most of these problems have major implications for the nursing service; however, the policy changes needed to eradicate them go well beyond the nursing arena. It will be seen that the alienating features of hospitals affect patients not only directly but also indirectly through the effects experienced by staff. Alienation may arise from three main sources:

● Living and working within a bureaucracy
● Presence and extensive use of advanced technology
● Issues related to professionalisation by health workers

Living and Working in a Bureaucracy

Weber (1947) first described a bureaucracy. He suggested that it has two main features: a division of labour and a hierarchical structure of management. Each individual with the system has a precise idea of each task he has to perform and to whom he is accountable. Power is invested in accordance with the position a person holds in the bureaucracy.

The existence of a high division of labour, whereby staff with specific skills carry out particular aspects of care, produces a large number of specialist workers with whom the patient may be confronted. In consequence, care may be fragmented to a needless degree through poor co-ordination of services and a lack of careful consideration being given to the distribution of responsibilities among the members of the ward team. Within nursing a high division of labour is seen with task-orientated practices, and often in practice those methods of assignment believed to be more patient orientated may perpetuate this situation for staff and patients.

Binnie's (1988) ethnography of the working lives of staff nurses found evidence of Watson's (1987) concept of the alienated worker. Staff were deprived of job satisfaction and effectively deskilled by the existence of a division of labour which required them to shift from being a care giver one day to managing the ward on another. Frustration arose from the difficulty of not being able to give the individual care they wanted to on any continuous basis. They lacked the freedom to make decisions related to a specific group of patients or to observe more directly the benefits of their labour.

Earlier, Brown (1966: 195) drew attention to the problems confronting nurses working within large bureaucratic organisations consistent with Binnie's findings 22 years later: '. . . this system is scarcely conducive to meeting the psychological needs of staff nurses for social approval, recognition of the importance of their work, sense of accomplishment, emotional support in anxiety evoking situations . . . .'.

The complex system of rules within a hospital bureaucracy may also contribute to alienation, although the problem of regulation is only one of degree. Excessive external control of ward-based activities may threaten the ability of staff to respond effectively to the needs of the individual because they lack the authority to operate with flexibility within policy guidelines.

Standardised and fragmented care has a tendency to lead to routinised nursing and medical practices. In his book *Hospitals in Trouble*, Martin (1984) analyses incidents of the 'failure of caring' from hospital inquiries over the last 15 years. Most hospitals analysed were those providing care for the chronically sick or disabled; these appeared to be at highest risk of the problem of routinisation. Regimented and impersonal practices often arose when staff had lost sight of their goal when there was little hope of cure. The preservation of order often then became paramount. These incidents represent the extreme case; however, they highlight the factors leading to dehumanised care. It is perhaps justifiable to speculate that this problem may also arise in any ward when demands to provide more care in less time leaves staff with a continuous feeling of never being able to give the care they believe patients need.

The size of hospitals alone may be alienating to patients, visitors and staff. The current tendency to centralise hospital care is seen as a rational attempt to utilise the costly resources of advanced technology and expertise economically. Large units where direct care is received, whether ward or bay, may be experienced as impersonal and alienating to patients, visitors and staff despite the fact that the hospital itself may be relatively small (Henderson, 1980). The size, layout and organisation of some hospitals may also interfere with the clear flow of information between staff and patients. This has to be seen in the context of the significance for patients of receiving clear and lucid information and the anxiety which may be caused when difficulties arise, as often occurs (see chapter 12).

It is not only the structure and organisation of hospitals which may have dehumanising consequences, but also the nature of the work performed. The dramatic proliferation of the use of medical technology has been a feature of the NHS since its inception.

Presence and Extensive Use of Advanced Technology

Technology is a dominant feature of our lives which is perhaps never more intrusive than when we receive hospital care. Despite the obvious and important benefits offered by technology, this feature of our world may induce a feeling of alienation from natural life (Marcuse, 1964). In hospital, both those who live and work in the organisation may be affected. The challenge is for staff not to become complacent about the extent and nature of its use and to consider the ways in which each individual responds to its presence. Henderson (1980) draws attention to the conflict nurses face in trying to provide humane nursing in a technological age. The problem is illustrated by reference to a friend she visited in intensive care. He was found to be cold, in a stark physical environment, with outrageously cheerful nurses who appeared no more busy than usual. When asked why he had not called the nurses he said he felt that they were too busy to ask. This example highlights the potential dehumanising effect of the interplay between the social environment created by staff and the physical environment. Consideration will now be given to the possible alienating effects arising from the behaviour of health workers with particular reference to the process of professionalisation.

Issues Related to Professionalisation by Health Workers

The process occupations progress through to achieve professional status is termed professionalisation. It is often a long process involving the attainment of certain attributes characterised in traditional professions such as medicine and law (Wilensky, 1964). It has been said that 'medical sociologists . . . and nurses themselves have tended to assume that the history of nursing is primarily a story of attempted professionalisation and that the goal is implicitly desirable' (Salvage, 1988a: 517). Illich's (1976) thesis maintains that professionalisation of medicine has had an adverse effect on the provision of health care. The medical profession has been said to have a tendency to withhold information about health from patients and in doing so exerts a form of social control.

The 'trait' approach to identifying where professionalisation occurs, as used by Wilensky, places emphasis on the attainment of certain attributes which reflect professional status. This approach has been said to be ' . . . uncritical, superficial and ineffective' (Schrock, 1987: 23). Hence the debate about the professional status of nursing may be seen equally sterile. Furthermore, it cannot be assumed that nursing is an occupational group that is a unified whole undergoing the move towards professional status. White (1984) and Melia (1987) suggest that nurses are not a homogeneous group but rather is composed of several different groups each with their own ideologies, some of which are directed towards achieving professional status in different ways. White (1984) proposes three groups. The generalists value experience in the ward situation, and it is suggested that they either do not want or will never achieve professional status. The specialists derive their status from attempting to develop a knowledge base through educational development and research. The managers' professional status is acquired from their ability to hold power and control within the system.

Primary nursing could be said to foster professionalisation through placing emphasis on a higher level of accountability by some nurses at the clinical level. The greatest focus within the system to account for decisions made may increase the pressure for the development of knowledge on which to base decisions about nursing. The decentralisation of authority will result in more nurses at the clinical level having a higher level of authority for action than they would otherwise have under team or task assignment unless they were a charge nurse. Primary nursing is frequently described as providing a 'professional model' of nursing; this belief is explored later in this section.

It is in the nature of groups undergoing professionalisation that they will attempt to secure a powerful position in their sphere, often through the control of knowledge or expertise (Friedson, 1970). This may conflict with the intent of nurses actively to share information with patients in order to help them. Despite the value of giving patients information, there is the risk that in practice nurses may actually withhold information, excluding patients from decision making and fuelling passivity and dependence. In criticising the exercise of this form of social control by the medical profession, nurses may fail to recognise their own, perhaps more subtle, practices, which may lead to this end. This is illustrated by nurses' use of controlling language when attempting to rehabilitate the elderly (Lanceley, 1985). In consequence patients may experience uncertainty, anxiety and lose the ability to cope with their situation effectively. These effects have been described as dehumanising features of hospital care (Leventhal, 1975; Howard, 1975).

It was argued earlier in this chapter that historically nursing's occupational strategy has not sought to gain greater autonomy and control over others (Davis, 1976). However, it has been suggested that the subsequent nature of nursing reform indicates that the strategy has now become a traditional professionalising type (see Historical overview). This process may lead either to a situation in which nurses may actually exacerbate the alienating effects of hospital care or to one in which the effects may be countered and the patient benefited.

Humanising Hospital Care: a Nursing Response

The nursing service has significant opportunities to ensure that the experience of living and working in a hospital is a humane rather than an alienating one. However, there are limitations to a strategy that relies only on the organisation of nursing. The good intentions of health workers to humanise the workplace can all too easily be compromised by the encroachment of social, economic and political factors which affect the nature of the workplace (Langrish, 1977). However, the approach nurses develop in providing and supporting direct clinical care may itself go some way towards offsetting the problems of providing humane hospital care.

Considering the alienating features described it would seem that two broad areas of reform are desirable when considering the response of the nursing service:

● Democratising working practices such that individual staff and patients have greater capacity to control or regulate decisions about their work or welfare, respectively (Wiedenbach, 1964; Davis and Trust, 1974; Watson, 1977a).

● Identifying and developing nursing practices that complement the above in providing a counterbalancing human response to the alienating factors described. (Gieger, 1975; Henderson, 1980; Naisbitt, 1982).

A fundamental issue confronting the nursing service is to identify the best way nurses can give patients greater control over their lives while in hospital, in a way which is desirable and acceptable to them. This may require nurses to be allowed a degree of authority which permits them to have greater freedom and flexibility to make decisions in their practice.

From Hierarchies to Networks

The creation of autonomous or semi-autonomous jobs can yield a high quality of service and a high level of satisfaction (Davis and Trust, 1974). In practice this will require a degree of devolved power such that the responsibility of individual workers remains within their level of competence. This will involve the development of more lateral or network staff structures to allow staff to relate colleagially rather than in a hierarchical structure based on largely power relations. Naisbitt (1982) argues that the development of networks in society represents a major direction of social change. He believes that networks have arisen from the failure of hierarchies to meet social need and their inability to respond to the high degree of selective information exchange required in modern organisations.

The authority of nurses at ward level may be dissipated. Nurses are subject to two sources of authority which regulate their activities; that which formally exists within the hierarchical structure (the administrative line) and that which emanates from the medical profession – a source of authority not specified formally but direct and persuasive in effect (Argyris, 1957). Pearson (1988) refers to the authority and status that has been largely vested in the person holding supervisory and administrative positions. Lack of devolved authority has left nurses in the unreasonable position of having to account for actions which they have little clinical freedom to control to their satisfaction.

Henderson (1980: 248) argues that alienation in hospitals may be countered by 'an organisational structure that gives nurses the same professional responsibility and accountability for patient care that is given to other health care providers'. Furthermore, this complements Binnie's (1988: 92) conclusion of the need to give qualified nurses greater control of their work through a system, such as primary nursing, to reduce alienation from their work due to the lack of control they have over it.

Opportunities to Benefit Patients?

Once greater authority is devolved to the practice level the nurse is in a more favourable position to help patients take more control of decisions about their health. This may counter the alienation patients may experience in hospital as well as promoting greater independence. The nurse may enable the patient to exert his influence in decisions related to his welfare and develop confidence in skill in caring for himself. The notion of 'partnership' is often sadly reduced to something of a cliché now. This approach to nursing involves the adoption of a non-directive style whereby the nurse attempts to give the patient greater choice to help him become a more active participant in his care, to a degree which accords with the individual's negotiated needs (Hall, 1969; Pearson. 1988). Such an approach has tremendous implications for nurses and patients, the complexities of which have not perhaps been addressed (Salvage, 1988b). Brooking's (1986) survey of 114 patients in two hospitals revealed that they had a positive attitude towards the idea of participating more in their care; however, despite claims by nurses that patient participation was encouraged, there was little evidence that patients actually did participate.

Fostering the independence of patients requires the nurse to impart knowledge and skills effectively and to help the patient to gain confidence. Patients will require nurses whom they can trust and who know their individual needs. Those nurses with whom the patient has most consistent contact will be most likely to fulfil these requirements. Primary nursing may facilitate this process by providing continuity of care. However, the process also depends on factors outside the organisation of nursing: the nurse's awareness of the patient's needs and how best to respond to them, her attitude to her work, and also her competence.

The understanding that nurses have about the nature of their work and their values as to what are considered desirable practice is of fundamental importance. Henderson (1980: 247) has said that 'humane service from all health workers is, in the last analysis, dependent on what society values'. We have described primary nursing as an approach to organising nursing; however, emphasis has also been placed on it being viewed as reflecting a philosophy of nursing by authors such as Hegyvary (1982).

Is There a Philosophy of Primary Nursing?

It remains unclear in what sense primary nursing is a philosophy of nursing in the sense that particular beliefs and values about nursing are intrinsic to a particular way of organising nursing. Rather it would seem that a design such as primary nursing serves as a framework, to some extent, enabling nurses to practise according to some nebulous but perhaps broadly shared values about nursing. For example, the individualised approach to nursing is seen by many nurses as desirable (Hayward, 1986). Some prominent writers on primary nursing believe that it is a vehicle for providing individualised care (Marram *et al.*, 1974; Manthey, 1980: 29).

Primary nursing could provide the opportunity to offer care in which the individual's needs are met and the involvement of patients in their care is encouraged. In this way it could give some practical form to the expression of values such as the respect of people as individuals and the right of patients to have maximum control over their lives. However, it would seem that there is nothing inevitable about this since primary nursing will only provide a framework from which nurses' varied beliefs are expressed.

Wilson-Barnett (1988) has argued that the exploration of nursing values is justified in order to ensure that development of practice takes place in areas of need. She also observes that central values are rightly being expressed more overtly in nursing, giving the examples of 'holistic principles' and 'individualised care'.

The adoption of a method of work organisation designed to promote patient-centred care takes place in a context in which features of humanistic thinking in nursing are promoted. Explicit reference is made to the broad humanistic and holistic principles underlying, for example, nursing models (Pearson and Vaughan, 1986). The promotion of such principles takes place both in the nursing literature (for example Styles, 1982: 61) and in conferences and curriculum statements (such as Bevis, 1983).

The term 'humanism' has been used loosely in nursing to reflect the value of the human being who is the patient. This relates closely to other recent statements about nursing in the UK, such as the RCN's (1987) reference to respect for person, equity and caring as fundamental values of the nursing service. Humanism itself has been said to be more of an attitude than a philosophy which has been discernible in literature since the Renaissance (Graham, 1986; Blackman, 1968). It advocates the development of human awareness and potential, concern about human and personal values and responsibilities, such as the importance of freedom and choice (influenced by existentialist thinkers such as Søren Kierkegaard and Jean-Paul Sartre (representing Christian and atheistic positions respectively), and the unique experience of the individual.

A prevalent belief related to the discussion of primary nursing is that it is synonymous with 'professional' nursing care (Manthey, 1980; Pearson, 1988). Hegyvary (1982: 181) has said: 'Primary nursing does not meet all the criteria of "professional" practice, although it comes closer than any other form of nursing in institutions'. She also suggests that primary nursing is often used interchangeably with 'professional nursing practice' (Hegyvary, 1982: 5). Kramer (1980: 6) supports this, saying that primary nursing is a 'vehicle for providing professional nursing care'. She goes on to say that professional practice may be 'taking responsibility for one's actions and being accountable for the results' (1980: 7), which is a feature of this approach. It is our belief that primary nursing, in isolation, does not necessarily constitute professional practice unless nurses practise competently. As Pembrey (1984: 541) suggests 'the need for competent nursing is the whole reason for professional practice'.

Competency is both a complex concept to define and a difficult quality to measure. It involves the development of knowledge, skills and attitudes appropriate to an occupational group. Jarvis (1983: 37) considers the notion of competency as too complex to define objectively but suggests that ' . . . competency is viewed as a level of professional practice which provides service appropriate to the wants, needs and expectations of clients'. It could be said therefore that primary nursing may be viewed as an organisational method which enables competent nurses to practise in a professional manner.

Earlier reference was made to the legitimate concern with the potential dehumanising effects of the professionalisation of nursing. Such a process typically involves social control through the exercise of power largely on the basis of the control of knowledge (Freidson, 1970). This would, at least in theory if not in practice, be in direct conflict to a nursing ideal of humanising hospital care through empowering patients by readily sharing information with them. However, it is a fallacy to believe that the nature of professionalisation in nursing may inevitably follow this path. Pembrey (1984) has said that we can derive professional nursing as a partnership with the individual, with the nurse working primarily as a teacher with a clear purpose of transferring some of the specialised knowledge possessed to the individual to enable him to increase his own competence and control. Schrock (1987) suggests that it is only appropriate for nurses to strive for professional status if it means that they are able to control events rather than be controlled by them. She speculates that the power gained through professionalising could be used constructively to benefit society. It has been said that it should be the wishes of the public that are fulfilled by nursing (Wilson-Barnett, 1988).

Primary Nursing and Patient Advocacy

Is it desirable for the nurse to adopt the role as advocate to the patient and, if so, what is the relationship of primary nursing to this role? Nelson (1988: 136) has said that advocacy has always been an integral part of nursing but the nature of the role has changed with time: 'Advocacy has moved from a posture of interceding, supporting or pleading a case for the client and acting as a guardian of the rights to autonomy and free choice'. It would seem that primary nursing may enhance and shape the practice of patient advocacy and bring nurses up against all the implications of adopting such a role.

The promotion of the nurse as a patient advocate is embodied in the UKCC (1984) *Code of Professional Conduct* and the *Code of Nursing Ethics* of the International Council of Nurses (1973). Advocacy has been seen as a means to help patients towards independence (Nelson, 1988). However, Fagin and Diers (1983) express concern that the patient may be made passive by advocacy.

The extent to which the practice of patient advocacy is achievable is another issue of concern. The nurse's attempts to ensure that patients have sufficient resources and that their rights are upheld may create significant problems. A nurse may lack authority and power when decisions conflict with those of medical staff with whom the nurse works interdependently; this may also arise with the managerial line of authority which is the nurse's employer (Webb, 1987a,b; Nelson, 1988). Porter (1988) argues that the advocacy role of the nurse is impractical on the basis that nursing has a tendency to exercise social control as it professionalises, which may lead to the creation of passivity in the sick role. As argued previously, this may not be inevitable. Further, Porter fails to recognise the significant growth of consumerism within health care and the potential value of nursing practices which may place the nurse in a position of authority to act with greater freedom on the patient's behalf, such as primary nursing. There have also been recent warnings for nurses to be aware of the legal issues when adopting a proactive role and the need to ensure that they are sufficiently equipped to give patients information (Tingle, 1988).

If nurses believe the advocacy role is necessary to counter the alienating aspects of hospital care and to develop the independence of patients, the question remains as to how the system is best established. It would seem that primary nursing is an approach which may at least support a patient advocacy role. Primary nurses are in a position to have detailed knowledge of the patient and his viewpoint; they have direct access to communicate with team members, and have sufficient authority to challenge decisions which impinge on the patient's rights or to support patients in their decisions. There may still, however, be ethical difficulties for the nurse when her beliefs and values conflict with those of the patient. It could be argued that primary nursing could exacerbate this position because the patient may have more limited access to staff who may be sympathetic to his position.

The Contribution of Primary Nursing

● Patient assignment, rather than task assignment would do more to preserve the essence of nursing in a technological age than any other administrative characteristic

Henderson, 1980: 250

Reflecting on the administrative changes necessary to humanise nursing care Henderson (1980: 248) spoke of the value of 'the assignment of patients or clients to nurses, rather than the assignment of tasks, functions, duties or activities'. Pioneers in the development of primary nursing in the USA have expressed their desire to bring about such change. For example Manthey (1980: xvii) described 'rehumanisation' of hospital care as 'the goal that has been my strongest motivation'. Although of course there is no certainty that the scope afforded by primary nursing would be achieved, it would seem reasonable to conclude that the system may provide a framework for buffering some of the alienating features of hospitals in addition to the therapeutic opportunities it may provide.

Primary nursing provides opportunity for:

● Developing a workable advocacy role for the nurse
● Gaining insight into the patient's perspective on his hospital experiences through the openings provided by the consistent contact
● Helping to reduce the alienating effects of uncertainty by freely offering information, which the primary nurse is in a valuable position to acquire

Attempts to improve hospital care in this way need to be viewed in a wider perspective. For example, despite nurses' attempts to reform the ward organisation of nursing it would seem inescapable that hospitals as we know them will continue to be of a highly bureaucratic nature. Furthermore, reforms would have to extend to all health and managerial workers within the organisation. A significant feature of the nursing service is the unique proximity and continuity of contact by nurses to patients, which in effect largely presents the 'human face' of the organisation. However, change in the structure of the organisation does not ensure that attitudes change. This has been illustrated with case studies (Carter, 1983). It is interesting that the RCN's (1986) *A Manifesto for Nursing and Health* states:

● We want to see . . . the philosophy of caring being presented in the midst of high technology, high pressure, high turnover and acute medical care.

The issue of reducing the alienating features of hospital care is an important one because it is likely to be a significant factor influencing the total welfare of the patient in hospital. It would seem likely that those alienating factors may affect both the degree to which the experience is generally therapeutic (or otherwise) for the patient and the patient's satisfaction with the care received. The importance of primary nursing may be that it will help nurses to provide a framework for practice in which the 'human' quality of a stay in hospital can be restored and sustained, and hopefully grow.

2

Introducing and Managing Change – The Move to Primary Nursing

Christopher Johns

The successful implementation of primary nursing involves managing a complex change process by altering the way nurses think about nursing, how they practise nursing, and how nursing is organised. The use of Ottaway's change strategy (1976) is advocated as a framework for organising and leading this change process. Those accounts of change that have involved implementing primary nursing have to some degree utilised this strategy (Pearson 1985a; Wright 1985a; Johns 1990a).

OTTAWAY'S CHANGE STRATEGY

Ottaway's approach focuses on change as a social process, the movement from one set of work norms to a new set. Lewin (1958) identified three stages to this movement which neatly summarise the main events in any change process:

- *Unfreezing* the old norms
- *Moving* towards new norms
- *Refreezing* the new norms

The seven major steps of Ottaway's strategy can be fitted into this scheme:

1. Unfreezing
   - contracting
   - diagnosis
   - design of change tactics
2. Moving
   - implementing tactics
   - skill training
3. Refreezing
   - reinforcing new norms
   - replicating to other sites

Contracting

Contracting refers to the relationship between the person bringing about change, commonly refered to as the change agent, and those being affected by the change. Ottaway (1982) cites Beckhard's (1969) definition of change agents as: 'Those people, either inside or outside the organisation, who are providing technical, specialised, or consulting assistance in the management of the change effort.'

Mauksch and Miller (1981) define a change agent as 'A person in a system whose role is to assist members of the system in making alterations to themselves or to the system.' The success of change to a great extent hinges on this relationship (Bennis, Benne and Chin 1976).

The Mauksch and Miller definition emphasises the agent's key role in helping people to make changes to themselves; Ottaway refers to this as adopting a 'bottom-up approach' to change.

Bottom-up approach

A bottom-up approach involves 'worker participation'. The rationale is that if people who will be affected by the change process are involved in it, it is more likely that they will adopt it as their own. This approach enables people to have some control over events and, in itself, becomes a new work norm. Primary nursing is a process whereby the traditional hierarchy of wards is dismantled in the process of devolving authority for managing care to primary nurses. Primary nurses in their new roles will be expected to make decisions about care which may, for many of them, involve learning new skills. Helping people to make decisions can be facilitated by a bottom-up approach to change, where the responsibility for change is shared. The primary and associate nurses are the people who will have to make the new norms work. A bottom-up approach facilitates the expression of resistance and its resolution. Consensus in decision-making can help to foster cohesiveness and high levels of morale and trust (Manthey 1980). Pearson (1985a) cites Sandford:

"There is no point in planning for people who will upset all such plans as soon as they find out they have not been party to the planning process."

Change in nursing has normally been associated with a 'top-down' approach from either management or education sources, an approach which can impose change on people, often without preparing them for what it will entail. Where the change implicitly disrupts existing norms, it is likely to encounter considerable resistance and result in compliance rather than real change.

However, a bottom-up approach needs management support (Manthey 1980), without which bringing about change is a frustrating business. The essential difference is that the control of the change process is with the practising nurses rather than with the management team.

Needs of the change agent

Beckhard's definition of the change agent suggested that this person could come from within or outside the change area. The writer's experience of change strongly suggests that the change agent should work from the inside. In many areas of nursing practice this person is likely to be the ward sister.

The reasons for this suggestion include:

1. Having legitimate authority to make changes. Where change agents lack this authority, they have to depend on being able to influence the staff who are affected by the change. It is important to appreciate that a bottom-up approach is compatable with a democratic style of leadership where the change agent actively involves staff in decision-making. The risk with an authoritarian approach is that the change is just pushed through when the going gets sticky.

2. Being a member of the ward team helps the change agent to maintain a high profile to encourage and support people during the change process. Being around helps to prevent people from reverting to previous norms in the agent's absence.

3. It enhances clinical commitment and motivation for the change. The change agent must support the changes fully and be able to articulate clearly and concisely why the change is important. Moving to primary nursing is not merely changing the roster system, it is a revolution in terms of thinking and doing nursing that will have a considerable personal effect on nursing staff. Motivation is essential for success.

4. The change agent has to have both personal and technical support for the changes. Having colleagues around to 'bounce ideas off' is useful, as is an empathic shoulder to lean upon in times of frustration.

5. The inside change agent is likely to know the strengths and weaknesses of other nurses, the likely foci of resistance, and the key issues. A problem with outsiders is that they are often identified as representative of management which, in itself, may lead to a conflict of authority and subsequent resistance. Outside change agents may also have a predetermined strategy (Ottaway 1982) that has little affinity with the needs of the change area or, as Rogers and Shoemaker (1971) quaintly put it, 'they scratch where others do not itch.'

6. The change agent needs considerable facilitation skills to help colleagues feel informed, to create opportunities for discussion, to set the pace of change, to raise awareness of key issues, and to fuel the change process with energy. Motivating staff that the change is worthwhile will help to address many of these issues; for example, people may then decide to come to meetings in their own time.

DIAGNOSIS AND INTERVENTION

The primary role of the change agent is to inspire colleagues to feel and understand the need for primary nursing.

There seems no obvious benefit in bringing about change for changes's sake in view of the conflict it always creates. Hence, the change agent has to establish a rationale for the change to primary nursing that will be understood and supported by colleagues. In areas of nursing that have not changed for many years the argument that primary nursing will lead to improved standards of care or more individualised care may well be questioned.

Philosophy for practice

A positive approach is to ask staff to identify what they believe and value about nursing and what the nursing unit is trying to achieve. This can then be compared with what the unit actually achieves and lead to discussion on how care could be better organised to meet the desired outcomes.

Clark (1978) comments: 'What people define as work is something to be reckoned with. When thinking about change, it cannot be assumed that people will necessarily start thinking differently about what is work when working conditions change.'

This comment reinforces the significance of understanding the nature of nursing work and the beliefs and values of nurses, when changing the system of work to primary nursing.

The change agent's role is to raise awareness of how primary nursing can benefit patient care, and this has been done through developing a unit philosophy for practice (Johns 1989a; 1990a).

It may be difficult for some nurses to share their values and beliefs and the results may not necessarily reflect what they truly believe because of a tendency to give socially acceptable statements about the nature of nursing. The change agent needs to feed in ideas that help to support the idea of change and primary nursing. Wright (1985a) describes this as a 'subtle background role'. These ideas should reflect a clear understanding of the principles of primary nursing (see Chapter 1).

Raising awareness may involve bringing in experts to talk to the staff, and visiting other units in order to understand their successes and difficulties with primary nursing. Ottaway (1976) describes the role of the pilot site as a place of change experimentation from which others can learn. An important consideration is that primary nursing needs to be designed for each location or, as Ottaway describes it 'made to order'.

Made to order

Each nursing unit is different and has its own culture and organisation. A primary nursing structure that is successful in one place has no guarantee of success elsewhere and planning for implementing primary nursing has to be tailor-made for the particular circumstances. Obvious examples of differences in structure are:

● establishment
● skill mix
● competency of staff
● budget authority
● type of patients
● nurse – doctor relationships

There is no right way of primary nursing (Manthey 1980). Units that have attempted to replicate another's practice have foundered through lack of understanding of the real issues (Johns 1989b) and of how to adopt the practice to meet their idiosyncratic needs.

Change can be defined as the process by which alterations occur in the function and structure of society (Mauksch and Miller 1981). A nursing unit can be described as a micro-society within the broad context of health provision. Nurses need to visualise the changes in their micro-settings in relation to wider changes in health and society. It is important, therefore, with change to consider the significance of culture.

Culture and change

It has already been suggested that traditional unit hierarchies need to be flattened to promote the change to primary nursing. Primary nursing is not conducive to pyramidal organisational structures that will inhibit the ability of the newly-fledged primary nurse to exercise her new responsibilities. Relationships within the primary nursing unit need to change from the hierarchical to the collegial (McMahon 1990); however, to change this structure is easier said than done. An understanding of some of the dynamics involved will help the change agent to construct suitable tactics to undermine the old norms.

Norms and values within the workplace can collectively be described as the culture of a unit. These have been developed over time and serve a real function in maintaining the status quo, which can be described as a state where staff anxiety is at a minimum. These cultures are maintained through a self-validating process that has to be invalidated and replaced by new ones (Ottaway 1982). Existing norms are maintained through the use of rituals (Turner 1969) that convey, in symbolic form, key values of that society, for example, how different people address each other and behave within specific relationships.

The Ward sister as a symbol

A strong symbol that needs particular attention during the process of changing to primary nursing is the ward sister. Traditional ward cultures have largely been built around her role so any redefinition of it is likely to cause a major upheaval in roles and relationships, not just for the unit staff and the sister herself, but for all workers affected by this change and for society in general.

A case-study of a unit that had implemented primary nursing illustrated how relatives continued to expect to see the sister for information about patient care, irrespective of the primary nurses (Johns 1989b). This same case-study highlighted how difficult it was for the sister to let the primary nurses deal with telephone calls, and discuss care with other workers. The problem stems not only from the sister's own expectations of her role but the expectations of others, for example, relatives and doctors.

A second case-study (Johns and Kingston 1989) highlighted the consultants' expectations of how the sister should act, and their subsequent difficulties in accepting a change in role with this unit's move towards primary nursing.

These internal and external expectations of the sister's role may result in a tension between 'keeping control' and 'letting go'. The success of primary nursing is dependent on sisters letting go to enable primary nurses to take the authority to make decisions about the care of their patients. Research already indicates that this can lead to discomfort and role-loss, even where the sister believes that the change is necessary (Johns and Kingston 1989).

Various symbols of the sister's control can be removed: for example, the blue uniform, the sister badge, who holds the keys in the morning. One of the sisters at Brackley was loathe to lose the title 'sister' when becoming a primary nurse: she felt she had earned it. A compromise was agreed – primary nurse sister. It may sound petty but such things are important to staff. In bringing about change, staff may well experience feelings of loss. The change agent needs to recognise and deal with these feelings on a personal level. The change agent has a significant role to help people to find meaning in new roles. Without this continuity of meaning, the people who are affected will have difficulty in looking ahead progressively as they are distracted by their feelings of loss (Marris 1978).

Where people are threatened by change, the likelihood is that values will be restated through reinforcement of the various rituals (Turner 1969) at the very time the change agent is attempting to undermine them.

Identifying new norms with primary nursing

Traditionally, the sister has shared the head of the hierarchy with the doctor, their roles complementing each other and reflecting nursing's Victorian household heritage (Carpenter 1978). The nurse training Florence Nightingale promoted stressed character, and an attitude of obedience rather than reasoning. In this way, to the doctor the nurse became an extension of his good wife with all the virtues of obedience and subservience (Buckenham and McGrath 1983) and subordinate to her husband, the doctor (Whittaker and Oleson 1978). The socialisation of nurses within such hierarchies has resulted in nurses generally adopting a handmaiden role. This role has been shown to be characterised by three themes: of loyalty to the doctor or health team as opposed to the patient, a consciousness of subordinate status, and a sense of powerlessness (Buckenham and McGrath 1983). These themes have a significant effect on the nurse's behaviour, particularly in being unable to carry out that function of patient advocacy that she and the profession acknowledge as a vital component of her role. This is particularly pertinent when moving to primary nursing within a philosophy of patient-centred care that directly challenges nurses who value medical tasks and routines (MacGuire 1980) and resort to communication tactics that reinforce this subordination (Stein 1978) and need approval from doctors for what they do. With primary nursing these old norms are replaced with new ones (Table 2.1). The emphasis on assertiveness may be critical.

The type of care provided by a unit is also culturally bound: traditionally, this has been organised through delegation of tasks or patients by the ward sister. Pearson (1985a) measured staff values prior to implementing changes that included the introduction of primary nursing at Burford Hospital. He found that staff valued the

Table 2.1

Old norm	New norm
values medical tasks	values nursing care *per se*
submissiveness to doctors	assertiveness with doctors
handmaiden role	collegial role
loyalty to doctors	loyalty to patients

medically-related and physically-orientated aspects of work and saw the psychological aspects as being less important. In this case study, work was organised through the execution of tasks, commonly described as functional nursing, and was primarily performed by untrained staff. The norms were that patients were expected to be dependent on nurses, with emphasis on completion of tasks and getting through the work.

These old norms, and the new ones suggested as being valid for primary nursing, are listed in Table 2.1.

Table 2.2 demonstrates a desirable shift in the norms of nursing practices which may be achieved through development work. The new norms described may assist the nurse in meeting patients' psychosocial needs.

The culture of the traditional ward team has been its allegiance to harmony (Johns 1990b). Johns comments:

'The harmonious team is concerned with maintaining a facade of togetherness or teamwork. It does not talk about difficult feelings between its members and seeks to protect its members from outside threat.'

Besides the difficulty this team has in supporting its members, it is also unable to deal effectively with conflict. The management of the change process is the management of conflict. A bottom-up approach to change presents an opportunity to challenge this 'harmonious team' by exploring conflict created within it by the change process. If the change agent can create a team where the exploration and resolution of conflict becomes a new norm, this team will then be likely to be better prepared to support its members in their new primary nursing roles.

Table 2.2

Old norms	New norms
emphasis on completion of tasks	emphasis on meeting patient need
emphasis on nurse control	emphasis on patient control
predominantly physically-orientated care	psychosocial and physically-orientated care in balance
untrained staff make decisions and give 'basic' care	untrained staff support nurses in giving care

Style of leadership or facilitation

The change agent can act as a role model by using a democratic style of leadership, as opposed to the autocratic style that tends to be more directive than facilitative. The democratic style is comparable to what Chin and Benne (1976) describe as a 'normative-educative approach to bringing about change'. This approach recognises that individuals have values, attitudes and beliefs that direct behaviour. The normative-educative approach aims to encourage people to examine these values in light of desired goals and to review their cognitive, attitudinal, individual and group behaviour (Hersey and Blanchard (1977)) (Figure 2.1).

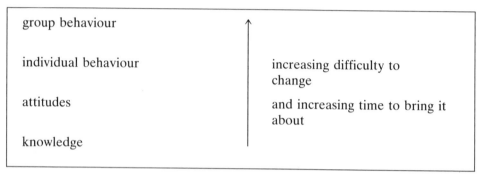

group behaviour

individual behaviour   increasing difficulty to
                                            change

attitudes   and increasing time to bring it
                                            about

knowledge

Fig. 2.1   Different levels of change in relation to difficulty and time (Hersey and Blanchard 1977)

Hersey and Blanchard's work is a useful reference for understanding the difference between what nurses say they believe in and what they practise. Very few nurses would claim that they do not value seeing patients as individuals but how many actually practise in a way that truly reflects such a thought or attitude? The way nurses practise has been through a powerful process of socialisation that needs to be unlearnt to enable new learning to take place.

Hersey and Blanchard's work picks up the issue of individual and group behaviour. Certain members of staff may begin to practise at a new level that will be frustrating for them if others fail to do so. These people need particular support to sustain them whilst others strive to reach a group behaviour level and without it they may be made scapegoats; for example, the nurse who is assertive amongst others who are not becomes threatening to the team.

IMPLEMENTING THE INTERVENTION

In many instances there will have already been a shift away from functional nursing towards patient allocation and team nursing that the change agent can build upon. In moving towards new norms in primary nursing, the staff involved will need considerable time to discuss these issues and to move forward at their own pace. The key to managing this pace is to capture the tension between working at the staff's preferred pace of change and proceeding at such a pace that staff feel the pressure. A problem for the change agent is that different people proceed at different rates, from keen change adopters who want the changes now and active resisters who, it seems, will do anything to prevent the success of the changes.

The change agent is wise to single out both these groups of people for special attention; the keen change adopters to foster their support, and the active resisters to understand the nature of their resistance and to plan tactics to help them to embrace the changes.

Involving doctors?

The change agent must also consider involving doctors in the change process. Their involvement would seem desirable, particularly as the new norms will alter the relationship between doctor and nurse. Issues of professional dominance suggest that doctors will resist developments in nursing as a natural process of asserting their control over the performance of all medical work, refusing to allow other professional health care workers to perform such work except as subordinates and insisting on jurisdiction on all matters, however vague, related to health care (Friedson 1970). As nurses suddenly become more assertive and stop playing the doctor-nurse game (Stein 1978) conflict with doctors socialised in their 'superior' professional role may result. Doctors can be good allies or great adversaries. Hunt (1987) reports that nurses were surprised at doctors' willingness to be involved in action research projects. What they need to see is, firstly, how the new norms will benefit them and, secondly, how they will benefit their patients. The argument that primary nursing improves patient care will need to be supported with empirical evidence, much of which is of limited value (see Chapter 12).

In designing appropriate interventions it may be useful if the change agent breaks down the change plan into stages and objectives so that the staff do not feel overwhelmed. Hegyvary and Hausmann (1981) state:

'Setting goals helps to keep the project on track and gives a point of reference for evaluating the change. Lack of specific direction gives a feeling of muddling through, that is frustrating and dissappointing.'

One hopes that this approach will offset the fact that change is in many ways unpredictable and difficult to plan for. The bottom-up approach gives shared responsibility to the team where failure to reach any objectives cannot so easily be blamed on the change agent.

Much of the unpredictability of change is due to resistance.

Resistance to change

A useful framework for considering resistance to change has been described by Breu and Dracup (1976), who apply Klein's (1968) eight principles that are endemic in change situations and represent forces to deal with in change.

1. There is an almost universal tendency to seek to maintain the status quo on the part of those whose needs are being met by it.
2. Resistance to change increases in proportion to the degree to which it is perceived as a threat. Mauksch and Miller (1981) have identified various reasons why staff might resist change:

- behaviour of the change agent
- unclear change programme
- lack of knowledge/lack of information
- past experience of change
- not believing in the change
- insufficient resources; for example, the adequacy of staffing is always a major question (Hegyvary 1981). In a description of the impact of introducing primary nursing into a nursing unit, failure to adjust to new norms was blamed on a shortage of staff; this tendency to identify scapegoats became a norm itself (Johns 1989b).

Changing practice can threaten experienced nurses because it implicitly challenges what the staff have been doing for years, rendering it valueless (Duberly 1977). A significant psychological barrier to primary nursing is that of status. Many experienced nurses work part-time due to personal commitments: these nurses may find it difficult to accept their limited decision-making role as an associate nurse. (Johns 1989b).

3. Resistance increases in direct response to the pressure for change. The change agent may become a driving force in this equation, with the resultant increase of resisting force.

4. Resistance to change decreases when it is perceived as being reinforced by those who are trusted and whose judgements are respected, and people of like mind. The success of the change agent lies in identifying and mobilising these people, both inside and outside the unit. This may prove difficult, as was demonstrated in the change process at Brackley hospital. The key 'adopter' (Ottaway 1982) was resisted by older staff due to her age and her apparent lack of credibility. These factors were exacerbated by her manner which alienated these older staff who percieved her as being disrespectful.

5. Resistance to change increases when those involved are able to forsee how they might establish a new equilibrium of resistance and change factors which is at least as effective as the balance of factors existing previously. The key to this factor is the change agent's role as clinical leader to create a sense of vision for staff to perceive a 'brave new world'.

6. Commitment to change increases when those involved have the opportunity to participate in the decision to make and implement the change, thus supporting Ottaway's change strategy.

7. Resistance to change, based on fear of the new circumstances, is decreased when those involved have the opportunity to experience the new norms under conditions of minimal threat. Lancaster (1982) states that a relatively safe environment is a significant issue, as change generates insecurity for people. At Brackley, the primary nurses were protected from being held to account for a period of six months in their new roles to enable them to experience these new and threatening roles.

8. Temporary alterations in most situations can be brought about by use of direct pressure, but these changes are accompanied by heightened tension and will yield a highly unstable situation.

Passive resisters in the change process can be very irritating. They do not turn up to meetings, nor do they say what they feel, at least not in public, and in general they are an unsupportive influence. They are nigglers and try to sap the change agent's confidence and so have to be identified and confronted, and the nature of their resistance exposed. They tend to undermine change, especially when the change agent is absent, creating massive role confusion (Zander 1977).

However, not all resistance should be viewed negatively, for it can actually help the change process by forcing the change agent to clarify the purpose of change (Olson 1979), or to rethink change interventions that turn out to be inappropriate. It is a foolish change agent who ignores resistance to change.

SKILL TRAINING

Ottaway (1982) comments: 'If change is seen as moving from one steady state to another steady state one can see that a vast amount of learning must take place.'

An earlier part of this chapter focused on interventions that highlighted the extent of training and development that nurses moving to primary nursing need. The success of change will be dependent on these learning opportunities, an essential reason for the need for management support. Manthey's (1980) belief that primary nurses can only learn within the role fits in with Ottaway's strategy that training follows change.

Various practical strategies that offer a framework for identifying and meeting development needs of staff, both during the implementation period of primary nursing and as an ongoing staff development programme have been developed.

1. Defining roles and relationships
2. Developing resource nurses
3. Developing standards of care
4. Performance review
5. Using reflection on practice, with supervision
6. Role modelling
7. Peer review and presentation of case material

1. Defining roles and relationships

Moving to primary nursing involves defining various roles and the relationships between these roles – definitions that provide signposts to guide people's actions. The process of writing these descriptions will help to reduce anxiety by identifying the skills associated with each role. The negotiation of roles should be part of the philosophy of the bottom-up approach to change.

2. Developing resource nurses

If primary nurses, in particular, are to be held to account for care outcomes then clearly they must make effective decisions. In the real world, time is always at a premium – hence, primary nurses need quick access to knowledge to help them to make those decisions. This can be achieved by creating resource files that are managed by different nurses who can also act as consultants or resource people for their colleagues. The library at Burford now contains 76 resource files and their use in the change process has been described by Johns and Kingston (1989). The advantages of developing resource people are that they

- involve all staff in the development of practice;
- encourage members of staff to pursue particular areas of clinical interest;
- the work of developing resources of information and skill is shared;
- create an effective learning resource.

3. Developing standards of care

The process of developing standards of care is, in itself, a framework of change (Johns 1991). The many problems that arise from the change process can be solved if the standards are written by members of a standards group. Such a group should meet regularly, ideally monthly, facilitated by the change agent. The standards are agreed by the nursing staff on the unit to ensure that they match the concept of a bottom-up approach to change.

4. Performance review

A key issue in implementing primary nursing is creating opportunities for primary nurses to demonstrate their accountability. This feedback is important in enabling them to monitor how effective they are in meeting the needs of their patients and in fulfilling the primary or associate nurse role. Identifying their strengths and weaknesses against a set of criteria developed from the job description enables both clinical leaders and nurses to focus on areas of appropriate development.

5. Using reflection on practice, with supervision

Supervision is a formal opportunity for primary nurses to derive support and development in their work in such a way that it benefits primarily their patients rather than themselves (Atherton 1986). Research at the Burford Nursing Development Unit indicates that supervision is an ideal medium for preparing nurses for new roles. The research method involved an associate nurse in collecting critical incidents from her daily practice and reflecting upon them under supervision (Johns 1990c).

6. Role modelling

The change agent can facilitate learning by acting as a role model (Felder 1983); even if she is primary nurse to just one patient, her credibility and influence may be significantly enhanced (Zander 1977). The planning, giving, and evaluation of care provides a rich material source for subsequent discussion and teaching. An advantage of this approach is that it enables the change agent to experience this role and its relevant problems but the disadvantage is that it requires her to be competent in the practice of primary nursing, which for many units will not be the case.

7. Peer review and presentation of case material

This method of learning encourages nurses to present their work to each other for critical review. It overcomes the difficulties the change agent may have by not being an expert practitioner and, in particular, facilitates skills in giving and receiving feedback, both of which are necessary if primary nurses are to monitor their effectiveness of action.

Staff capability and commitment

The effectiveness of primary nursing depends largely on the skills and commitment of individual nurses. As a result of the learning strategies just described, some nurses may realise that they have neither the capability nor the commitment to function effectively as a primary nurse (Hegyvary and Hausmann 1981). Where nurses clearly are struggling, they can be counselled about their future careers, either at a performance review or during supervision.

REINFORCING NEW NORMS

This is possibly the most difficult stage of Ottaway's change strategy and the process of change. Just when you think you have got there you realise that, for whatever reasons, things are not working out.

The strategies for learning become, in effect, the strategies for reinforcing the new norms. The bottom-up approach strategy can become a new norm for making decisions about the organisation of the unit. Monthly or bimonthly staff meetings are a useful forum for discussing issues of concern and agreeing on solutions.

Monitoring standards is another effective way of reinforcing new norms in practice. Feedback from monitoring gives the staff information on whether the changes are working. Probably the most important tactic the change agent can use is simply to be there, to support people in their new roles and practices, to troubleshoot problems as they arise, and generally support the new norms on a daily basis. The experience at Brackley Hospital was that being away from the hospital created an opportunity for the resisters to undermine the new norms and revert to previous ways of working. The fieldwork diary of this experience has many entries about this phenomenon.

The process of change itself becomes a new norm for the workforce, replacing the old norm of maintaining the status quo, replacing the 'static' with the 'dynamic'.

REPLICATING TO OTHER UNITS

This takes the discussion on change back to raising awareness and using sensibly the expertise of other units. The message is: use the experience and lessons of other people, particularly where units have attempted to evaluate the changes honestly. Ottaway's concept of the pilot site is that it should enable others to learn from the unit's experience. Wright (1985a) comments: ' . . . the pilot site becomes a source for change in other places. . . . where trained staff from other settings come for experience to refresh their own knowledge and return at some stage to their own place to act, in turn, as agents for change.'

CASE STUDY

Much of the work presented in this chapter emerged as a result of the author being a change agent both at Brackley and at Burford hospitals between 1987 and 1990, and from carrying out research into some aspects of the changeover to primary nursing in other units.

The Brackley experience is offered in summary form to help the reader visualise how different interventions were planned. Brackley is a community hospital with 13 in-patient beds providing for the needs of acutely ill people in the local community who do not require high-tec medical intervention but do need nursing: terminally ill people, respite care for carers of dependent people, and rehabilitation following major surgery or illness. This wide diversity of patients gives an indication of the broad range of knowledge needed by nurses who work in community hospitals.

Nursing work had been organised in the traditional manner around a matron who delegated work downwards through the staff nurses to the nursing auxiliaries, who read the workbook before proceeding to deliver basic care. The hospital had lost its maternity service in the previous year and this had resulted in midwives, reluctant to travel 20 miles to work in a maternity unit, having to care for generally elderly people without any clear purpose. My appointment followed the matron's retirement. It is interesting to note that it was expected, and, indeed, written in my job description, that primary nursing would be implemented.

Plan of action

This was split into two stages (Table 2.3):

● planning stage – 6 months
● implementation stage – 6 months

Within this loose framework it was useful to plot the various factors that supported change and those that resisted it, because identifying specific resisting forces helps to focus the tactics of change. These factors or forces (Lewin 1958) are shown in Table 2.4.

If one uses the analogy of a force field, in which the status quo is simply the balance of positive and negative forces in a state of equilibrium, the status quo in human terms is seen to be one of comfort or minimal anxiety. Where additional forces are introduced into this equation, the balance is lost and the status quo is disrupted. Activity is then focused on returning to the status quo or position of minimal anxiety. People are strongly motivated to reduce anxiety or disharmony within themselves.

Table 2.3

	Target

Planning stage

1. To establish relationships with staff.   1 month

   Key issues in this process were
   ● clinical credibility
   ● leadership
   ● creating a sense of vision.
   Major advantages were
   ● a background in community hospital nursing
   ● staff's perceived need for leadership
   ● no obvious obstacles to deal with.

2. Generating a felt need to change the type of care the
   hospital offered to use the beds more effectively to meet
   community needs, based on belief in individualised care.   3 months

   Raise awareness of primary nursing and the assessment
   of patients.

   To write a philosophy of care.

   Analysis of resources
   ● structural, eg. skill mix
   ● staff capability and commitment.

3. Formulate a working structure for implementation of
   primary nursing.

   Key issues included managing conflict
   ● job design
   ● planning the development of staff.   6 months

4. Agreement by staff to proceed.   4 months

Implementation stage   6 months
1. Writing policies and standards to guide action:
   ● policy for assigning patients to nurses
   ● communication style policy.

2. Developing a performance review tool and defining
   accountability.

3. Introducing staff meetings to reflect on the process of
   change and staff development.

   Key issues
   ● decision-making
   ● peer relationships.

Table 2.3 *(continued)*

	Target

4. Challenging all practice in the light of the new
    philosophy of care. Trying to solve the problems of the
    incongruence between the practices of staff and their beliefs
    through developing standards of care.

5. The use of the methods QUALPACS and/or of Nursing
    Audit many provide a baseline measure for identifying
    subsequent improvement of care.

6. Create nursing auxiliary development group to support
    and develop this role.

7. Specific skill training.

Table 2.4 Change force field (after Lewin, 1958)

Driving forces	**Resisting forces**
Staff need for direction	Existing hierarchical structure
Low morale due to need for change	Low morale due to loss of maternity services
High expectations of change agent	Dependence on change agent
Good skill mix	Lack of nursing process skills
Key change adopter	Powerful status resisters
Strong management support	Doctors very resistant
Democratic leadership style	Perceived lack of authoritative leadership
Well planned strategy	Change introduced too quickly or taking too long
Using standards to solve problems	Change agent unable to maintain a constant high profile
Shared beliefs about care	Nursing auxiliaries loss of status and satisfaction

SUMMARY AND CONCLUSIONS

Ottaway's seven-stage strategy for change has been described in relation to moving to primary nursing using empirically-derived knowledge and the literature about change theory. It is impossible to say that Ottaway's is the best strategy for change, and it has been stated that an eclectic approach using various models may be just as effective, Mauksch and Miller (1981). What is essential is to approach change in an organised way if the results are to be more than haphazard. The design of change is unique to each setting, and primary nursing is itself a complex concept.

3

Educational Preparation for

Primary Nursing

Mary Fitzgerald

This chapter has four parts:

- A résumé of the philosophy underpinning and linking professional nursing and professional education
- An examination of educational theory and methods using the work of Knowles (1970) describing the adult learner, and of Jarvis (1983, 1987) and Schön (1987) considering education for professional practice
- An attempt to clarify nursing practice and locate concepts worth exploration, such as caring, communication and interpersonal relationships in order to find content for learning
- A brief description of a formal educational course for primary nurses and a learning programme running for nurses on one ward which is preparing to change to primary nursing. Both are based on the principles outlined in the chapter but are quite different in structure, academic depth and content.

It would be difficult and indeed suspect to suggest a blueprint syllabus for the preparation of primary nurses. Nurses about to take on this new role have a range of abilities, past experiences and motives, and acknowledgement of these differences is required if nurses' individuality is to be appreciated.

These individual differences can be accommodated if the correct method of teaching or learning is chosen. An ability to learn independently is important for the professional practitioner, who is expected to make knowledgeable decisions regularly, and whose statutory education is complete. Independence is fostered by teaching methods that centre on students and acknowledge their individuality.

An analogy can be drawn between the maturational path to independent nursing practice and that toward independent learning. Independent nursing practice in this instance relates to the primary nurse who is capable of accepting responsibility for a client group, establishing a close professional relationship with each member of the group and choosing an appropriate nursing therapy with them, without deferring to a higher authority; but at the same time this nurse is aware of the obligation to account for the decision made in practice and the outcomes of the work undertaken. The independent learner is able to identify personal learning needs, mobilise resources and learn without deference to a teacher. Like the independent practitioner, the independent learner is responsible for the actions chosen and the results accrued. The two concepts of independent nursing practice and independent learning sit comfortably together; both are founded on beliefs about the value and potential ability of the individual, requiring from participants core skills such as self-awareness, integrity and confidence in their own potential. When nursing practice and education are both moving in the direction of independence there is harmony, with the one supporting and motivating the other (see figure 3.1).

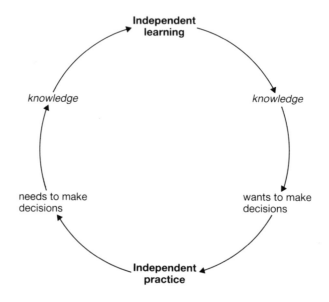

Fig. 3.1 Mutual support of independent learning and practice.

The choice of subjects to study is wide. A review of the literature that describes preparatory courses for primary nursing reveals a range of material, all of which the potential primary nurse might find relevant. On consideration of this literature, one is left with an overriding feeling that the material is not specific to primary nurses but would be useful to nurses in general. This is interesting, and it might be suggested that nurses who have not continued to learn actively since qualification can get by in many areas of practice by constantly deferring or postponing decisions. The primary nurse, however, cannot do this and therefore needs knowledge (both theoretical and that borne from experience) to make decisions and justify them. As Manthey (1980) points out, primary nursing exposes the good and the poor nurse. Manthey has found, in her long experience of introducing primary nursing, that nurses new to the role typically identify the following learning needs:

● Specialist medical knowledge
● Skills for using the nursing process
● Communication skills

Each of these subjects will be considered later in the chapter; however, to elaborate the subjects it is useful to link specialist medical knowledge and communication skills with the work of an American nurse theorist Jean Watson. Watson (1985) has described what she calls 'core' and 'trim' nursing fields. The trim refers to knowledge required for a speciality, such as interpretation of ECGs or pharmacology, and the core refers to skills that all nurses need in order to care for people. The caring components described by Watson are mainly interpersonal skills. The trim can be linked to what Manthey (1980) described as specialist medical knowledge and the core to the development of communication skills.

The thoughts and ideas presented in this chapter are offered to readers for their consideration when choosing an appropriate learning experience for potential primary nurses.

PHILOSOPHY

In contemporary education and nursing thought, humanistic thinking is to some degree a valued philosophical stance (see chapter 1). This is confirmed in the writings of modern nurse theorists such as Orem (1985) and Watson (1985) and is apparent in discussion papers (e.g. RCN, 1987). Rogers (1983) and Knowles (1970) are influential educationalists who emphasise the centrality of the individual.

Humanistic philosophy concentrates on the individual, recognising the uniqueness of each person. Although the philosophy is complex and open to differing views, humanists share certain assumptions. They believe that the person is intrinsically worthwhile and that all human values should emanate from a respect for this worth. All humans are potentially intelligent, which once realised allows them to exercise freedom and make choices to control their lives (Blackham, 1968).

These beliefs find expression in many of the modern trends in nursing (Pearson 1988):

- Individualised care
- Holistic care
- Patient education
- Nurse–patient partnership
- Promotion of independence, adaptation to stress or self-care for patients
- Autonomous nursing practice

Current trends in education are also centred on the client (Jarvis, 1983; Rogers, 1983):

- Student-centred learning
- Self-evaluation
- Student autonomy
- Education as a lifelong, self-directed process

These developments all convey to some degree an acknowledgement by modern nurses and educationalists of the worth of the individual and concern for the individual's potential to develop in order to exercise the right to control his or her own life.

These notions converge in the idea of the ideal nurse: well-educated people capable of acknowledging their own worth and using their knowledge and skills to help patients reach their potential; nurses who are aware of their responsibilities for making decisions and are accountable for the consequences of their actions.

However, difficulties arise because this discussion has concentrated on ideals; education and practice for nurses are in a transition phase, and as yet neither has achieved the modern ideal. Generally nurse education does not foster independent learning (RCN 1985; UKCC, 1986). Students are required to attend lectures, timetables are packed leaving little time for reading and investigating topics of particular relevance to individual students, and in some schools learning resources, such as the library, are poor. Practice shows more evidence of pragmatism than humanism; there is a concentration, because of scarce resources, on 'getting the work done' by the least number of nurses, leaving no time for developing important relationships with patients. An appreciation of the real situation and the stress this places on nurses is important if change agents, in education and practice, are going to help develop nurses' abilities. Time spent exploring the beliefs and values underpinning modern nursing's preferred ideology will help nurses to understand and appreciate the need for development.

If nurses develop educationally at the same time as accepting changes to primary nursing, they should find the transition comfortable because the two are philo-sophically compatible and mutually supportive. However, nurses who have been persuaded to change practice without developing as independent learners may find themselves lacking knowledge and skills essential for independent practice, and may be unable to redress the imbalance. Considerable frustration and stress may also be experienced by nurses who have developed new knowledge skills and attitudes but are not practising primary nursing. They find that these new skills are redundant in traditional practice, where decisions are made by the nurse in charge for the day.

EDUCATIONAL THEORY AND METHODS

Adult Learning

Adult learning (andragogical) theories are a useful guide when considering the educational opportunities appropriate for nurses preparing for professional prac-tice (Knowles, 1970; Jarvis, 1986).

Adult learning is based on four main assumptions about adult learners (Knowles, 1970). These are related to:

- *Changes in self-concept* As people grow and develop, their self-concept changes from one of dependency to one of increasing self-directiveness. People expect to make decisions about their own life and face the consequences. Knowles (1970) suggests that adult learners therefore need to be treated with respect; an environment that is not compatible with their self-concept as automonous individuals will be treated with resentment and resistance.

- *The role of experience* Adults have accumulated a whole range of experiences which are a rich resource for learning. This experience is unique to the individual and is so personal that if it is not acknowledged or encouraged this may be taken as a sign of rejection of the person.
- *Readiness to learn* The need to learn is associated with social roles; for example, parent, wife or nurse. Learning needs to be seen as relevant to life's roles.
- *Orientation to learning* Adults like to be able to apply learning to immediate problems in life.

With these assumptions in mind it is expedient to allow nurses preparing to be primary nurses to reflect on their own competencies and identify their own learning needs. They need a learning environment in which they feel safe and respected and can evaluate their own progress.

Acknowledgement of each nurse's past experience and a commitment to using it will enrich group learning and give the person a feeling of worth.

Nurses need to see the learning experience as relevant to their practice. Difficulties will be encountered if individuals are resistant to primary nursing or will not have a chance to practise as primary nurses because the knowledge, skills and attitudes gained will have no immediate practical use.

Not all adults feel comfortable with learning experiences based around these assumptions (Knowles, 1970) because they still expect conventional teaching and feel safer if someone else makes decisions and gives them direction. Indeed, Jarvis (1986) suggests that Knowles has overestimated the adult's self-directiveness. Northedge (1981) suggests that it is inappropriate to expect students to make the leap from dependent pupil to independent scholar without some support and direction, otherwise students may waste time doing inappropriate things or nothing at all because they don't know what is expected. Many, but by no means all, nurses preparing for primary nursing will need help to accept the shift in responsibility from teacher to student, because all their past experience of education has been teacher directed. At the same time they will be accepting a shift in responsibility in practice from the sister to themselves. The educationalist should be prepared to be flexible and accommodate individual differences in the students.

Professional Education and Learning

It is understood that professionals have expert knowledge and skills to offer the public (Baly , 1975). This assures them privileges in society, but these privileges are accompanied by responsibility to provide a competent service. In a rapidly changing profession, practitioners need to develop their knowledge and skills continually, to keep up-to-date with new developments. Jarvis (1983, 1987) makes the case for learning to be a lifelong process for all professionals, and describes (1987) a useful distinction between lifelong professional education and lifelong professional learning. He defines lifelong professional education (1983: 5) as:
- any planned series of incidents at any time in the lifespan, having a humanistic basis directed towards the participants' learning and understanding.

Lifelong professional learning is a continuous process which is self-directed (see figure 3.2).

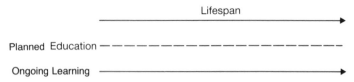

Fig. 3.2 Lifelong professional education and learning.

Both these concepts are relevant to the educational preparation of primary nurses. The educational event can be planned to give nurses some concentrated work before taking on the responsibilities of a primary nurse. The lifelong learning process is a skill and attitude to be fostered so that, as primary nurses practise professionally, they have the ability to learn independently what is required in order to offer a quality service. The educational event can be used to help nurses acquire study skills and explore the notion of lifelong learning.

Jarvis (1987) explains that lifelong learning can be both proactive and reactive. Proactive learning is the more familiar concept; the learner identifies a learning need, mobilizes resources and meets the need. It is a deliberate and planned action. On the other hand, reactive learning occurs on reflection of action. After the event the learner thinks about the action and attempts to explain it. This is an important idea for practitioners because it means that knowledge is being generated from practice rather than practice conforming to theory. Schön (1983) suggests that reflection on activity helps professionals to understand the complex and highly contextual situations they encounter in practice. Clarke (1986) stresses that this approach is appropriate for nursing because it makes practice and the theories arising from practice the focus for education, as opposed to externally generated theories applied to practice. Nurses can be helped to reflect on actions by allocating time to thought, encouraging retrospective discussion with colleagues and patients, and encouraging the use of reflective diaries. Benner (1984) successfully uses exemplars of nursing practice to identify expert nursing in context; by asking nurses to relate examples of their practice they were able to highlight clinical knowledge accrued through experience. Benner also expresses concern that nursing knowledge is practical as well as theoretical and that reflection on practice can generate the 'knowing how' of nursing.

CONTENT

It may seem inappropriate to suggest the content for learning after a discussion favouring student-centred learning. However, nurses in the transition from dependent to independent learners may welcome some advice and direction. It is also difficult for nurses to identify learning needs specific to becoming a primary nurse before they have had actual experience of the work. This can be made easier after the role and responsibilities have been explored.

Expansion of the link between the requests for learning made by Manthey's (1980) nurses, who had experience of practising as primary nurses, and Watson's (1985) ideas for a nursing curriculum, mentioned at the beginning of the chapter, may be helpful.

Specialist Knowledge or 'Trim'

Manthey's nurses' first request was for increased medical knowledge of the specialty, which is akin to Watson's trim field of nursing. Specialist knowledge is vital, because nurses are expected to understand what is wrong with their patients, the treatment required and potential complications that could arise. On the whole, nurses have no problem in relating this knowledge to their work (Lathlean *et al.*, 1986; Rogers, 1983), especially if they are accepting responsibility for planning nursing care.

Communication Skills or 'Core'

Watson believes that core nursing is relevant to all nurses, whatever their specialty. The core relates to nursing actions that are intrinsic to the nurse–patient relationship and to nursing therapy. Watson suggests that nursing therapy is concerned with caring more than curing, and she identifies ten 'carative' factors in order that they can be clarified, understood and mastered to the benefit of the partnership between nurse and patient.

Watson proposes that caring is an interpersonal process. I believe that nurses who recognise that they need to develop their communication skills may have appreciated the potential therapeutic value of a good nurse–patient relationship and be ready to explore and develop nursing skills, such as listening, counselling, instilling faith and hope, and empathy. If specific actions are chosen, caring can become a deliberate process initiated with the specific purposes of helping the patient achieve goals. This kind of development raises the level of basic nursing skills from something most 'kind' people do naturally to a subject field requiring sophisticated manipulation of advanced knowledge, skills and attitudes. Of course it is not suggested that all nurses reach this level before becoming primary nurses; indeed, some may strive to achieve it all their working lives. However, the core of nursing is worth highlighting for nurses hoping to progress with their particular patients.

The Nursing Process

Primary nurses need to be able to explain decisions rationally to their patients and associates to gain their support and co-operation. It is more likely that the plans will be used if they have been written down, and if the plans have not been used the primary nurse has evidence that she had left instructions.

The nursing process notes can be used by the primary nurse to account for her actions. Within one document, the nurse can demonstrate an assessment of the patient and his circumstances, what was hoped to be achieved, what was done, why it was done and what the results of the actions were. Hence the nursing process becomes an important communication, an accountability document vital to primary and associate nurses.

Work Role and Responsibilities

To practise confidently, primary nurses need to understand their new role, responsibilities and accountability mechanisms. Boundaries need to be agreed within which the nurses are free to make decisions.

PREPARATION FOR ASSOCIATE NURSES

Associate nurses may be newly qualified registered nurses, part-time registered or enrolled nurses, enrolled nurses, or student nurses under direct supervision.

Educational preparation for nurses who will take on the associate nurse role deserves a separate mention, as sometimes these nurses feel undervalued because the emphasis seems to be on primary nurses and their patients. Of course associate nurses are important members of the primary nursing team, ensuring a continuity of care for patients. The associate nurses support the primary nurse and contribute knowledge and experience in solving clinical problems. They are also quality controllers monitoring the primary nurse's work and when appropriate challenging decisions made. They, like primary nurses, need to be skilled practitioners and therefore their education needs to be along the same lines as that of the primary nurse; they are simply at a different point along the continuum. Given the knowledge and skills gained during enrolled nurse training there is considerable scope for developing associate nurse skills among this group of nurses. For newly qualified registered nurses the associate role can be seen as excellent experience in preparation for a primary nurse role. The experienced part-time registered nurse may well need to extend knowledge in a specialist area and become the ward consultant for this area in order to find an outlet for her considerable skill and experience.

Programmes in Current Use

Primary Nursing Module

This course was designed to help nurses wishing to practise as primary nurses and who preferably come from areas practising primary nursing.

The course is run three times a year in term time and comprises 12 study days spaced as shown in table 3.1. The curriculum planning team included practising nurses, teachers and managers. On discussion and reflection, the team recognised shared beliefs in a humanistic nursing service, professional practice, and theories of professional and adult education.

Table 3.1 Primary nursing module timetable

Date and venue	Time	Topic
Thursday 27.7.89 Post Grad Seminar Room	09.30	Introduction to course and course assignment information Meet all tutorial staff
	10.30	Coffee
	11.00	Professional nursing practice/autonomy
	12.30	Lunch
	13.30	Role theory Work boundaries
Friday 28.7.89 Post Grad Lecture Room	09.30	Case study approach to sources of knowledge
	14.00	Identification of clinical problem for investigation How to do a literature search How to critique an article
Thursday 3.8.89 Post Grad Seminar Room	09.30	Comparison of current nursing roles with those in a primary nursing system To be arranged (G. Lawrence)
	12.00	Seminar assignment information
Thursday 10.8.89 Post Grad Seminar Room	09.30	Study day – free
Thursday 16.8.89 Post Grad Seminar Room	09.30	Seminar presentation: Exploration of theoretical and personal concepts of primary nursing
Thursday 23.8.89 Post Grad Seminar Room	09.30	Seminar presentation: Establishing therapeutic nursing relationships
Thursday & Friday 30/31.8.89 Room 6, Level 3 Post Grad Seminar & Lecture Room	09.30– 16.00 both days	Interpersonal skills development

Table 3.1, continued

Date and venue	Time	Topic
Wednesday 6.9.89 Post Grad Seminar Room	09.30	Seminar presentation: Clinical team roles ● Extended/expanded ● MDCT ● Legal aspects
Wednesday 13.9.89 Post Grad Seminar Room	09.30	Seminar presentation: ● Clinical nurse specialist ● Ethical issues
Wednesday 20.9.89 Conference Room, Level 3	09.30 11.30	Workshop: Presentation of care plans to fellow students Prerequisites for further development Job descriptions Peer review
Wednesday 27.9.89 Room 6 Level 3 JRII	09.30 11.00 13.00	Coping with change Evaluation Lunch – all course staff

The aims of the course (Burns *et al.*, 1988) are:

● To promote an understanding of the implications of professional nursing practice within the context of an organisation
● To identify areas of responsibility and accountability of a primary nurse
● To use knowledge for skilled practice
● To recognise the relevance of self-awareness in respect of developing helping relationships with partners in care, including patients and associate nurses

After consideration it was decided that, although predetermined aims may seem directive, some course members not used to independent study might find them a useful guide. The students are given information about the course and its aims in advance and are welcome to make suggestions according to their particular needs.

A variety of educational methods are used in the course; however, there is a predominance of student-centred activities such as seminar presentations, tutorials, group discussions, workshops and experiential learning. All students write a literature review related to their specialist practice, which gives them added specialist knowledge and skills such as literature searching, critical reading and analysis. The students also keep a diary of practice for reflection, making daily notes about incidents at work and recording anything that seems appropriate to them – the event, their interpretation, other people's reaction, their feelings. This encourages them to reflect on their practice regularly, hopefully helping them to make sense and increasing their repertoire of practical knowledge.

Formative evaluation of the course is undertaken in an informal manner; members are encouraged to make suggestions and give constructive criticism at any time during the course. Summative course evaluation is undertaken using a nominal group technique (Delbecq *et al.*, 1975) to accommodate a broad range of views and gain a consensus.

The course is considered as an educational event that equips the nurses with an understanding of the work they will undertake as primary nurses and an ability to find and use critically information useful to their practice. It is hoped that nurses are motivated to continue the lifelong professional learning process.

Contract Learning

This method has been chosen by a team of nurses on a medical ward which is planning to change to primary nursing. The team already has a well developed, working philosophy of nursing which complements primary nursing. It stresses the importance of the nurse–patient partnership, and the need for nurses to make knowledgeable decisions within a supportive rather than a hierarchical organisation. Nurses chosen to be primary nurses are experienced in the specialty and have shown an ability to learn independently. The team has chosen to use Orem's self-care model as a guide to nursing practice.

Contract learning involves a transaction between two people (Jarvis, 1986) with mutually agreed needs and learning objectives. Each nurse spent time with the lecturer-practitioner or senior staff nurse (who were jointly working as facilitators) discussing the individual's strengths and weaknesses, and the proposed role change, and identifying areas for development. Goals were then set and the actions of both the nurse and the facilitator were planned bearing in mind the resources available. A completion date was agreed and time was set aside to evaluate progress and make more plans. This was all recorded on a contract form and signed. This work was undertaken with all the nursing staff, both potential primary nurses and associate nurses.

There were problems with this method of learning. The students have individual programmes and therefore seldom join together for tutorial work, which meant that the facilitator has a heavy commitment to tutorial work. Nurses have found it difficult to keep up to date with the work because tutorials are hard to arrange and study is not easy after a long shift. However, the work is being completed and found to be relevant to practice.

Examples of work undertaken for the contract work were completion of a learning pack on Orem's model of nursing, specific work to refine the use of the nursing process, attending a communication skills workshop, and reading current literature on primary nursing and discussing it critically.

This contract work will continue when primary nursing is introduced. It is anticipated that the contract contents will become more diverse when the nurses have a clearer idea of what the work entails and how they cope with new responsibilities.

CONCLUSION

The educational preparation for primary nurses is not specialised. Primary nurses need to be mature, expert practitioners, with a well defined notion of nursing, fully conversant with the role and its accompanying responsibilities, and able to learn on their own and to seek appropriate educational opportunities as the need arises. It can be argued that these are attributes and skills that all professional nurses should aspire to, but that they can get by without in a system that seldom requires that they make decisions on their own or holds them to account for their practice.

How much each nurse needs to learn before practising as a primary nurse will depend on her starting point, the social setting of her work and the patients she will serve. Until basic nurse education is designed to prepare nurses for professional practice there will be considerable work for most nurses to do in order to work as a primary nurse.

A humanistic approach to learning (paying attention to the particular nurse, valuing each individual's unique contribution and appreciating knowledge) links with humanistic nursing and will help nurses to appreciate the individual and confirm belief in each person's ability to learn and control their own lives, be they teacher, nurse, student or patient. The methods of learning chosen and the attitudes generated among all participants are possibly more important than the subject matter.

Lastly any course of study in preparation for primary nursing is just an event in the continuum of lifelong professional education.

4

Accountability and Legal Issues in Primary Nursing

Julie Goulding and John Hunt

This chapter examines what it means to be held accountable and the legal position of the nurse within a primary nursing system.

Responsibility, authority, autonomy and accountability are terms frequently used in nursing today. They are often used interchangeably; however, each denotes a specific concept. The understanding of primary nursing requires an appreciation of these concepts:

1. *Responsibility* is a charge for which one is answerable. The focus is on the charge, not on how or to whom the answering should occur.
2. *Authority* is the rightful (legitimate) power to fulfil a charge (responsibility). Authority in nursing derives from at least three sources:
   - Authority of the situation
   - Authority of expert knowledge
   - Authority of position
3. *Autonomy* means self-determination, self-direction, freedom to design a total plan of nursing care and to work on an independent level with other professionals, being left on one's own to work (Batey and Lewis, 1982).
4. *Accountability* is examined in detail in the text.

Until recently it has been difficult to hold a single nurse accountable for her actions; however, in the system of primary nursing, the line of accountability is clear. Inextricably linked with issues of accountability are the legal issues about which each responsible nurse should be aware. Accountability will now be examined in greater depth, followed by an overview of relevant legal principles.

ACCOUNTABILITY IN PRIMARY NURSING

According to Manthey (1980), accountability is the cornerstone of primary nursing. The *Concise Oxford Dictionary* defines accountability as 'bound to give account, responsible (for things to persons)'.

Simms (1967) felt that the concept of accountability should be equated with a type of responsibility or more specifically being answerable for one's actions. Murray and Zettner (1974) extended this definition of accountability as being responsible for one's acts to include being able to explain or define them, and being able to measure in some way the results of decision making. This approach is supported by Schweiger (1980), who stated that, in nursing, accountability is concerned with what was done as compared with what should have been done. It is a measure of efficiency and productivity of a person as judged against professional or nursing standards. However, Claus and Baily (1977) clearly distinguish between the two concepts of accountability and responsibility. They regard accountability as a sense of overriding concern for nursing care, and responsibility as the sense of duty in performing specific tasks. Barret *et al.* (1975) maintained that the essential difference was that responsibility was delegated whereas accountability was not.

Manthey (1980) in her four elements of primary nursing talks of the acceptance as well as the allocation of responsibility by the nurse for:

● Decision making of a group of patients
● Quality of care 24 hours a day, seven days a week

Bergman (1981) concluded that responsibility was the key component of accountability but was nevertheless only a part of it. She suggests that there are three preconditions for accountability:

● *Ability* The primary nurse cannot be held accountable unless she has the required knowledge, skills and values to act on specific issues.
● *Responsibility* The primary nurse is responsible for the care she provides for her patients; continuous responsibility is demonstrated through an appropriate up-to-date care plan.
● *Authority* A nurse cannot accept accountability for patient care unless she is given the authority to make decisions that affect care.

The Code of Professional Conduct for the nurse, midwife and health visitor (UKCC 1984) states clearly that each registered nurse, midwife and health visitor is accountable for her own practice. In a traditional nursing system it is not always clear who is to be held accountable for certain aspects of care. However, in a primary nursing system the location of accountability is often clearer.

The relationship between the exercise of accountability in nursing and the legal principles involved are now explored. This is highlighted using the code of professional conduct (UKCC 1984).

LEGAL PRINCIPLES

Code of Professional Conduct and the Duty of Care

A code of professional conduct for the nurse, midwife and health visitor is published by the statutory body for nursing – The United Kingdom Central Council for Nursing, Midwifery and Health Visiting (UKCC, 1984).

The Code provides guidance on nursing standards which all nurses working in a traditional or primary nursing system should uphold. Failure to do so could be relevant or significant in the event of any legal action. The following should be of particular relevance if accidents, injuries or unsatisfactory outcomes have to be examined in the course of complaints or legal action by or on behalf of patients:

- Act always in such a way as to promote and safeguard the well-being and interests of patients/clients (clause 1).
- Ensure that no action or omission on his/her part or within his/her sphere of influence is detrimental to the condition or safety of patients/clients (clause 2).
- Acknowledge any limitations of competence and refuse in such cases to accept delegated functions without first having received instructions in regard to those functions and having been assessed as competent (clause 4).

All of this emphasises the fact that the nurse is morally and legally accountable to the patient/client for her professional behaviour and actions. In particular, she owes a duty of care to the patient/client. This means that she takes responsibility for the direct care that she gives (and the advice and training that she offers), and will avoid taking unreasonable risks. In other words, she must be a safe practitioner. The standards of knowledge that would be applied would normally be those expected of a person in that position, with those qualifications and that experience.

Both employer and employee have a responsibility towards the patient. In the words of Lord Justice Denning (*Cassidy* v. *Minister of Health* 1951): Whenever health authorities 'accept a patient for treatment they must use reasonable care and skill to cure him of the ailment. They cannot of course do it by themselves . . . they must do it by the staff they employ; and if their staff are negligent in giving the treatment, they are just as liable for that negligence as is anyone else who employs others to do his duties for him . . . once they undertake the task, they come under a duty to use care in the doing of it'.

Negligence

In a perfect world, patients will be completely satisfied with the standard of care, the treatment they receive, and the outcome. They expect no harm to occur. In the real world, though, mistakes, accidents and injuries can sometimes occur, and while there may be a host of seemingly plausible reasons why those have arisen (e.g. pressure of work, shortage of staff), their occurrence is always unfortunate and in some cases may be very serious.

When mistakes and other untoward incidents occur, patients or their relatives can understandably feel aggrieved. It may be that with discussion at the time with the staff involved on the ward, this can be explained and the position clarified. It may be that this could be the subject of a more formal complaint or investigation subsequently. But it may be that the patient or relative resorts to legal action because of the seriousness of what has gone wrong. In doing this, the plaintiff (the person bringing the action) may feel that there has been a negligent act or omission, and that one or more persons is responsible.

In law, negligence is a 'tort' or civil wrong: a breach of duty imposed by law whereby a person acquires a right of action for damages. Negligence 'is the omission to do something which a reasonable man, guided upon those considerations which ordinarily regulate the conduct of human affairs, would do, or doing something which a prudent and reasonable man would not do' (per *Alderson, B-Blyth B*. v. *Birmingham Waterworks Co*. 1856).

A plaintiff must demonstrate three things if he is to succeed in an action:

● The existence of a duty to take care which was owed to him by the defendant (so, for example, a nurse would clearly have a duty to care for a patient on her ward).
● Breach of such duty by the defendant.
● Resulting damage to the plaintiff (the patient must show that he has suffered some loss or actual harm as a direct result of the act or omission).

So negligence can occur if professional duties are performed in a negligent manner, or if tasks are undertaken which are beyond the capabilities of those concerned because of inadequate training or experience, or lack of the necessary skills and ability. This may arise if, for example, a nurse undertakes a job normally undertaken by a doctor. The standard that applies is the same for a person who has trained to undertake the task.

Concept of Vicarious Liability

One of the most important duties imposed on all employees by employers is the duty to take reasonable care when carrying out his duties at work. If the employee is negligent, his employer will be able to take disciplinary action against him, and his employer has the right to sue him for the resulting loss. If he has acted reasonably, however, he will not be liable.

In addition, individual employees are held to be bound by disciplinary codes and disciplinary procedures. In the context of the nursing profession, the UKCC's national code is clearly relevant here. It is supplemented by local codes and procedures published by the health authority. Notwithstanding any legal consequences following on from any breach of these codes and procedures, health authorities as employers can take disciplinary action, which can be, at worst, dismissal but which depending on the circumstances could be suspension (usually on full pay while investigations take place), warnings or reprimands. The statutory body for nursing, the UKCC, may remove the nurse from the professional register.

So what happens when something goes wrong in the working environment? In particular, who is responsible? The principle of vicarious liability is important in this context. This means that one person or body is responsible for the actions of another because of their relationship (e.g. an employer could be liable for the actions of an employee). The plaintiff can sue either, or both, of them. If something goes wrong with the treatment of a patient, and the patient feels that there has been negligence, the patient as the plaintiff is within his rights to bring a legal action against the members of staff concerned and/or their employing organisation. If he fails to prove that there has been negligence, his case of course will fail, but if he succeeds it would be relevant to determine who is responsible for the acts of the negligent person (it could be a more senior person or the employing authority itself).

Health authorities, as well as individual staff, have a duty of care – to provide care for the patients under their care, and to the staff employed by them. This means, among other things, that they should ensure that staff are properly qualified and adequately instructed to care for those in their charge.

Invariably, it is the health authority that would be named as the defendant in any legal action that could involve nurses, so a health authority will be vicariously liable for injury caused by negligence or incompetence of any members of its staff. However, it should be noted that the negligent person is also liable, and the health authority technically has a right at common law to claim indemnity against that person.

IMPLICATIONS FOR NURSING

Changes in Traditional Nursing: Accountability and Legal Implications

The question often asked by nurses when considering primary nursing is how the exercise of accountability within primary nursing differs from that within a traditional nursing system. This was introduced in chapter 1, but is explored further here.

In the traditional nursing system the nurse is viewed as a servant of an institution, or as an 'organisation man or woman'. The nurse is seen to draw authority from the organisation, an authority delegated downward through the hierarchy of superior–subordinate relationships and validated by the occupancy of a position in the chain of command. In this system major accountability is to representatives of the organisation who occupy senior positions, and this accountability is for the performance of designated functions in accordance with the regulations. Provided these are adhered to, the organisation will accept vicarious liability for the nurse if there is any question of litigation (Davies and Francis, 1976). This bureaucratic structure is still evident in nursing today, with the ward team often being led by the sister or charge nurses, who are accountable to their senior nurses if something goes wrong. The staff nurses, enrolled nurses, students and auxiliaries all carry out instructions from above, with little authority to make key decisions. The staff nurses in the traditional setting are often not expected to make decisions regarding total patient care. They have no delegated authority to act and if problems arose they would be dealt with by the ward sister.

There have been numerous changes in the command structure within nursing in recent years, and this may have caused some confusion about accountability.

If things go wrong, it is through the ward sister or charge nurse that matters are taken, and enquiries or investigations made. She is the focus. If the matter relates to one of the nursing staff on her ward, she is the person who would normally take the matter further with that member of staff. She has some direct responsibility for the actions and behaviour of her staff (although obviously much depends on the precise nature of the enquiry – for example, whether she was on duty at the relevant time, whether she allocated a specific responsibility to a particular nurse, or whether she saw the notes or a report on the matter, and the sequence of events thereafter).

As the manager of the ward, the ward sister or charge nurse may, therefore, have a managerial or professional responsibility for the acts or omissions of her staff. This responsibility could well be shared by other nurses as a group or by nurse managers higher up the nursing management hierarchy. This means that nurse managers may not be exempt from claims for negligence. This would depend on the circumstances, obviously, but they could have contributed to the negligence even if they were not directly involved. For example, there may have been failure on their part to ensure adequate instruction in new nursing techniques or in the use of new equipment. A nurse manager could also be liable vicariously if she should have undertaken a task herself, or if she should have supervised the work of a more junior nurse more carefully while it was being carried out.

In the traditional setting it is often the enrolled nurses, the students and the auxiliary staff who perform nursing care or various parts of care for each patient, making it nearly impossible to hold one person responsible or indeed accountable for omissions of care or care that is inappropriate.

Issues Arising from the Interdependence of Medicine and Nursing

Accountability also needs to be considered from a medical viewpoint as nursing is often seen to be legitimised by medicine. Nursing maybe seen as part of the medical division of labour, an auxiliary occupation drawing authority from medicial protocols. High status is attached to technical skills which are often handed down from doctors. The nurses role may be perceived as that of a doctor's assistant and not that of a practitioner in her own right. In this view of nursing the nurse is seen as being accountable to the doctors for the decisions made and care performed.

Doctors, like other professional practitioners, have personal responsibility for their work. They can be held liable in law for their actions or advice, and it is a requirement of their employment with a health authority that they have their own insurance with a medical defence organisation for this reason. In the event of legal action in connection with treatment of patients, doctors or their health authority are much more likely to be sued than nurses. Historically doctors have been seen to have the responsibility to treat, whereas nurses have a lesser responsibility of 'merely' caring, with perhaps less risk in the event of things going wrong.

With the introduction of primary nursing, medical staff will certainly be aware of some fundamental changes in nursing practice in the wards. Consultants and junior doctors will need to become used to the fact that they should liaise with the primary nurse in charge of the nursing care of the patient over whom they have responsibility for medical care. Previously, consultants expected to liaise with the sister (or senior nurse in charge of the ward) for all of the patients on the ward. This will probably take some getting used to, but the benefits should become clear to the medical staff when they realise that the primary nurse will have much more detailed knowledge of the patient.

In recent times there has been a trend towards greater levels of responsibility assumed by nurses in general and primary nurses in particular. There is sometimes a fine dividing line between where the responsibilities of the doctor end and those of the nurse begin, and vice versa. For example, there is the issue of how compatible the nursing care plan is with the medical care planned. Hopefully, there will be no contradictions or inconsistencies. If there are, it will be necessary to have a mechanism whereby this can be resolved – probably with the involvement of the senior nurse. In practice, however, nurses may be experiencing difficulties, when their planned care differs from the medical decisions about care. This is demonstrated in a recent example related to the individual's right to be told the truth. The primary nurse and the patient involved had a close, professional relationship and the nurse attempting to fulfil her professional responsibility helped the patient to face the truth about his terminal illness. This was against the wishes of the medical staff. The nurse was asked to account to the doctor concerned and indeed was able to do so. It highlights the very complex nature of the changing relationships and the recognition of accountability within the primary nursing system.

Primary Nursing – the Changes

Changed Responsibilities and Greater Delegation of Authority

It is implicit that, with the introduction of primary nursing, there would be a greater delegation of responsibility for decision making from the sister to the primary nurse herself, and to an associate nurse in her absence. Although this devolution of responsibility is probably welcomed by all concerned, it is of importance that guidelines for safe practice should be followed. Here are some examples:

- If new work is accepted, the nurse must agree that it is a reasonable commitment, in relation to the nurse's present responsibility.
- If the nurse delegates work, she must ensure that staff are not asked to perform tasks for which they are not fitted, or from which they are prohibited by legal enactment.
- The nurse should acknowledge any limitations of her competence, and should not accept responsibility for work she does not feel prepared to undertake.

The differences between the work and responsibilities of the staff nurse and the work and responsibilities of the primary nurse are considerable. Ideally, these differences should be made explicit to staff nurses who become primary nurses. If the staff nurse is not willing to become a primary nurse, with all that it entails, or does not feel competent to take on those responsibilities, there should be an opportunity to practise as a staff nurse in a more traditional environment or ideally as an associate nurse. This would allow more time to appreciate what is involved in the transition to becoming a primary nurse, and perhaps give opportunity for further development if this is identified as a requirement.

It could be, though, that former staff nurses who become primary nurses will not feel comfortable with their new role, will not feel competent to carry out extra responsibilities, or will in fact not be competent to carry out this changed work.

The primary nurse may not feel comfortable with the new role. There is often apprehension over change itself. The responsibility here lies with the senior clinical nurse or senior nurse manager in handling the situation and taking time to ensure appropriate explanation, discussion, training and development, throughout. The ward team should be able to offer peer group support, as well as the support offered by the senior nurse.

The primary nurse may not feel competent to carry out the extra responsibilities. Again, the responsibility lies with the senior nurse to identify this and to determine whether there is a basis for this feeling. If it is without foundation, the primary nurse should have the chance to discuss this and for her confidence to be restored, possibly with peer group support or by support from the senior nurse. If there is some cause for concern, it may be possible to improve matters with appropriate continuing education and development.

There is also the more serious issue of whether the former staff nurse is competent to carry out the extra responsibilities of the primary nurse. The primary nurse is expected to offer the same high standard of clinical care to her patients as the staff nurse, but by accepting responsibility for the overall quality of care her patients receive the primary nurse will also need particular skills in decision making, communication and care planning. Although there may be no differences in the competence between the primary nurse and the staff nurse, the expectations of them will be different. The ward sister no longer holds direct accountability for patient care. If things go wrong with aspects of nursing care and treatment given by nurses, the primary nurse is the key person who will be answerable in the first instance, and who retains overall nursing responsibility for the care of the patient. The senior nurse on the ward will probably not have had the same involvement with the patient, and will not have the same supervisory function or vicarious liability as did the sister formerly. Let us now examine the roles more closely.

Changed Responsibilities: the Primary Nurse

In the system of primary nursing the primary nurse is seen as a professional practitioner, contracted to provide total nursing care to her client group. Responsibility here is for the care one contracts to provide and primary accountability is to the client. The authority to act comes from a sound knowledge base and the claim of expertise in prescribing and delivering nursing care. This system of nursing also demands accountability to society, to the profession and to other members of the multidisciplinary team for the quality of care provided.

The primary nurse takes responsibility for a client group from admission through to discharge. She is responsible not only for planning care but for implementing and evaluating the care given. Once the primary nurse has accepted responsibility to care for a patient or group of patients she immediately becomes accountable for any commissions or omissions of care; she cannot pass the buck to the ward sister or senior nurse. For a primary nurse to practise at this level she must have a high degree of professional competence, the need for continuing education becomes crucial and again the primary nurse must accept responsibility for continuing her own education. She will, however, need support to continue her education: support from her clinical leader/senior nurse to plan off-duty time to allow time away from work, and support and guidance with courses being undertaken. The implication is that by endorsing primary nursing the health authority should be prepared to accept responsibility for funding courses. Without continuing education it is impossible for a primary nurse to make appropriate decisions about care. It may even be dangerous for the patient and the nurse could easily find herself facing a professional conduct committee.

The Plan of Care

A fundamental part of the role of the primary nurse is the writing of the nursing care plan for each patient. It is important that the plan is appropriate for the patient's needs and is clearly communicated. The care plan becomes an essential element in extending decisions about care in the absence of the primary nurse. In this respect the primary nurse remains accountable for the plan, as has been explained previously. What happens if this care plan does not result in the desired outcome? There may be, of course, good reasons why favourable results cannot follow all the time, but if those results are unsatisfactory there is always the chance that the patient will feel aggrieved. There are several approaches available ranging in seriousness from a point of clarification being raised and discussed with the patient at the time of attendance, right through to court proceedings.

It may be that the outcome is not favourable to the patient for reasons quite beyond the control of the nurse; for example, because of the seriousness of the patient's condition, or because the outcome relates to aspects of treatment and cure that are more dependent on the actions of the doctor. However, it may be that the nursing care plan is not felt to be entirely satisfactory for the patient. The primary nurse initiates this plan. What if she fails to identify the problem correctly with the patient or to establish an achievable goal? What if she outlines incorrect nursing action? There could clearly be difficulties if there are errors of judgement and errors of fact. The difficulties may not be perceived by the patient (or his relatives), or if perceived may not be serious, but if they are serious what would the position be, and who would be liable? Much would obviously depend on the circumstances of each particular case. The primary nurse, as the author of the document, is accountable for its contents. She may say that she has drawn on facts and opinions expressed by others, but she would be expected to have analysed these to the best of her ability, and be satisifed that, to the best of her knowledge, the resulting plan is appropriate. In undertaking this, she will have received training (failure to provide such training before undertaking this could in itself be negligence – and presumably a defence that could be offered by the primary nurse). Also the quality of that plan will be judged in accordance with standards expected from a 'reasonable' primary nurse.

Although not usually directly involved in the formation of the nursing care plan, the senior nurse has the responsibility of monitoring the standards of plans and ensuring that they are of acceptable quality. If she is aware of difficulties that any of the primary nurses are experiencing in this work, she is under an obligation to take action to rectify matters. Failure to do so would be an omission amounting to negligence, as well as not being in accordance with professional standards.

Changed Responsibilities: the Senior Nurse

The differing roles of the ward sister in the traditional model of nursing and the senior nurse in the primary nurse model can best be appreciated by contrasting the job descriptions of these two posts. The ward sister has a direct managerial responsibility for the more junior nurses on her ward (and in some places for the non-nursing staff too). The responsibility the sister has over the staff nurses within the traditional systems of organisation is one of a supervisor. As such, she is normally responsible for their actions on the ward, and will usually be spokesperson for them in the event of any complaint or legal enquiry, in that she will, as 'ward manager', usually be the contact point and the co-ordinator of any enquiries.

In comparison with the traditional ward sister the senior nurse within the primary nursing system is responsible for leading and managing the ward team. She is responsible for ensuring that the primary nurses have the skills and ability required to be responsible and accountable for their own actions. The senior nurse is accountable for the overall quality and standards of care on the ward; the individual primary nurses are accountable for the care their patients receive and in the event of a complaint or legal enquiry the primary nurse would be expected to deal with the situation, to account for her actions, supported and advised when necessary by the senior nurse.

Having said this, primary nurses, associate nurses, staff nurses and other nursing staff on the ward are clearly responsible for their own actions and will remain accountable for them. The primary nurse is clearly accountable for the overall direction of the care planned for the individual patient, and in the event of something going wrong will be responsible for providing statements about the circumstances. The standards that will be applied would be those expected of nurses with their experience and training.

Primary nursing demands a high level of clinical expertise from all the team members. Team work is still a vital element, and perhaps the most important person to the successful implementation and continued development of primary nursing is the team leader. Manthey (1973) describes the role of the senior nurse on a primary nursing unit as ' . . . the factor most critical to the success of primary nursing'.

The senior nurse on the primary nursing unit has a number of roles:

- She acts as an expert adviser on clinical nursing. To fulfil this part of the role, the senior nurse must be an experienced clinical nurse who has continued her own education and professional development. She may be approached by the primary nurses for advice related to clinical issues. She also has a responsibility for being a resource person, and acts as a facilitator for the primary nurses to help increase their own knowledge and develop their skills by arranging courses and encouraging conference attendance.
- She ensures that patients are allocated to primary nurses with the appropriate skills and knowledge to care for the patient safely and appropriately. She must know her nurses well, be aware of their strengths and weaknesses, and play an active role in their development.
- She is responsible for ensuring that high standards of care are achieved on the ward and for setting up quality assurance programmes, an area until recently largely ignored by nurses. When the senior nurse notices that care planned is inappropriate or that there is more recent research evidence to suggest a different way of organising care, it is her responsiblity to discuss this with the primary nurse concerned.

- She acts as a manager. This role is potentially the most time consuming. This includes managing staff on the ward/unit, employing staff with the primary nurses, disciplining staff where appropriate, record keeping and generally ensuring the smooth running of the department. The role itself requires extensive skill and knowledge; many senior nurses on wards today may be ill prepared for the managerial component of their role.
- She is accountable to her managers and the health authority for the budgetary control usually vested in the senior nurse.
- She should strive to continue her development as an expert practitioner, carrying out clinical care. It is usually not possible for the senior nurse also to adopt a primary nurse role because of the significant content and potential incompatibility of the two roles. In such a case one role may be neglected. The senior nurse often works as an associate nurse in the absence of the primary nurse. She is then responsible and accountable for the care implemented. She is also responsible for keeping the primary nurse informed of any changes in planned care during the absence of the primary nurse.

In acute units where changes occur rapidly, it is often not practical or desirable for the primary nurse to be consulted about all changes in care (when off duty). In this situation the senior nurse will often make the changes with the associate nurse involved, but informing the primary nurse of the changes and the reasons for those changes immediately on her return to duty. In some units for the care of the elderly, where changes in care may occur less frequently, or can often be anticipated, the primary nurse may agree to be contacted 24 hours a day seven days a week, within reason. This area of who should alter plans of care needs to be negotiated in the planning stages when setting up a primary nursing unit (see chapter 1).

Pembrey (1989) believes that the senior nurse is crucial to primary nursing, with the specific task of leadership and management of a team that will provide excellent patient care over 24 hours. She believes that the team leader's role is still vital to nursing, but that the content of the role changes, with the role of leader and manager having different components, each vital to the primary nursing system.

The Absence of the Primary Nurse

One of the difficulties inherent in the introduction of primary nursing is that the primary nurse cannot be available at all times and the responsibility for nursing care must therefore be shared with associate nurses.

The primary nurse does not work in isolation. When she is off duty her patients are cared for by one of her associate nurses. The associate nurse may be an inexperienced registered nurse or a part-time registered nurse. She may be an enrolled nurse, and in some areas with student nurses this role is performed by students. The associate nurses are important members of the nursing team. They are responsible for carrying out prescribed care for patients. Once they accept this responsibility they will also be expected to account for care given, although they cannot be held accountable for care prescribed. The associate nurses are supervised by the senior nurse. Any changes to planned care in the absence of the primary nurse would be discussed with the senior nurse or other primary nurses; they would never be made by a student nurse.

In handing over responsibility for nursing care to associate nurses, the primary nurse should take all measures reasonable in effecting this transition. This means that there should be a clear understanding of the current state and condition of the patient and the expectation of the nursing care to be given in the period following the handover. It means that appropriate information about this should be documented in the plan, and that the overall plan of care should be understandable and adhered to. Failure to communicate this effectively could be serious, and could even be deemed to be a negligent act or omission.

Likewise, in handing back to a primary nurse at a later shift, the associate nurse is expected to communicate effectively and to a reasonable standard. With written care plans this will include a written statement in the evaluation section about the revision to the plan necessary in the light of the patient's changed condition. It is the primary nurse's prerogative to review this revision. The primary nurse and the associate nurse should be expected to strive to achieve the highest standards of care within the confines of their role.

The senior nurse may be directly involved in this process (if, for example, she is covering for a primary nurse). More likely, though, she will be indirectly involved. As the most senior nurse on the ward, she is responsible for monitoring the care of the patients on the ward, and this includes the necessity for ensuring that there is continuity in the provision of such care.

The Care Assistant's Role

The role of the care assistant/auxiliary in the primary nursing unit is to provide maximum support to the nurses, to allow the nurses maximum time to be involved in patient care. The care assistant's key role is to assist the nurses in patient care, and she is responsible to them, with overall accountability to the senior nurse. In some units when not assisting the nurses the auxiliaries have total responsibility for keeping the ward clean and serving patients meals.

CONCLUSION

Primary nursing demands a level of accountability never before seen in nursing at a clinical level. The primary nurse will be expected to account for her decisions and actions, the associate nurse will also be expected to account for the care that she gives, and the clinical leader is responsible and therefore accountable for the overall standard of care. The code of professional conduct (UKCC, 1984) states very clearly that the nurse is accountable for her actions and indeed may be called upon to do so. For professional and legal reasons the nurse would at all times be expected to be able to support the claim that she acted in the best interest of her patients and in doing so that she had taken all reasonable care.

Primary nurses, and indeed other nurses working within the exciting system of primary nursing, thrive on the opportunity to exercise greater responsibility.

However, it is very difficult in the bureaucratic structure that still dominates nursing today to take responsibility and to be allowed the authority to act. This needs to be delegated from above. This area needs to be carefully considered and addressed before a primary nursing system can be successfully implemented.

The knowledge and skills required to plan effective nursing care and to make intricate ethical decisions are highly advanced, and basic nurse training does not prepare a nurse for the complex nature of the role of the primary nurse. Therefore it is essential that the primary nurse, and indeed all of the nurses working in the system of primary nursing, are actively encouraged to continue their education at an advanced level – an area that often receives only lip service in practice.

Finally, primary nursing by itself does not improve the standard of nursing care. As a system, though, it facilitates the provision of a very high level of quality by enabling individuals to perform at their maximum capacity. Whether they do so or not depends on them, the support they receive, their preparation for the role, and their starting competency.

ACKNOWLEDGEMENT

We would like to thank the Legal Department of the Royal College of Nursing, London, for checking the accuracy of legal statements made in this chapter.

PART 2

Primary Nursing in Practice in the

United Kingdom

5

Primary Nursing in a Surgical Unit

Chris Allsopp

WHAT PRIMARY NURSING OFFERS SURGICAL PATIENTS AND THEIR NURSES

Surgical wards are characteristically busy places. The patient's average length of stay is short (approximately 4–5 days on the unit). What could primary nursing offer patients and their nurses in a surgical unit? For patients it could offer a great deal more continuity and co-ordination in their care. Even though a stay on a surgical ward may be short, this kind of continuity could be very comforting for a patient. His primary nurse would provide direction and collaborate with others to ensure that appropriate care was given to him, so the patient would not find that a different person was caring for him each day and feel that no one nurse really had any full appreciation of his problems. Thus there is a greater likelihood that optimum care would be given to the patient and his family, because the primary nurse is in a better position to focus care on the patient's individual needs (Marram Van Servellen, 1982).

Primary nursing may also lead to the development of a close relationship, which could give the patient a sense of being a participant in his care (Pearson, 1988; Zander, 1980). The possibility of such a relationship would be a particular breakthrough in the surgical setting, where the emphasis is often on doing things to and for the patient, rather than allowing informed choice and active involvement. Furthermore, the primary nurse may be in a better position to develop a deeper knowledge and understanding of her patient, through focusing on a smaller group of patients, and so may be better equipped to meet her patients' individual needs.

Primary nursing, with its highly patient-centred orientation, could also lead to less fragmentation of care for surgical patients. This individual but consistent approach is also vital in building up trust in one person; it is this which may help him to cope through an often frightening and bewildering run up to surgery and then through postoperative recovery.

It would also seem that a system of care which has the potential to improve the quality and humanity of nursing is of particular value in the surgical ward areas which are swamped with technology and where length of stay is short. Also, in an area where the medical model flourishes, there is the risk that a patient's fuller range of health needs may not be met by nurses. The reductionist approach of medicine, which separates the mind from the body and has a tendency to reduce the patient to a set of organs to be treated, has in the past impeded the development of nursing and a broader-based health assessment (Pearson and Vaughan, 1986).

The nurse's motivation, which is often hard to maintain under the workload of acute surgical nursing, may be improved by the practice of primary nursing because of the opportunity for nurses to have a greater degree of automony – freeing them to become more creative in care planning and to have a greater voice in decision making in multidisciplinary discussions.

Job satisfaction may also improve as the nurse moves back to the bedside, rather than being solely an overseer of care, 'in charge' of the ward. Primary nursing also offers the nurse scope to develop clinical expertise in surgical nursing. A highly patient-centred approach to care may be allowed to flourish in an environment in which responsibilities such as the doctor's rounds and the bed state may dominate; aspects of nursing that are necessary but which take the nurse away from the patient. Primary nursing may also create an opportunity for nurses to strip away the often stifling effect of the nursing hierarchy, where the sister gives out instructions for nursing care and nursing work is carried out by routine.

THE PRACTICE SETTING

The surgical area described in this chapter comprises two 20-bedded surgical wards, within a large British teaching hospital (see figure 5.1 for layout). The specialty

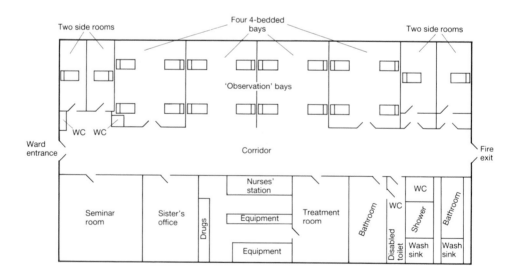

Fig. 5.1 Layout of one of the surgical wards within the unit.

within the unit is vascular surgery although general surgical patients are also nursed on the wards.

Primary nursing has been practised on the unit for almost two years and a great deal of preparation for change was necessary to facilitate this.

PLANNING FOR CHANGE

The idea for moving toward primary nursing was put forward by Alison Binnie, who as Senior Sister was the unit's nurse manager. Discussions in earnest began a year before the actual introduction of primary nursing, although Alison had been preparing herself for the changes for much longer.

It was felt that there were serious inadequacies in the existing system of nursing on the unit. For instance, no one nurse was responsible for the management of a patient's nursing for more than the span of an 8-hour shift, so care was often fragmented and ineffective because of this discontinuity. Also, only the sister had the authority to make long-term decisions about a patient's care, and so other qualified nurses were denied the satisfaction of following care through, and there was little encouragement to be creative or innovative.

In the light of these failings in the existing system, the idea of primary nursing was discussed. Although many of the new thoughts were welcome, there were also reservations expressed about the organisational difficulties of such a system on a busy surgical ward. This resulted, over the next year, in heated discussion about the pros and cons of primary nursing. During this time, a few people who felt they could not adapt to the new system left the unit and the recruitment policy was to look for nurses who would flourish given the chance to practise primary nursing.

Three key areas were considered in the planning of the changes:

- The ward philosophy
- Organisational concerns
- Educational preparation

These three areas will now be discussed.

The Ward Philosophy

It was felt necessary to consider the beliefs and values of all the nurses on issues such as health, the patient and professional nursing. Deliberations concerning these issues had already begun through weekly ward meetings at which primary nursing was discussed. The results of these meetings and a final discussion session enabled a unit philosophy to be written detailing the nurses' shared beliefs and values about nursing practice on this ward.

The written philosophy incorporated beliefs such as holism and values which included emphasis on a person's rights to be informed, have choices, be treated with dignity and respect, and be cared for by trained, competent nurses.

Beliefs about health included the notions that it was a subjective state of well-being, in which a person adapts comfortably to biological, social and emotional pressure and is free to grow towards his full potential.

The nurses also believed in the value of attempting to work in partnership with patients; that nurses should show sensitivity and support to patients and be able to teach and give advice about self-management, using the nursing process. It was felt that nurses occupy a unique position within the health care team and that respect and concern for each other was all-important. In addition, it was stated that nurses have educational needs, with a personal responsibility for continuous learning. It was also acknowledged that nurses are accountable and responsible for any care they provide for patients.

An open atmosphere was also considered important; nurses should have permission to make mistakes and should feel supported. In addition to commitment to change, it was felt necessary to foster an environment in which people were free to express their personal feelings.

Organisational Concerns

The structure of the organisation also had to be tackled. Alison Binnie, as Senior Sister, had control of the budget and so was able to decide what mix of nursing staff the unit would have. A skill mix was arrived at working within the budget limitations allocated to the surgical unit, where the quality of nurses was seen as important, rather than simply numbers of nurses (Binnie, 1987). Therefore, at the present time, one ward has trained nurses only and the other has trained nurses and student nurses. Neither ward has nursing auxiliaries as it was felt that previously this had led to fragmentation of care. Therefore the only support to nurses are non-nurse workers. Each ward has a part-time ward clerk carrying out administrative duties, plus a part-time ward auxiliary. The ward auxiliaries' role does not incorporate nursing care, but involves supporting the nursing work by taking responsibility for items such as stocking up equipment, taking messages and making up beds.

Managerial support was also sought as this was deemed to be vital to the success of the development. This involved the Senior Sister meeting with the Director of Nursing Services and the Chief Nurse to discuss primary nursing with them.

The fact that the sisters were able to choose their own nurses was also felt to be necessary to ensure that they were employing people with beliefs and values compatible with those of the unit.

Job descriptions for both primary and associate nurses and the ward sister, whose role it was predicted would change enormously, were developed over time. A performance review programme was also established as change got underway. This appraisal system involves setting personal targets and a development plan for each nurse, in such areas as their primary/associate nursing role, co-ordinator's role, team role and mentor role with student nurses, and was designed to allow time for discussion and consideration of each individual's progress.

New ways of formulating the off-duty rota were experimented with, in an effort to improve continuity of care for associate nurses and their patients. (Associate nurses had previously been allocated patients on a day-to-day basis). This included experimentation with the introduction of different lengths of shift. However, these were generally disliked by the nursing team, as they proved tiring and stressful. Continuity of care for the associate nurses therefore remained a problem until eventually the idea of teams was initiated. This involved working the off-duty rota around three teams of nurses, each headed by their primary nurse. This ensured that constructive relationships could be built up between the primary nurse and her group of associates, and also enabled the primary nurse's patients to get to know the same group of associate nurses.

Educational Preparation

Educational issues also had to be addressed. Opportunity was taken for preparatory workshops to be organised during the temporary summer closure of one of the wards. This allowed three days for each trained nurse to think about what primary nursing would mean and what roles she would play. Roy's adaptation model (Roy, 1976) was introduced by the sister as the model on which the unit's nursing care would be based.

Books and articles were made available on the wards and were readily available for the use of everyone, including student nurses. The collection was added to as the unit developed. Handouts were written for the use of students and new nurses to the unit; these included an introduction to primary nursing, a summary of Roy's model and a copy of the ward philosophy. At present two introductory study days are run for all new trained nurses on the unit. It is envisaged that learning packages will also be available in the future. Time out for study is seen as a priority in order to prepare people for the new roles and expectations that primary nursing produces. A minimum of five study days per year for each nurse is the unit's standard to work towards.

Liaison with Medical Colleagues

The need to discuss the introduction of primary nursing with the unit's surgeons was also seen as vital for its success. This was achieved by arranging for discussion time with the surgeons, and this was organised by the senior sister. The idea that primary nursing might improve the quality of nursing care was well received by the Professor of Surgery. As time has passed, the initial fears and reservations of the other surgeons have given way to a more positive view of the new system.

Once the ground work in developing the philosophy of nursing, addressing the organisational concerns and providing educational preparation was accomplished, a date for the start of primary nursing was set. Despite problems and setbacks, primary nursing has developed over the last two years and indeed continues to do so in a constant effort to improve practice.

THE PRIMARY NURSE IN A SURGICAL WARD

When nurses are employed by the unit they function first of all as associate nurses and then, when experienced enough and educationally prepared, they decide with the ward sister when they will take up the role of a primary nurse. A primary nurse will have her own case load of patients, which may consist of three or four patients on the ward with trained nurses only, and six or seven on the ward which has students as well. Within this case load the primary nurse will be responsible for assessing each patient and formulating a care plan in the first 48 hours of admission. She also liaises and collaborates with the associate nurses so that care and necessary arrangements to facilitate care can be followed through.

Since primary nursing began on the unit, nurses have expressed the opinion that it does allow them to be closer to their patients, enabling them to readily develop relationships. It appears to have re-emphasised the satisfaction that can be gained from clinical nursing. It appears that, because primary nurses are making their own decisions within a supportive environment, they feel more motivated and are enthusiastic about the care they provide for their patients.

Inevitably, however, continuous accountability and responsibility does bring additional stresses, which may not be encountered in a usual staff nurse's role. There is no longer anyone to pass the buck to if you are the primary nurse. There is the uncertainty that one may have made the wrong decision about care; that one may not be able to cope with the close involvement of some patients and the frustration of finding that the planned care may not be followed through as you had hoped. We have found therefore that an open atmosphere is vital, in which people can voice their frustrations and anxieties, and do have permission to make mistakes. In this capacity the role of the sister is most important as a support and resource person, to be used as a consultant for nursing care and to provide someone who will listen to the nurses and give active support.

THE ASSOCIATE NURSE IN A SURGICAL WARD

Within the unit, associate nurses are enrolled nurses, student nurses and registered nurses who have not yet developed the skills or experience to practise as primary nurses. This also includes those who do not wish to take on the role, or who work less than four days per week. The unit emphasises the great value of the associate nurse's role and she is not seen as a second class of nurse. The primary nurse is not on duty 24 hours per day and she has to value the associate nurses contributions and liaise with them in the planning of care.

Those associate nurses who are trained do change care plans in the absence of the primary nurse, as the nature of surgical nursing means that a patient's problems can change very rapidly, and it is not felt that primary nurses should be contacted at home to change care decisions. The primary nurses are, however, expected to leave care instructions to cover foreseeable problems, and on return to duty have the right to make the final decisions in discussion with the associate nurses.

The primary nurse has to be able to listen and take advice from the associate nurses. An attitude of possessiveness over care planning does little to foster collegial relationships between the primary and associate nurses. There is therefore an awareness that open communication is essential to allow primary and associate nurses to work interdependently towards the individualised care of the patient.

Student nurses learn to use Roy's adaptation model to assess patients and to formulate care plans under the supervision of their primary nurses. Each student nurse has a registered nurse mentor, who assesses and advises them throughout their placement, and who will usually do night duty with them. The student nurses are usually anxious about working in an area that practises primary nursing, but at the same time interested to find out what it can offer them. It does seem to enable them as associate nurses to take more responsibility and to become more involved with their patients. In our experience, they generally find the experience stimulating and exciting. Statements such as the following are frequently heard:

- I have found the way I want to nurse
- I'd like to come back here when I've qualified and try being a primary nurse
- It's brought everything together for me [working with primary nursing]

Full-time associate nurses and primary nurses rotate onto night duty, approximately every 5–6 weeks. All nurses act as associate nurses when on nights, with the primary nurses winding down their case load as night duty approaches. This is usually possible considering the short length of stay of the surgical patient. However, some patients such as those who have experienced a limb amputation may have a longer length of stay and will be handed over to another primary nurse. This is seen as a break in continuity, and it is envisaged that eventually primary nurses will not rotate onto night duty.

Associate nurses work with the same primary nurse for a few weeks at one time; continuity is at present interrupted by rotation onto night duty. The continuity that is achieved means that good working relationships have a chance to flourish between members of nursing staff and that the 'team' have a good idea of the skills of the student nurses within it.

THE PATIENT IN THIS WARD ENVIRONMENT

Patients are admitted to the wards either via the waiting list for cold surgery or through casualty as emergency admissions. Once on the ward they will be allocated to a primary nurse for their stay in hospital. This potentially provides patients with the opportunity to experience continuity of care and the chance to build up a caring relationship with the primary nurse and the associate nurses. Many of the patients with vascular problems will have repeated admissions as their disease progresses, and we try to allocate the same primary nurse to these patients. On one occasion the off-duty rota was arranged at the request of a patient who wished to have his primary nurse there when he was readmitted to one of the wards.

As the patient has the opportunity to get to know his primary nurse well, the nurse is able to follow through problems, support the family, and start arranging discharge from the first few days of admission. This is important because the surgical patient's problems rarely consist solely of his recovery from surgery. Although surgery can offer cure, the wards are still places where people die; where people suffer the loss of a limb or breast or have to come to terms with the fact that they have cancer. Hopefully the opportunity to develop a close nurse–patient relationship, facilitated by primary nursing, will help to support the patient and his family through such problems, so that the achievement of caring is seen to be as important as that of curing.

Spontaneous comments from patients about how they feel about primary nursing are heard:

- I was surprised when Mary came up to me and said she would be responsible for my care while I was in hospital
- I think that primary nursing is a wonderful idea. I like the idea of one nurse knowing everything about me

Also it has become noticeable that patients will often write to their primary nurse rather than to 'sister' when they write with thanks and news to the ward. For example, a letter thanking a particular primary nurse and her team, reads:

- My grandmother being almost totally deaf, blind and also lame really benefited from having nurses who knew her problems . . . Primary nursing is obviously a wonderful idea, and especially for old people who may be confused.

Therefore it appears that patients and their families are noticing and appreciating what an individualised approach to care can offer them.

CO-ORDINATION OF CARE

In a busy surgical ward, the primary nurse as a direct care giver is not always able to engage in direct person-to-person communication with all those concerned with a patient's case, because of the high degree of disruption that would be involved. The primary nurse would, however, endeavour to be present for all key communications related to her patient group.

The co-ordinator role involves co-ordinating the ward's activities, such as joining ward rounds, liaising with physiotherapists, occupational therapists and social workers, and carrying out other functions which are supportive to nursing care. It must be emphasised that the purpose of this is to support and feed back information to primary and associate nurses who are unable to attend discussions. The primary nurses, in particular, will use the co-ordinator as a 'go-between' to carry out instructions from the primary nurse involving her patients (for instance, arranging transport and finding beds), which will then free more of the primary nurse's time to care for her patients. If a particular problem arises the primary nurses will speak to the appropriate member of the health care team themselves and this may involve a detailed discussion rather than just a superficial word on a ward round.

In this setting, the primary nurses may also act as co-ordinator for the ward, as may senior student nurses in their professional development module and associate nurses who are Registered General Nurses.

It has to be emphasised that the co-ordinator is not carrying out the role of 'being in charge' of the ward. She is able to facilitate co-ordination of the activity of the ward but is not expected to hold in-depth information on each patient, because the primary or associate nurse is available if discussion about a problem is necessary. The co-ordinator is also not necessarily the most senior nurse on duty. The role is often taken by junior staff nurses who need to learn the skills that the job entails, while being supported by more senior colleagues. The ward philosophy underpins the fact that, as the most experienced and skilled nurses, the primary nurses should be providing direct nursing care where possible.

BENEFITS AND DISADVANTAGES OF PRIMARY NURSING

In my experience on the unit, primary nursing has created the chance to give more individualised care and a greater level of continuity of care. The use of the nursing process has improved dramatically. The use of Qualpacs and Phaneuf's Nursing Audit (quality assurance tools) was applied during the development of primary nursing and there appear to be general trends of improvement in the quality of care, with particular improvements in the areas of individual psychosocial care, communication and initiative, and responsibility indicative of the professional nurse, and minimal improvements in the areas of psychosocial care of a group of patients, and physical care.

Nurses appear to feel more job satisfaction and motivation with primary nursing, while patients seem to appreciate the individualised approach to care. These opinions are monitored through discussion and ward meetings with nurses and through conversation and correspondence to the ward from patients and their families, as described earlier.

However, within the type of surgical ward environment, the fast turnover of patients and restrictions of the service, such as shortages of nurses, sickness and deterioration in support services, can all affect the continuity of care. These difficulties are hopefully overcome by staff continuing to maintain the principles of primary nursing, while having to be flexible to accommodate the stresses and strains found in the Health Service generally today.

Stress is also a problem as nurses take on more responsibility, and often get closer to their patients and more involved with their problems. There is also sometimes a lack of understanding of primary nursing from other nurses or members of the health care team who do not work on the unit. This highlights the need for nurses to communicate the benefits of primary nursing, and to support each other as we have learnt through our own experiences.

WHAT THE MOVE TO PRIMARY NURSING HAS BROUGHT
TO THE UNIT

I feel that primary nursing has created a greater awareness of the need to appraise and develop practice continually. From this awareness has arisen the use of research and information on which to base our practice in many areas; for example, the use of more advanced and diverse wound care, adopting temperature taking procedures based on research, the use of therapeutic massage, music and relaxation, natural juice therapy and more importance being placed on psychosocial aspects of care.

The change has also heralded the use of our own appraisal system, which is essential in order to monitor the professional practice of nursing. It has succeeded in flattening the hierarchical structure of nursing, and the two ward sisters have continued to develop their democratic styles of leadership. Primary nursing has also created more awareness of the need to support each other as it becomes all too obvious that change and development create many stresses and doubts, however enthusiastic the participants.

Primary nursing has also seemingly resulted in increased assertiveness among our nurses, although through our active recruitment policy we may well have attracted this type of personality! I hope that, despite all these positive progressions, the most important change has been an improved experience of surgery and surgical nursing care for our patients.

6

A Change for the Better – Primary Nursing in a Medical Ward

Sue Chilton

In October 1986, we moved from a pre-war hospital into a brand new hospital in Redditch, belonging to the Bromsgrove and Redditch Health Authority. At the time, I was working as one of two sisters on a busy mixed medical ward, accommodating 28 patients.

We had previously decided to introduce a modified form of primary nursing onto the ward on the day we moved, believing that this new method of work organisation would be more readily accepted then as there were various changes all taking place at the same time.

Before the change, we used to organise our work on a 'patient allocation' basis with little or no continuity in the allocation of nurses to specific patients on consecutive days. Under such a system, it was felt that our patients were not receiving individualised care and that the nurses were becoming disillusioned with their role and gaining little job satisfaction.

It was felt that we needed to reorganise nursing on the new ward to:

- foster the development of more effective nurse–patient relationships;
- improve the quality of nursing care;
- develop the knowledge and abilities of the individual nurses through encouraging accountability and getting qualified nurses to give care;
- base nursing practice on a model of nursing and apply the 'nursing process';
- promote a more democratic style of leadership, allowing all nursing staff and members of the multidisciplinary team to contribute ideas towards improving nursing.

Shortly after completing the Open University 'Nursing Process' course, I began to consider the different methods available for organising nursing on the ward. As an acute medical ward, we needed a system of work organisation that was flexible enough to cope with the heavy demand of the ward, easy to manage and, above all, conducive to improvements in standards of care. Primary nursing appeared to fulfil most of our requirements.

THE PHYSICAL SETTING

Our ward is a 28-bedded mixed medical ward, designed on the 'nucleus' principle (figure 6.1). It is a very busy ward and, in theory, we accept acute admissions from the Accident and Emergency Department on an alternate day basis. However, in practice, it is not unusual for the ward to take such admissions every day because of the demand for beds. In addition, we accept a few routine admissions. The average length of stay of patients on the ward is 10 days.

The ward is served by four consultant physicians, each with two junior doctors working for them. There are nine formal 'consultant' ward rounds held each week and, in addition to this, there are several informal medical ward rounds.

Our part-time ward clerk helps to free nurses from some clerical duties, which is vital on a busy day. She works 20 hours a week and is present on the ward Monday to Friday from 9 am to 1 pm.

We operate a system of open visiting. Relatives and visitors are typically welcome onto the ward at any time.

The ward is extremely spacious. It is divided into four large six-bedded bays and four individual side rooms. Two of the four six-bedded bays are for the acutely ill and are situated in view of the nursing station, providing good observation.

STAFFING, STRUCTURE AND ROLES

When we first introduced our modified form of primary nursing on to the ward, our funded establishment was four full-time RGNs and one part-time RGN, five full-time enrolled nurses, three full-time auxiliaries and one part-time auxiliary nurse.

In this section the key features of the modifications will be described; most keep intact the principles of primary nursing as described by Manthey (1980).

The four full-time RGNs, two sisters and two staff nurses became primary nurses. Our part-time staff nurse at the time was newly qualified and it was felt that she needed extra guidance and support before taking on this role. She was allocated to one of the groups, spending her time learning to become a primary nurse and also gaining experience as a ward co-ordinator (see p. 90).

With primary nursing, we found that the sister/staff nurse became a more independent practitioner, developing greater accountability for her own decisions and actions.

On admission to the ward, each patient is allocated to a primary nurse, who is then responsible for assessing his problems, and planning, implementing and evaluating appropriate care until the patient is discharged. This ensures, hopefully, that the nurse in greatest contact with the patient is also the nurse who makes the major decisions regarding the patient's nursing care.

Manthey (1980) describes four elements which outline the principles behind primary nursing (see chapter 1).

It was felt impractical in our situation for the primary nurses to assume 24-hour

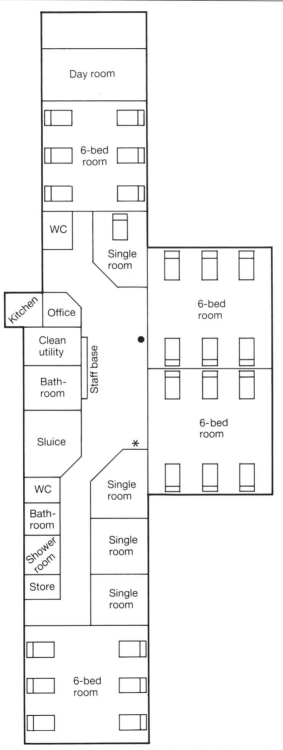

Fig. 6.1 Our ward: * Primary nursing board, ● Information board.

responsibility of their patients in practice and so, in their absence, associate nurses take on responsibility for making alterations to the patients' care plan. Whenever possible, enrolled nurses take over this responsibility in the absence of the primary nurse. However, on occasions, learner nurses or auxiliary nurses become care givers under the close guidance and supervision of the ward co-ordinator. The primary nurse does have the prerogative to change the care plan on her return.

Owing to the 'modular' system of nurse training in operation in our hospital, the number of student and pupil nurses on the ward at any time varies greatly from three to as many as eight nurses.

After much deliberation, it was decided to divide our 28 patients into four primary nursing groups with seven patients in each group. Ideally, we would have preferred smaller groups but staffing levels did not permit this. The seven patients in each group are identified by a number clearly visible on the bottom of their beds. The groups are numbered 1, 2, 3 and 4. Patients in each group may be situated anywhere on the ward. The groups are of mixed sex and consist of some acutely ill patients as well as some patients improving in health.

The ward co-ordinator is the person who decides on the allocation of patients to particular groups. It is important that the groups have an equal dependency wherever possible. Often beds need to be moved around the ward so that patients are situated in the most appropriate position to suit their specific needs. It is sometimes the case that one group may have a slightly more demanding workload than the other groups. In this instance, any 'spare' nurses would be allocated to the group with the greater need. Although it is preferable for nurses to work in their own groups, it is inevitable that they are moved from time to time.

Each of the four primary nursing groups has its own set of nurses. The skill mix of a typical group of nurses is shown in table 6.1.

Table 6.1 Example of a skill mix of a primary nurse's associate nurse group

RGN (sister/staff nurse)	Primary nurse
Enrolled nurse	Associate nurses
Senior student/pupil nurse	
Junior student/pupil nurse	
Auxiliary nurse	

In theory, the same group of nurses cares for the same seven patients from admission to discharge, promoting continuity of care. As already explained, this cannot always be the case in practice as associate nurses are sometimes required to move to other groups.

The Co-ordinator's Role

In addition to the nurses giving hands-on care to the patients on a daily basis, one nurse is appointed as co-ordinator for each shift. The co-ordinator is responsible for the management and administration of the ward as a whole and also provides support for those nurses delivering care.

There are three main functions within her role:

- *To allocate nurses to patients*   She decides on the most appropriate group for a patient to join, taking into account the existing workload of the group as well as the skills and abilities of the nurses within that group.
- *To provide information*   She assists the primary nurses by providing appropriate information and also attempts to provide research-based knowledge if required to do so.
- *To give support*   She discusses with the primary nurses any problems they may have in planning patient care. At the same time, she may be required to provide emotional support for nurses, who often find nursing under the primary nursing system more stressful, possibly due to the closer interaction they have with their patients.

There is a sign above the nursing station indicating (by Christian name) who is the co-ordinator for the shift.

The co-ordinator must be a qualified nurse or a third-year student/final-year pupil nurse working under the close supervision of a trained nurse, who is not responsible for giving any patient care.

We try to ensure that the nurse acting as co-ordinator has worked on the previous day shift so that she has a knowledge of the patients as well as events planned for that particular day. Thus, it no longer follows that if one of the sisters is on duty that she will automatically act as co-ordinator. With our previous system, it was ludicrous to have nurses acting as co-ordinator after days off on holiday just because they were most senior in rank.

The Co-ordinator's Job Description on our Ward

1. To allocate nurses to appropriate primary nursing groups (where possible), ensuring that auxiliary and junior nurses are well supervised.
2. To inform the Nursing Officer if the ward is understaffed.
3. To conduct the drug round with a student or pupil nurse for the whole ward. (Originally, we thought of each group doing their own drugs, but levels of trained staff per shift did not allow this. We appreciate that often some tasks need to remain despite primary nursing; this sometimes leads to greater efficiency.)
4. To advise student/pupil nurses on care planning in the absence of the primary or more experienced associate nurse.
5. To order all supplies and stores.
6. To conduct the whole medical ward round, enabling the nurses from the different primary nursing groups to discuss their particular patients with the doctors.
7. To communicate the information gained on the ward round to the nurses in their different groups if they were unable to be present.
8. To monitor the 'bed state', liaising with medical staff regarding admissions.
9. To liaise with other disciplines/departments if the primary nurse is unable to

do this or, if required, to contact, for example:

● a porter to take patients to Radiography,
● a dietician if several patients need to be seen.

10. Be present at the 'handover' of reports to nurses coming on the next shift, acting as chairperson and contributing where necessary.

11. To work closely with those student/pupil nurses who wish to gain ward management experience, teaching by example.

12. To monitor and direct staff meal breaks, ensuring that nurses are aware of the needs of the patients they are covering for.

13. To assist with nursing care as an associate nurse if time allows or the need arises due to lack of qualified staff.

A copy of the co-ordinator's job description is pinned to the wall behind the nursing station.

An ideal number of nurses for the early shift is nine – two nurses on each of the four groups and one nurse acting as co-ordinator. The two nurses on each group will care for a number of patients each and work together if a patient requires two nurses for his care. A total of five nurses is ideal for the late shift – one nurse per group and one co-ordinator. In practice, staffing levels vary greatly but a typically early shift has seven nurses and a typical late shift four or five nurses.

The off-duty rota is fundamental to the success of primary nursing. We try to ensure that there are always two qualified nurses working together on each shift, including one RGN, so that meal breaks are covered. We like to have a trained nurse or senior learner nurse on each group for each shift during the day. An attempt is made to allocate learners with their 'personal' nurses. We also like to honour off-duty requests if possible as it is felt this helps staff morale and job satisfaction (see figures 6.2 and 6.3).

The Ward Sister's Role

My role as ward sister has changed quite markedly with the advent of primary nursing. It has enabled me to become a more clinically active member of the ward team, working closely with patients and nursing staff in giving direct care. My fellow sister and I both elected to become primary nurses, with a group of seven patients each. In this way, we are able to share our clinical expertise more easily with other nursing staff. However, we continue to manage the overall ward development and are in a better position to promote holistic patient care and facilitate the development of our nursing staff.

Having seriously reassessed my own priorities, I have come to the conclusion that the ward sister is of greater value giving hands-on care than constantly adopting the role of co-ordinator. The role of the ward sister within primary nursing is described later in this chapter and in chapter 17.

Staff	Group	Monday	Tuesday	Wednesday	Thursday	Friday	Saturday	Sunday
Sister	1	E©	L©	E©	L	E	DO	DO
Sister	2	L	E	DO	DO	L	E	L
Staff Nurse	3	DO	DO	L	E	E	L©	E
Staff Nurse	4	E	E	L©	E	E	DO	DO
Staff Nurse (PT)	2	E	L	E	E©	DO	L	DO
Enrolled Nurse	1	L©	E©	E	DO	DO	L	E©
Enrolled Nurse	2	DO	DO	L	L©	E©	E	E
Enrolled Nurse	3	E	L	E	DO	DO	E	L©
Enrolled Nurse	4	E©	DO	DO	L	L©	E©	L
Enrolled Nurse	1	E	E	DO	DO	E	E	E
Senior Student Nurse	3	E	E	DO	DO	L	E	L
Senior Student Nurse	4	DO	DO	E	E	L	E	E
Student Nurse	1	L	L	L	E	DO	DO	E
Student Nurse	2	DO	DO	L	E	E	L	E
Student Nurse	3	DO	DO	L	E	L	L	E
Student Nurse	4	E	E	L	E	E	DO	DO
Auxiliary Nurse	1	DO	DO	L	L	E	E	L
Auxiliary Nurse	2	E	E	E	L	E	DO	DO
Auxiliary Nurse	3	L	L	E	L	E	DO	DO
Auxiliary Nurse	4	L	L	E	DO	DO	L	E
L/E		9/5	8/5	9/7	9/5	9/6	8/5	9/5

Fig. 6.2 Sample off-duty rota: E, early shift; L, late shift; DO, day off; ©, co-ordinator on the shift; PT, part-time.

		Monday	Tuesday	Wednesday	Thursday	Friday	Saturday	Sunday
Group 1								
Sister		E	L©	E©	L	E	Do	Do
Enrolled Nurse		L©	E©	E	Do	Do	L	E©
Enrolled Nurse		E	E	Do	Do	E	E	E
Student Nurse		L	L	E	E	Do	Do	E
Auxiliary		Do	Do	L	E	L	E	L
	E	2	2	3	2	2	2	3
	L	2	2	1	1	1	1	1
Group 2								
Sister		L	E	Do	Do	L	E	L
Staff Nurse (PT)		E	L	E	E©	Do	Do	Do
Enrolled Nurse		Do	Do	L	L©	E©	E	E
Student Nurse		Do	Do	L	E	E	L	E
Auxiliary		E	E	E	L	E	Do	Do
	E	2	2	2	2	3	2	2
	L	1	1	2	2	1	1	1
Group 3								
Staff Nurse		Do	Do	L	E	E	L©	E
Enrolled Nurse		E	L	E	Do	Do	E	L©
Senior Student Nurse		E	E	Do	Do	L	E	L
Student Nurse		Do	Do	L	E	L	L	E
Auxiliary		L	E	E	L	E	Do	Do
	E	2	2	2	2	2	2	2
	L	1	1	2	1	2	2	2
Group 4								
Staff Nurse		E	E	L©	E	E	Do	Do
Enrolled Nurse		E©	Do	Do	L	L©	E©	L
Senior Student Nurse		Do	Qo	E	E	L	E	E
Student Nurse		E	E	L	E	E	Oo	Do
Auxiliary		L	L	E	Do	Do	L	E
	E	3	2	2	3	2	2	2
	L	1	1	2	1	2	1	1

Fig. 6.3 Individual nursing groups off-duty rota: E, early shift; L, late shift; DO, day off; ©, co-ordinator on the shift.

PREPARATION FOR CHANGE

Before the introduction of primary nursing on the ward, we organised a series of tutorials for all the ward nursing staff, refreshing their knowledge of the nursing process and introducing the principles behind primary nursing. It was felt that if we were to implement the stages of the nursing process successfully, the nurse who admits the patient and takes his nursing history needs to care for that patient throughout his hospital stay. This would help to maintain continuity and avoid fragmentation of care. The primary nursing system seemed to be the most effective in achieving this end.

We arranged six sessions in all, each relating to a different aspect of the nursing process. A useful teaching package was prepared by a post-basic nursing tutor.

We felt that it was important to involve as many of the staff as possible and members of the School of Nursing and ward nursing staff all contributed by giving talks. The enthusiasm and commitment of all those taking part was impressive.

Staff present at these meetings were encouraged to pass comment and ask questions, and in this way we were able to pool all our ideas, which we later put into practice.

As Blanchard and Johnson (1983: 5) state in their book, *The One Minute Manager*: '. . . the symbol – a one minute readout from the face of a modern digital watch – is intended to remind us to take a minute out of our day to look into the faces of the people we manage. And to realise that *they* are our most important resources!'

We believe, from our own experience, that a democratic style of leadership is more conducive to the introduction of change generally. It is of vital importance to consider and value the staff's comments and suggestions.

A booklet on primary nursing was also produced and circulated among the staff at this preparatory stage, explaining in detail:

1. Different styles of work organisation
2. Skills required to implement individualised care:
   - Organisational skills – including different styles of leadership
   - Decision-making skills
   - Interpersonal skills – including the key elements of the helping relationship as described by Carl Rogers (1961) and the personal approach within the nurse–patient relationship
3. Methods of communication:
   - Written records and reports
   - Verbal handovers
   - Discussion between nurses about patient care
   - Transfer letters to other departments and hospitals
4. The potential constraints when implementing primary nursing
5. The concepts of primary nursing
6. The role of the co-ordinator

Within the booklet, we included a comprehensive bibliography to encourage further reading around the subject. By preparing our staff in this way, we felt that they gained enthusiasm and became motivated towards the forthcoming change.

Six months after our move to the new hospital, primary nursing was functioning well and all the staff seemed to have adapted admirably to the change. The RGNs had accepted their greater level of responsibility well, and were beginning to show signs of personal development and were taking greater pride in their work. Most of the nurses were happier to be allocated to their own groups, felt more secure and were more aware of of their own roles within the system. The ward sisters felt greater job satisfaction and less disillusionment within their roles.

As a result, we organised a study entitled 'The implementation of primary nursing in practice', with the aim of sharing our experiences with colleagues from other wards, the School of Nursing and colleagues from a neighbouring hospital. We invited a guest speaker, George Castledine, principal lecturer in Nursing from Wrexham College. He was followed by a video describing the ward geography and how we divided the patients into groups. Methods of communication were also illustrated. We then went on to describe the implementation in greater detail, outlining problems and comparing the advantages and disadvantages of the system as we saw them. To finish, we formed a panel of nurses, representing each grade of staff, for a question and answer session with the audience.

On that day, we stressed the importance of preparing staff for the change to primary nursing and that it is impossible to adopt the system overnight. Those of our colleagues who later introduced primary nursing successfully themselves appeared to be those who spent time with us on the ward, listening to our comments and taking note of our teething problems.

In conclusion, we adopted a normative re-educative approach to introducing change, as described by Filkins (1986) (see chapter 2).

We discussed primary nursing with other members of the multidisciplinary team working on the ward in a more informal manner. The majority of them found little problem in accepting the new system. The consultant physicians from our ward invited us to a medical seminar to discuss our new system. No objections were raised to primary nursing and there was a fair degree of interest.

Initially, it was felt that the consultant physicians preferred to communicate mainly with the ward sister whilst on the ward. We wondered how they would react to the changed role of the ward sister. However, after a relatively short time, the doctors were happy communicating directly with the primary nurses and ward co-ordinator because they gained more comprehensive information in this way.

METHODS OF COMMUNICATION

Written Documentation

The nursing notes – including the nursing care plan and charts – are kept with the patient's drug chart in a folder at the end of the bed. This allows the patient to read his own documents and become actively involved in his care and care planning. It also allows the nurses to make changes to care plans at the bedside, where most of the nursing care takes place.

A group decision was made to keep the nursing history sheets at the nursing station (the staff base) to preserve confidentiality. For example, it was sometimes felt by the medical staff that it was inappropriate for a patient to be aware of his true diagnosis. However, the nursing staff did not always agree with this. We keep the history sheets in four separate folders, providing easy access for all disciplines.

The primary nurses are mainly responsible for planning and updating nursing care which is documented in the care plan. However, associate nurses take over this responsibility at times, as explained earlier. Student and pupil nurses write in the care plans if supervised by a trained member of staff, who must countersign and approve what is written.

We have found that the nursing care plan is a much more valuable document under our new system as it is essential in communicating information about the patient's care, not all of which may be relayed at verbal handovers.

Verbal Handovers

All nurses of the early shift listen to a full report on all the patients given by the night nursing staff. Reference is made to the nursing history sheets. This is a fairly brief report, giving personal details about patients and outlining their main nursing problems and the care given.

After breakfast, the primary nurse or associate nurse conducts a bedside report with the other nurses in her group for their seven patients. They discuss problems with each of their patients, referring to the care plan and charts as required and plan the nursing care for the morning.

Before the nurses arrive for the late shift, the primary/associate nurse conducts a further bedside report, teaching junior nurses at the same time, ensuring that care plans are up to date and have been amended appropriately throughout that shift.

To inform the late shift, a nurse from each of the four groups provides a brief verbal report about the patients she has cared for that morning to all other nurses. After this report, the primary/associate nurse from the morning shift hands over her patients at their bedsides to the nurse who is to continue the care of that group in the evening.

Just before the end of the late shift, the nurses ensure that their care plans are up to date. The primary/associate nurse, from each group verbally reports on her patients to the night nurses. The co-ordinator for the shift oversees this report session yet again and supervises any junior nurses.

There are often only two nurses on duty for the whole ward at night. At present the night nurses feel it is impractical for them to practise primary nursing. However, they have adapted well to the idea of the groups and write in and update care plans as needed throughout the night, relaying important changes to the appropriate primary nurses in the morning. There are plans to implement internal rotation in the future, which should lead to a greater continuity of care over 24 hours. At present, the night staff feel that a form of task allocation is the most efficient method of organisation because of low staffing levels.

It was hoped that, in the future, we might introduce 'care conferences' at least weekly on the ward, including members of the multidisciplinary team, with each primary nurse representing a group of patients under her care.

Ensuring Continuity of Care

When patients are transferred to other wards or departments within the hospital, the primary nurse escorts the patient herself whenever possible. On arrival, the primary nurse gives a comprehensive verbal handover to the staff. The nursing notes are also transferred with the patient.

When a patient is transferred to another hospital the primary nurse provides a written outline of the patient's problems and gives an evaluation of the care given so far. A telephone call may also be made, which also proves very beneficial in promoting continuity of care.

The primary nurse is the main person responsible for planning the patient's discharge home. We try to ensure that primary nurses go on home visits if possible and liaise with relatives regarding proposed plans. In her absence, she delegates these arrangements to her associate nurses.

Primary Nursing Board

Positioned centrally on the ward is our Primary Nursing Board. All the patients from each of the four groups are identified by name here. Each consultant physician is represented by a different colour, and the patient's name is written in the colour of his consultant. So we can see at a glance, how many patients each consultant has under his care at any one time. This method helps the nurse to prepare her patients and herself for each of the consultants' ward rounds.

The set of nurses for each of the four groups are listed by name (including Christian names) below the patients' names (see figure 6.4).

Group 1	Room	Group 2	Room	Group 3	Room	Group 4	Room
1. Elsie Moore *	A	1. Debbie Jones ¶	A	1. Roger Lovell *	B	1. George White §	D
2. (Peter Wright) *	B	2. Reg Smith *	B	2. (Paul Farmer) §	B	3. (Melanie Dunn) *	A
3. Billy Davies §	D	3. Lucy Boswell §	F	3. Michael Green *	H	3. David Austin ¶	D
4. Jane Page ¶	C	4. George Dean *	D	4. Peter Gordon ¶	D	4. Penelope Rose *	C
5. Mark Woburn †	D	5. Simon Smart †	G	5. Nellie Taylor †	A	5. John Thomas †	B
6. Rose Walters †	C	6. Ruby Albutt §	C	6. Bert Rogers †	B	6. Susan Pearce §	A
7. Robert Simons §	E	7. Sarah Downs ¶	C	7. Joan Blackwell §	C	7. Louise Watts ¶	A
Sr Mary Walker		Sr Ann James		SN Ivy Grace		SN John Smith	
EN Jean Simmons		EN Pam Lowry		EN Vicky Lowe		EN Paul Webb	
StN Jenny Major		StN Ivan Walker		PN Sue Lambert		EN Jean Butt	
PN Ian Wallace		PN Sarah Tow		PN Iris Small		StN Liz Barber	
Aux. Pat Moran		Aux. Ivy Tongue		Aux. Lucy Scott		Aux. Bev Cross	
* Dr Midway		† Dr Grange		§ Dr Large		¶ Dr Reynolds	

Fig. 6.4 Primary Nursing Board: underlined names are patients due to be admitted, names in brackets are patients due to be discharged. In practice, the patients of each doctor would be indicated by the use of a different colour on the board; for printing purposes, they are indicated here by the use of the symbols * † § and ¶. Sr, sister; SN, staff nurse; EN, enrolled nurse; StN, student nurse; PN, primary nurse; Aux., auxiliary nurse.

Information Board

We also have an Information Board, situated in a prominent position so that everyone entering the ward will notice it. It includes details of visiting times, canteen facilities, and names and ranks of staff, for example.

STAFF DEVELOPMENT

As a teaching ward, we are responsible for basic and post-basic learners. Student and pupil nurses on their first ward experience are allocated to a 'personal nurse', who may be an RGN or an enrolled nurse. Wherever possible, we try to ensure that the learner nurse and her 'personal nurse' work the same shifts and are in the same primary nursing group to promote optimal supervision and opportunities for teaching.

We have found that primary nursing enhances clinical learning. The learner nurses relate closely to their personal nurse and benefit from sharing in the patient's care from admission to discharge. They also seem to develop deeper nurse–patient relationships.

Third year student/final year pupil nurses are given plenty of opportunity to undertake the role of the co-ordinator in preparation for ward management assessments.

Since introducing primary nursing, individual staff nurses and enrolled nurses take on more direct responsibility and are regarded as being accountable for their own actions. All trained staff are given the chance to adopt the role of co-ordinator.

Nursing auxiliaries are now more involved in feeding information back to the primary or associate nurses and, in this way, contribute to decision making.

SUPPORTING THE SYSTEM

Fortunately, we gained full support from our Nursing Management team and the School of Nursing when we introduced primary nursing. Many people have shown great interest in the venture and this has helped the staff to continue making improvements to the system.

Manthey *et al.* (1970) suggest that primary nursing needs an environment:

● in which individuals feel free to learn, to risk, to make mistakes and to grow. Nurse leaders must trust individual nurses whose attempts at comprehensive patient care lead to unorthodox activities.

It was felt that our nurse managers allowed us the necessary amount of freedom to introduce and develop the primary nursing system. The tutorial staff have fairly recently introduced primary nursing into the basic and post-basic curriculum and ward staff have taken part in discussions with learners in school about the principles behind such a system. The teachers feel that our written documentation and continuity of patient care have improved with primary nursing. Roles seem more deeply defined and responsibilities more apparent.

Manthey *et al.* (1970) state that primary nursing presents a challenge to nursing education, which must seek to provide each nurse with a sound knowledge base, an ability to relate sensitively to others and an ability to determine priorities confidently and to make valid judgments.

We encourage an informal atmosphere on the ward and attempt to create a homely environment wherever possible. It is felt that the fact that nursing is organised on collegial rather than hierarchical lines helps to sustain primary nursing.

The ward sisters interview and help to recruit new staff who will easily adapt to a democratic form of leadership, are able to act on their own initiative, and are prepared to answer for their own actions.

RETROSPECTIVE REVIEW

It is now almost two years since we first adopted primary nursing as our system of work organisation. Along the way, we have encountered some minor problems, which we have mostly been able to solve.

Nurses initially found it quite difficult to understand the role of the co-ordinator. We have since compiled a job description for the role, which may need to be amended periodically.

The off-duty rota has posed several problems as we have attempted to adapt it to suit the needs of the primary nursing groups. At first, we encouraged each primary nurse to formulate the off-duty for her own group. However, because of the staffing levels and the effects of annual leave and sickness, this method did not always provide enough nurses to cover the ward as a whole. The ward sisters now formulate the rota for the ward, taking each group into consideration, and we have accepted that during periods of staff shortages nurses may be required to work on another group as associate nurses. This is not always well accepted, but is unavoidable.

At times, we have found that there is a need to support junior nurses emotionally, especially as they seem to become much more involved with their patients with primary nursing.

Another potential problem was the risk of a personality clash between nurse and patient. Although this has not occurred, if the situation were to arise, we would transfer the patient to another primary nursing group.

Medical staff and other disciplines, accustomed to the hierarchical system, sometimes found it difficult to communicate with the care givers instead of the ward sisters, whom they often falsely believed to be the only source of true information! However, they are now beginning to accept the changed role of the ward sister.

It is quite clear that the nurse–patient relationship is enriched with primary nursing as the patients can identify their particular care givers and the basis is there to create a trusting relationship with them. This relationship leads to a sense of belonging for both patients and nurses.

Feedback from the nurses demonstrates that they gain more job satisfaction from primary nursing because they are encouraged to develop their roles by improving their clinical, communicative and leadership skills. The staff are more motivated and their individual skills are more easily identified, which increases their feelings of self-achievement.

Teaching staff from the School of Nursing feel that our written documentation and use of the nursing process have improved because the nurses are giving more individualised, holistic care on a continual basis.

Learner nurses have generally had favourable attitudes to primary nursing. However, some of the learners do not like the way in which the patients are placed around the ward and would prefer to work in one bay. Also, some find it difficult to accept a greater level of responsibility for their own patients at times as this is new to them. Many learners resent being moved to work on other groups at times of staff shortages – which probably shows that they gain a sense of security and greater self-esteem and job satisfaction when working in their own group. Third year student/final-year pupil nurses enjoy the challenge of being a co-ordinator under supervision and feel that they gain invaluable experience for their future roles.

With primary nursing, the traditional hierarchical organisation where the care planner was not the care giver is eradicated. Runciman (1983) and Swaffield *et al.* (1987) describe the feelings of ward sisters and how the role of ward sister can often be filled with disillusionment. This is often due to the fact that ward sisters are ill-prepared for their roles, feel that too much is expected of them and that they have little time to become active members of the ward team. However, since the change to primary nursing, my fellow sister and I have personally felt more fulfilled with our roles as we have been able to teach by example as primary nurses – in an attempt to continually raise standards of nursing care.

Observations made by Ogier (1980) revealed that the ideal ward sister spent less time interacting with doctors than with learners, and had a leadership style that was approachable. Although we, as ward sisters, act as primary nurses, we appreciate that we are fully responsible for the ward management and development and we continually attempt to provide support and to give advice to all nurses and constantly monitor the care given in all groups.

I can imagine that many ward sisters might feel that they were losing control if they relinquished the 'hot seat' (the role of co-ordinator). However, I have personally felt more in control since working on the shop floor and feel I have more to offer the patients and nurses if I am seen to be able to carry a bed pan like all the rest! In addition, I feel it is easier to monitor standards of care as a primary nurse because, as co-ordinator, there are so many tasks that remove me from the patient and his direct care.

Evaluation of Primary Nursing

To evaluate our primary nursing system two years after its implementation, a questionnaire was circulated among ward staff, members of the School of Nursing and nurse management team. Out of a total of 30 nurses, 22 replied. All those who replied had an adequate understanding of the term primary nursing. Of these, 20 gained their knowledge of this system of work organisation from our ward. The majority of the nurses, 19, approved of the care plans being kept at the end of the patient's bed. This was considered to allow patient access to the care plan and encourage him to participate actively in his own care, and easy access for nurses to update the care plan if required. The majority of nurses felt that reference was made to the care plans at the start and end of each shift, at report times and on medical ward rounds. It was stated by most nurses that staff were always allocated to specific patients and that this allocation lasted from the patient's admission to his discharge. Comments from the majority of nurses indicated that each primary nurse (or associate nurse at times) always gives a report on her patients to the nurse who is to continue the care. From the results, it was apparent that trained nurses all participated at some time in all aspects of patient care, teaching and ward management.

The majority of learner nurses also gained similar experience. Auxiliary nurses were seen to contribute to discussions and verbal handovers about patients as well as to direct patient care. All those who replied felt that the style of leadership practised on the ward was democratic. Most learner nurses felt that they were supervised more closely under the primary nursing system and said they received equal support from all staff.

The questionnaire encouraged nurses to comment on the advantages and disadvantages of primary nursing as practised on the ward. Their comments have been summarised as follows.

Advantages

It was felt that primary nursing led to the development of a more fulfilling nurse–patient relationship. Individualised patient care was enhanced and continuity of care improved.

Some felt that communication was better under the new system and that standards of care appeared to have improved.

It was considered that individual nurses developed their own clinical, teaching and managerial skills more readily as their responsibility and accountability was increased. Thus, job satisfaction was enhanced with primary nursing.

Disadvantages

At times of staff shortages, individualised care suffered a little as nurses were allocated to other groups. Some nurses resented moving to work on other groups and felt disillusioned slightly with the system at these times.

Other nurses felt isolated within their own group and considered their knowledge of the rest of the patients on the ward to be inadequate. Some would have preferred to nurse one bay (room) of patients instead of having to move around the ward.

It was occasionally felt unfair that one group was sometimes more physically demanding than the others.

Personality clashes between nurse and patient was depicted as a potential problem.

Conclusion

Having carefully evaluated the results of the questionnaire, it would appear that the advantages of primary nursing outweigh the disadvantages. The implementation of this form of work organisation has proved to be a change for the better.

7

Primary Nursing in a Unit for the Young Disabled

Jan Dewing

This chapter describes the development of primary nursing from its inception through to the first year of its practice. The unit under discussion is a Young Disabled Unit within the Oxfordshire Health Authority. It stands in the grounds of one of the general hospitals, situated on the edge of the site, and is provided with the normal range of hospital services. In addition to providing a descriptive account, this chapter will offer some analyses of major events associated with the introduction and development of primary nursing for the reader to consider. Positive as well as negative aspects of the change process will be highlighted.

No pretence has been made that the unit and people involved in the change process about to be described are anything other than 'ordinary'. This chapter is not about describing excellence in nursing care, although that is an aim towards which primary nursing is moving. Every attempt has been made to present an objective account of events; however it should be appreciated that as with most retrospective accounts, especially where the author has been involved in the process of change, it will be tinged with subjectivity.

BACKGROUND INFORMATION

To facilitate reading this chapter some background information on the area in which primary nursing was developed will now be presented.

Layout

The unit offers a purpose-built environment for people with physical disabilities. It is a single-storey building where every effort has been taken to ensure that the clients have access to facilities and·plenty of space in which to move themselves around. Figure 7.1 shows a diagrammatic representation of the unit layout.

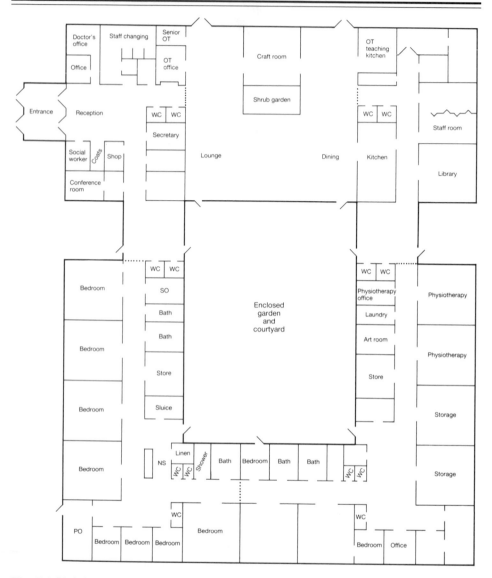

Fig. 7.1 Unit layout: bedrooms sleep one to three people; PO, Primary nurse's office; SO, Senior nurse's office; NS, Nurses' station; Bath, bathroom.

Client Group

The majority of people referred to the unit can, for ease of reference, be put into one of the following four categories:

● People with progressive chronic disorders such as multiple sclerosis, motor neurone disease and muscular dystrophies.
● People who have suffered from disabling congenital abnormalities in childhood and require care and support into adult life.

- People who have suffered from spinal injuries.
- People who have suffered brain damage in adult life, either through injury or through accident.

Referrals are accepted from any source. Following an initial assessment period, care packages are individually tailored to meet the needs of each client and their relatives and carers. This is then reviewed annually and adapted as required, or as the need arises. Clients are offered care packages consisting of either day care or residential care or a mixture of both. Care may be undertaken solely by the unit, but usually it involves professional and lay carers in the community as well. The number of clients admitted to the unit in any 24-hour period is regulated by monitoring the nursing care dependency levels. Theoretically, this ensures that demand for nursing does not exceed availability of nurses to deliver that care. In practice it also has the effect that primary nurses' caseloads are kept to a workable level, usually averaging around four clients who would be resident on any one day. Additionally, primary nurses have some input with clients coming in for day care. This level is more difficult to predict and can vary from day to day.

Staffing

Before introducing primary nursing the nursing establishment was composed of:

- 1 senior sister
- 1 sister
- 3 staff nurses on 37½ h week
- 2 staff nurses on 20 h week
- 3 enrolled nurses on 37½ h week
- 4 nursing auxiliaries on 37½ h week
- 2 nursing auxiliaries on 32 h week

Each night of the week the establishment allowed for:

- 1 staff nurse
- 2 nursing auxiliaries

There were and currently still are separate day and night staff. Many of the nurses on nights are part-time workers. Initially, night staff were not fully involved in the introduction of primary nursing. This was not intentional but simply the way events turned out. Moves have been made to enable the night staff to become more involved with primary nursing and also to initiate a degree of flexibility between working during the day and at night (i.e. some night staff worked some day shifts and vice versa). The system of separate day and night staff is an inherited one and by its nature is difficult to adapt.

Before the introduction of primary nursing the nursing structure was hierarchically organised. The functions of the two senior nurses were not clear and there was overlapping in some areas of their roles. Nursing work was organised around a system of task allocation. In practice this often meant that unqualified staff delivered nursing care with little or no supervision from nurses.

Two years on and with no increase in financial allocation to the nursing establishment the number of nurses has altered very little. However, some adjustments have been made to the skill mix between different grades of nurse and nursing auxiliaries. The skill mix is a dynamic feature. As staff leave and conditions in which nurses work change so the skill mix is adapted to take account of these events. Figure 7.2 shows the skill mix as it currently stands. The working relationships between the nurses are also indicated. As can be seen the relationships are organised on a collegial basis as required by primary nursing (Manthey, 1980).

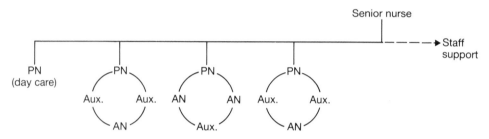

Fig. 7.2 Diagram to show the daytime skill mix on the unit: PN, Primary nurse: AN, Associate nurse; Aux., Auxiliary (Adapted from Pearson, 1974).

Other staff on the unit include a senior occupational therapist, two occupational therapists and a small team of unqualified staff. There is a senior physiotherapist, two physiotherapists and an unqualified helper, a social worker and a medical consultant who divides working time between two clinical units. The unit also has the services of an administrative assistant and a volunteer services organiser. The services of other agencies are available on a referral basis. All therapists, including nurses, aim to maintain and promote an environment that is conducive to personal growth and development of clients within the range of abilities they possess. This also means provision of a range of services, advice and support, as necessary for the maintenance of people with physical disabilities in the community with a quality of life both they and their family and carers are satisfied with. The main role of the unit is that of a respite care unit, therefore it differs considerably from a rehabilitation unit in its approaches to care.

ROLE OF THE SISTER

The sister was one of the two key people involved with initiating the move to primary nursing. It may be helpful to look at how frustrations with the traditional sister's role led to the introduction of primary nursing. It is difficult to say that the idea to introduce primary nursing into practice actually started with the sister. Certainly she had expressed a desire to change the way in which nursing care was organised and delivered, although this desire was not specifically focused in any one direction.

On the unit the sister represented nursing within the multidisciplinary team. She was responsible for assessing planning and evaluating care for approximately 130 clients. In addition to this she was expected, by the rest of the team to act as the major resource of information on matters relating to nursing care such as discharge planning and community liaison. It was clearly unreasonable to expect one person to hold accurate and detailed information on every member of a client group of this size and complexity. Other responsibilities involved managing nursing staff and the nursing administration of the unit. The major problem for the sister at that time was a lack of job satisfaction, partly because of the unreasonable expectations of the senior members of the multidisciplinary team on the sister. The sister also felt that the contribution of nursing to total client care was devalued by the rest of the teams on the unit. She wanted to reorganise nursing work in a way that would eliminate these two problems.

She decided to participate in a Ward Sister Development Course, run locally, to try to obtain knowledge and skills to be able to alter her practice. This particular course stemmed from the belief that sisters are instrumental in the way in which clinical nursing develops (Pembrey, 1980). Throughout the course alternative methods of organising and delivering nursing care were examined. This enabled the participants to examine their own areas of practice critically. As a result of this the sister decided to think about the feasibility of having a system such as primary nursing on the Young Disabled Unit. Following several meetings with a tutor, who was acting as a course facilitator, it was decided to approach the staff on the unit about actually putting it into practice.

As the sister had no experience of clinical development and little knowledge in the area of managing change, she looked to the course facilitator for support. With the full agreement of the sister they both negotiated with nursing management to make provision for the facilitator to adopt the role of nursing advisor to the unit. Rather than this simply being an informal role, overall responsibility for nursing on the unit was taken on by the advisor. Allowing a nurse educationalist such a degree of authority in a clinical area may be challenged. In this instance, given the nature of the proposed change and the personalities of the two nurses involved, it worked exceptionally well. The arrangement provided a high degree of clinical autonomy for the sister while providing a nurse who had expertise in management and specifically in managing change. It should be stated that it was possible for this arrangement to occur because the senior sister's post had been vacant for some time. It was not intended, at that time that the post would be filled thus modifying the existing nursing structure. The resource was to be utilised in a different way. Clearly during such a proposed development the sister and all the nurses required active and ongoing support. Looking back, it is now possible to say that the nursing advisor's role and knowledge proved to be an invaluable resource. This was especially so when discussing proposals with the other disciplines and with nursing management. This is an example of education and practice working in direct partnership to develop nursing practice in an effort to improve the quality of care provided for clients.

WHY CHANGE?

Nursing staff on the unit, in particular the sister, recognised a need to review their contribution to client care within the context of the unit as a whole. Several problem areas were identified:

- There were unrealistic expectations of the role of the sister.
- Lack of job satisfaction was expressed by the sister, who had felt powerless to try to resolve these difficulties on her own.
- The other nurses who were responsible for actually nursing clients were frustrated by the lack of opportunity to contribute to overall care planning and by the lack of information they needed to carry out day-to-day care.
- There was very little formal interdisciplinary care planning below the level of the senior members of each discipline, who met once a week. This allowed only an overview of each client, and the smaller more important details were often neglected.
- Nursing documentation was very poorly developed, with most of the written information pertaining to physical care. It was accorded a low priority and was often not up to date. There was no evidence of a problem-solving approach in nursing work.

MAJOR AIM OF THE DEVELOPMENT

The major aim of the development was to introduce an alternative method of organising nursing care with the specific aim of improving the quality of nursing care. It was also anticipated that there would be other benefits, such as increased job satisfaction, improved interdisciplinary communication, improved documentation and better links with community carers.

PREPARATION FOR THE INTRODUCTION OF PRIMARY NURSING

Preparation for the introduction of primary nursing involved nurses, clients and other disciplines. It turned out to be very time consuming as there was resistance, to a degree that had not previously been anticipated from the senior members of the multidisciplinary team. This will be expanded on later in the chapter. Planning involved a series of stages including education of nursing staff, consultation within the multidisciplinary team, preparation of clients, and practicalities of introducing a new working system, such as who would take on which roles and the allocation of clients to primary nurses.

Preparation of Nursing Staff

Initially the attitudes of nurses to the proposed development ranged from apprehension to hostility in a few nurses. They responded positively to the idea of changing the way in which they organised nursing as they wanted to become more involved in the overall planning of care. They also wanted nursing to be valued more and given recognition within the multidisciplinary team. However, they were not prepared for the extent of change proposed by introducing primary nursing. It is possible that it meant too much of a disruption to their normal routine or that they sensed that the senior members of the other disciplines were not in favour of primary nursing and that they had no desire for a conflict to develop. These were rational fears given the nature of the proposed change.

All nursing staff were involved in discussions and planning towards introducing primary nursing. Although they were at best apprehensive of the plans they were extremely confident in the sister. Their support for her was such that, although they were not committed to the idea of implementing primary nursing, they were prepared to try because she so clearly wanted to go ahead. In the early stages this made introducing new practices related to primary nursing difficult at times, as the nurses were very questioning in their approach. Therefore it was essential that an idea once implemented should be seen to work not only by the other disciplines but also by the nurses. Retrospectively, this has not had a negative outcome because change had been carefully planned by the nurses. Once fully supported by the majority of nurses an idea put into action has nearly always proved successful.

A series of study sessions were held once a week, which were open to all nursing staff. These sessions were seen as only the beginning of a programme of ongoing staff development. In total there were eight sessions based on the following themes:

- Patients or people?
- Views on nursing
- Methods of work organisation
- Models for practice
- Use of a named model
- Primary nursing in practice
- Assessment
- Planning

The final three sessions were specifically concerned with the practicalities of implementing primary nursing, as would be experienced on the unit. By discussing possible problems that may arise and potential coping strategies the nurses were able to manage the change process more effectively. During these sessions there was constant referral to how primary nursing may affect the other disciplines. The introduction of primary nursing was planned as if the multidisciplinary team members would be supportive towards nurses. Consequently, attempts were made to consider in what ways nursing would best be able to assist them from within a structure of primary nursing. The belief was, and still is, that primary nursing and multidisciplinary teamwork are not mutually exclusive activities.

Very minor difficulties arose when appointing primary nurses and associate nurses from within existing staff. The major difficulties during the preparatory stages were experienced with the senior members of the multidisciplinary team.

Preparation of the Multidisciplinary Team

Full consultations with senior members of the multidisciplinary team started as soon as the sister and nursing advisor were certain that the nurses were prepared to aim towards introducing primary nursing. They had anticipated some apprehension or even some reluctance about the proposals. What had not been expected was that they would perceive the development as dependent on their authorisation before it could be introduced into practice. The senior members believed they had executive powers of decision making on any and all matters affecting management of the unit. They made this very clear in the early stages of the consultation process. Nurses had been prepared to discuss plans with the senior members and listen to their views. Instead it emerged that nurses had to argue and assert their right to manage nursing. Some members of the multidisciplinary team believed that the purpose of such teams was to control the professional practices of each of the member disciplines, especially when it was not agreeable to their own beliefs or it was perceived as a threat to their position of authority.

Pearson (1988) argues that primary nursing promotes the development of a professional practice of nursing. This has now been demonstrated on the unit, but at the planning stages it was difficult for nurses to assert control over their own area of work let alone think about promoting professional practice. It was a real struggle and probably one that many nurses working in different areas still face and may eventually give up in order to avoid confrontations with other disciplines. During this time the nursing advisor was the major influence in determining nurses' right to manage nursing. Providing a knowledge base on which argument could be built enabled the nurses to have feelings of confidence about primary nursing.

The hesitant reception to the proposals by the multidisciplinary team was perceived by nurses as negativity towards the idea of introducing any change in nursing practices. The nurses believed that an overt demonstration of what primary nursing could achieve was justified. Much momentum had been built up and efforts could easily have been frustrated at this stage. While continuing to assert their right to manage nursing change, the nurses decided to continue with plans to introduce primary nursing, rather than expending energy on a direct confrontation at this stage. It was anticipated that at the end of the first year nurses would have available some indications as to whether or not primary nursing had achieved its aims.

Preparation of Clients

This was the area of preparation most poorly managed by nurses. Clients became aware of an impending change in the way in which the nurses were working. They were also aware of a state of conflict between nurses and the other disciplines, although not fully aware of the exact nature of this conflict. By the time consultations with senior members of the multidisciplinary team had ended and community meetings with clients had been organised, myths about primary nursing were well circulated among clients. Some of their beliefs reflected natural apprehensions about who would care for them when 'their nurse' was not there. Community meetings were utilised to provide clients with the opportunity to find out about what it was and how it would affect them and also to find out what they expected from primary nursing. They had time to ask questions and discuss it between themselves. Nurses also discussed issues with clients on a one-to-one basis.

With the benefit of hindsight, more discussion groups could have been offered. Carers in the community could have been better informed, as could the other professional agencies in the community. If these contacts had been more widely and formally established at this stage it might have lessened the difficulties that are still experienced by agencies outside the unit in attempting to liaise with primary nurses rather than the sister. In the effort to put primary nursing into practice these issues were somewhat neglected.

PROGRESS AFTER SIX MONTHS

Primary nursing was finally put into practice on a named day. The first six months were not without incident. Problems sometimes arose on a daily basis and sometimes there were no problems for at least a week! Some of the problems were related to the initial difficulties primary nurses had in getting other nurses to follow their care plans. Nurses had to learn to stand back and allow other nurses to do their work as they had planned with clients instead of all the nurses teaming up to try to get through the work as quickly as possible. Initially, one of the primary nurses and the associate nurses experienced difficulties with the ways in which they both worked. All the primary and associate nurses were given the freedom in which to develop the best working relationships possible for themselves. This was felt to be a priority as each primary nurse had named associate nurses, therefore they needed to be able to relate well with each other as they would be working together. The nurses were made aware that if they were unable to develop good working relationships then assistance was available from the sister and nursing adviser. Failing this, provision was made to alter formal relationships. However, such action has never been required. The nurses were also sensitive about comments made by some clients and members of the other disciplines in relation to primary nursing. In an effort to ensure that primary nursing was accepted the nurses had a tendency to over-react to comments. Perhaps this also reflected the anxieties of nurses about primary nursing at this early stage of implementing it into practice.

Some difficulties arose with documentation, such as how to organise the paperwork, where to store it and who should be writing in care plans and progress notes. These problems were, for the most part, anticipated and were dealt with relatively easily. Often they arose simply because nurses were learning to work within new boundaries and to relate to their colleagues and clients in a different way. These issues and others were discussed at weekly meetings. Any action decided on was always subject to review on a one, three or six monthly basis until a satisfactory outcome was achieved.

These meetings were also used to praise nurses where events or situations had been managed well. It was felt that this was very important as sometimes it seemed that nursing was responsible for all that went wrong on the unit. Retrospectively, it is easier to see that primary nursing was being used as a means of attributing blame where there were any negative changes on the unit. At this stage nurses were still lacking in self-confidence relating to some areas of primary nursing. Additionally the senior members of the multidisciplinary team were still not as supportive as had been hoped by the nurses. To evaluate the experience so far it was decided to organise a meeting with senior members of the other disciplines. The aim of the meeting was to present the progress to date and to allow for discussion of any positive and negative effects of primary nursing from their perspective.

Progress to Date

- Three primary nurses were introduced, to work with named associate nurses and nursing auxiliaries.
- All clients were allocated to a named primary nurse. Allocation was continuous with each admission.
- Primary nurses contribute to weekly care planning meetings in weekly rotation.
- Primary nurses undertake home visits, where appropriate, for those clients for whom they are responsible. They are also responsible for making contacts with services outside the unit.
- Nursing assessment is based on a named model with target dates being set for their completion.
- Care plans were introduced.
- Nurses pass on information directly during handovers about those clients they have cared for.
- The nursing documentation system was reorganised. Each primary nurse adopted a filing system for the nursing notes. In total there were 130 sets of notes; previously there had been only a Kardex system.
- Primary nurses held regular meetings with their associate nurses and nursing auxiliaries to discuss nursing care of clients and sometimes to discuss the way in which they were working with each other. Ideas for practice were fed back to nurses meetings for debate.
- Primary nurses identified a commitment to clients attending for day care.
- Monthly meetings were held with other therapists. This was at their request. General discussion on how primary nursing was affecting them occurred. They did, on occasions, offer positive suggestions that enabled the solutions to problems to be put into practice that provided positive outcomes for all.

It may be argued that primary nursing is only about nursing and the involvement of other therapists is not required. In practice, on a unit where all disciplines need to work together for the benefit of the clients, the involvement of the other disciplines is important when implementing primary nursing. Undoubtedly, they will experience some effects on their own areas of work and for this reason they should be included in discussions. It should be made clear that the nurses were receptive to their involvement on a positive basis, and that suggestions for change in practice conducive to primary nursing were seriously considered.

The progress to date had been achieved despite problems associated with nursing shortages, unfamiliarity with assessment and care planning formats, and the whole process of catching up on a new system of work organisation. In addition to the whole process being more time consuming simply because it was still new, nurses were more cautious about the way in which they worked as they perceived that they did not yet have the full support of the senior members of the multidisciplinary team.

The positive consequences at this stage were that nurses had an increased understanding of clients and their needs, on a holistic basis. Written information in terms of both assessment and care planning was felt to have improved. Positive feedback had been received from wards in the hospital and from some community services. Nurses stated that they were happier working with a system of primary nursing and they felt more committed to their work because of the closeness of their relationship with clients. All nurses recognised that the system was still new and therefore still presented some obstacles, but given the choice they wanted to work towards improving primary nursing rather than returning to their previous way of working. Points raised by the senior members of the other disciplines centred around three areas:

- Communication
- Allocation of newly referred clients to their primary nurses
- Presence of primary nurses in the day area, the main area for social contact and formal and informal activities

They were all areas that nurses had already identified as the weak links in the new system. Nurses were aware that improvements could be made. Senior members of the multidisciplinary team argued that nursing presence in the day area was non-existent since the introduction of primary nursing. Indeed it was, but it is possible to suggest that this occurred as a result of a nursing staffing crisis, which developed as those nurses resistant to primary nursing decided to leave. During this time all efforts were concentrated on keeping the basic structure intact. Therefore most of the plans to make improvements to the system had to be temporarily set aside until the staffing situation improved. It was anticipated that nursing presence in the day area would then improve. (It should also be stated that nursing presence was virtually non-existent before the introduction of primary nursing.)

Interdisciplinary communication was difficult as some of the senior members of the multidisciplinary team still insisted on channelling information through the sister rather than the appropriate primary nurse. They did not always prepare new staff in their departments for working with a system of primary nursing, and then individual therapists became confused over the aims of having such a system. Communication requires sustained effort from all involved parties for continued success (Smith and Bass, 1982). Primary nurses were inexperienced in dealing directly with therapists on the level of care planning, which could also have contributed to poor interdisciplinary communications. Nurses could have taken more initiatives in making use of tools such as the off-duty rota and in/out boards to let the other therapists know who on the nursing staff was on duty. It soon became clear that the other members of the team needed to know who to channel information through in the absence of primary nurses. Plans were formulated to try to improve the situation; for example, the use of a communication board for the doctor and introducing message books for written communications between the nurses and therapists. Primary nurses learnt to pass on information to their associate nurses on a more formal basis. Additionally, in the absence of a primary nurse, such as would occur with annual leave, another named primary nurse acted as a back up along with the associate nurse so that there was nearly always a nurse available for discussion of care with other members of the team.

Allocation of new clients to primary nurses reflected the anxieties of the administrative assistant in dealing with a system of primary nursing. It required a major reorganisation of the way in which the weekly care planning meetings were organised. Perhaps nurses had failed to appreciate how primary nursing would influence the way in which they worked. Although considering the needs of administrative staff is important, administrative staff should not be allowed to determine nursing practice.

Primary nurses found it difficult to divide their time between working with resident clients and working with clients coming in for day care. But, as previously stated this had been a problem before the introduction of primary nursing. Nevertheless nurses agreed to try to complete the nursing care needed by resident clients before 11.00 a.m., which was to enable them to spend time with clients coming in for day care. The introduction of primary nursing enabled the nurses to alter some of the ritualistic aspects of nursing such as all clients having baths or being bathed from head to toe on a daily basis. Despite this, mornings still proved to be a busy time. It became impossible for the primary nurses to work to this deadline. They reported feeling that they were being pressurised to work by the clock rather than by the clients' needs. Client dependency levels varied from week to week, which factor also made the 11 a.m. deadline even more difficult to meet.

In reality, nursing presence in the day care area had never been a nursing priority, and there had not been formal and effective communication networks between the different disciplines before primary nursing was introduced. There was a feeling that primary nursing was being 'scapegoated' as the cause of these problems. As the first year progressed it was important that nurses took this into account when evaluating the experience of primary nursing. Consideration of how primary nursing affected the multidisciplinary team was considered important with respect to planning developments to the system for the next year. However, it was equally important to put events into perspective and to appreciate that all the disciplines contributed to a less than harmonious working atmosphere, some of which had been in existence before the introduction of primary nursing. Introducing change will have positive and, perhaps, some negative effects on the rest of the multidisciplinary team. Nurses need to be prepared to consider that actions they take will affect others around them, but must be wary of being totally blamed for problems within the multidisciplinary team that were already in existence before primary nursing.

REVIEW OF THE FIRST YEAR OF PRIMARY NURSING

Working relationships between nurses and the rest of the multidisciplinary team became very strained around this time. This was probably a reflection of anxieties related to the change process in general rather than specifically to primary nursing. Relationships between different members of the team had been intermittently strained throughout the year, but it would not be possible to state that primary nursing was an independent factor. Nursing staff perceived that the senior members of the multidisciplinary team were still under the misapprehension that they had the right to decline their permission for primary nursing to continue. Nurses were understandably anxious about an impending confrontation with the senior members of the multidisciplinary team. They were given the choice of opting out of such a situation should it arise. They decided, with the support of the sister and nursing adviser, to assert their right to manage nursing and deal with any conflict that should arise in a direct and assertive way. Before the planned review, primary nursing was evaluated using the quality assurance tools Qualpacs (Wandelt and Ager, 1974) and Nursing Audit (Phaneuf, 1976) as well as nursing staff appraisals.

Baseline information had been collated before primary nursing was introduced. This enabled a comparison to be made at the end of the first year. Both the quality assurance tools demonstrated a significant improvement in the quality of nursing care. The initial Qualpacs evaluation indicated care to be in the range between average and poorest and average. Two years later the range was between best and average and best care. Likewise the initial audit indicated care to be predominantly in the poor range. Two years later this had improved to be comfortably in the excellent range.

Appraisals indicated all nurses to be highly satisfied with the primary nursing system when compared with a traditional system. Nursing auxiliaries expressed a preference for primary nursing. As they worked with the same primary and associate nurses they still felt that they were very much part of the nursing team, despite some restrictions on their clinical role. Baseline information on client's perceptions of nursing was started before primary nursing was introduced but it was never fully evaluated at that time. It was not repeated one year later. However, had it been appreciated at that time how severe the resistance from senior members of the multidisciplinary team would be, every effort would have been made to ensure that information from clients, as consumers of the service, was collected and evaluated. Although no formal evaluation had taken place attempts were made to ascertain the views of clients. In general their comments were favourable. As a result of the quality assurance reports and the appraisals nurses were confident that they could present a reasoned argument in favour of primary nursing having achieved its aims.

Despite the presentation of such an argument senior members of the multidisciplinary team continued to advocate the dissolution of primary nursing for a return to the way nursing had previously been organised. Although they were able to see some of the benefits of primary nursing for nurses and clients, they argued that problems outweighed any benefits from their perspective. Although they generally accepted that nursing care had improved and clients were receiving the care they wanted, they also considered how primary nursing had affected them. This is legitimate, but it occurred to such a degree that no matter how beneficial the outcomes were for clients, if they had not found it an agreeable system to work with they would not have approved it. Perhaps they had not been sufficiently prepared for the consequences of primary nursing on their practice. The nurses might have been able to do more during the preparatory stages to ease the transition of primary nursing for the other members of the team. It became apparent that the team members had anticipated more positive outcomes for their own areas of practice, where in fact primary nursing had the effect of highlighting some pre-existing multidisciplinary team problems.

The real issue for the senior members of the multidisciplinary team was that their assumed executive powers of management were being openly challenged by nurses. This had not been an intention of primary nursing. Indeed, nurses had looked towards the team for support in the initial stages. Nurses asserted their right to manage the organisation of nursing at the meeting. The senior members of the team were unable to alter this and were resolved to accepting primary nursing. Nurses agreed to have further meetings with the senior members of the multidisciplinary team to discuss how primary nursing could be adapted to meet the needs of the other disciplines. As a result of these meetings some areas of practice were altered. For example, daily feedback meetings with primary nurses and therapists were established to discuss care of clients on a daily basis and to talk about events that had occurred that day. Not long after the review a new primary nurse post was introduced and developed for clients referred for day care from within the existing nurse establishment. This not only put into practice the commitment nurses felt towards clients attending for day care, but demonstrated the nurses' commitment to working within the multidisciplinary team as partners in clients care.

EVALUATION OF THE EXPERIENCE

Primary nursing is still being practised on the unit. It is continuing to develop as can be demonstrated by quality assurance findings and the high level of job satisfaction expressed by nurses. Additionally the commitment to professional and personal development is high among the nurses. Using these criteria, the outcomes of primary nursing are positive. However, the system was difficult to introduce and develop in the first year. This would have undoubtedly have been made easier with the active support of the senior members of the multidisciplinary team. Perhaps their response to the introduction of primary nursing was a predictable reaction to the process of change being introduced into a large and generally inflexible organisation. Despite what seemed to be almost constant lobbying against primary nursing, the growing enthusiasm of nurses ensured its survival. Lessons learned from the experience have been utilised positively and have helped the nursing team to strengthen their commitment to what they now know is a more effective system of organising and delivering nursing care.

8

Primary Nursing in a Continuing Care Unit

Catherine Miller

The Royal Marsden Hospital is a specialist hospital which treats individuals with cancer. Treatment may include surgery, chemotherapy, radiotherapy or combinations of these. The Continuing Care Unit serves patients for whom active curative treatment is no longer appropriate, providing supportive, palliative care to alleviate pain and other symptoms. The prognoses of the individuals referred vary greatly, and therefore rehabilitation also plays an important part in symptomatic treatment.

The hospital is staffed by qualified nurses holding either a Registered General Nursing or an Enrolled Nurse General Certificate who have also attained the ENB Course in Oncology Nursing. A proportion of the staff in the hospital are nurses undertaking the oncology courses.

The Continuing Care Unit shift system is the same as that practised in the rest of the hospital. The shifts have been reviewed so that at present we maintain a three-shift system as follows: 07.30–15.30, 14.00–22.00, 21.30–07.50. This has substantially lessened the previous shift overlap, necessitating improved nurse handover time to avoid compromising the time available for nurses involved in direct patient care. Normal staffing numbers are four staff on an early shift, three on a late shift and two on night duty. Internal rotation to night duty practised on the unit maintains continuity of patient care. This British shift method of organising nursing differs from the American four-shift system which operates with a static number of nurses on duty, and initially it seemed problematic when considering primary nursing in an English setting.

A second consideration, as regards staff cover, was the grades of staff on the unit. The ward has two ward sisters, five staff nurses (one on permanent night duty), four enrolled nurses and a transient population of registered and enrolled nurses undertaking the oncology course whose ward allocation ranges from 5 to 8 weeks. One of the staff nurses is a 'consolidating' nurse, on a 12–week allocation following the final oncology course examination.

CHANGE FOR CHANGE'S SAKE?

The previous system of nursing employed on the unit was patient allocation. This was relatively successful in providing individualised patient care, but continuity proved erratic. Nurses were unable to maintain relationships with patients and their families when their patient allocation changed frequently. This shortcoming was reflected in the care planning; nursing instruction was not always structured, so evaluation was poor. This was attributed to the lack of a nurse co-ordinating the care for one particular patient. The results of Monitor (a quality assurance tool; Goldstone *et al.*, 1983) reinforced this view. Evaluation and documentation of nursing intervention required improvement as well as the need to rethink the way nursing is organised.

During ward closure for upgrading, the opportunity arose to change nursing practice on the unit. Regrading took 6 months and the ward reopened with an almost entirely new staff. Bed complement remained at 13, but the ward layout had changed. The unit now had one four-bedded ward, two two-bedded rooms and five single rooms. After discussion with the ward staff it was decided to consider various approaches to nursing care, and a formal staff meeting was convened.

The meeting generated both interest and consternation among the established staff, who felt that the old system had proved satisfactory and expressed doubts about 'change for change's sake'. Newly appointed permanent staff were generally open-minded. My role as unit Senior Nurse manager was to explain the concept of primary nursing and its practical application in the unit.

The established staff's reservations concerned the use of an American system in a British hospital, the lack of specialty knowledge of the new staff, and a lack of confidence among the staff nurses about expanding their role. Indeed the latter was a real concern for both ward sisters, who also felt threatened by this radical change. Their new role as co-ordinator and resource person was explained, but their doubts remained.

Another area of concern was the enrolled nurse's role. Primary nursing was seen as a form of demotion by some nurses who saw their role as associate nurses unsatisfactory. This was an extremely sensitive area, as previously the enrolled nurses' roles in practice had not differed greatly from that of the staff nurse. Although the value of the enrolled nurses was emphasised and explained, they expressed a fear that their organising and clinical skills would not be appreciated. Because of the sensitivity of the subject and the strong feelings voiced, enrolled nurses were encouraged to read relevant articles before returning to a further meeting to re-examine their reservations (see chapter 17).

When permanent staff had had the opportunity to read about the subject a second meeting was held. The role of the night staff was discussed. Their role was seen as one of 'caretaker' rather than primary nurse, as decisions taken about changes in care were usually taken during the day. The concept of the associate nurse was re-examined and time given to digest the relevant information.

The meeting brought to light other concerns about the implementation of primary nursing in the unit. One was the unit's U-shaped layout. Nurses asked how patients would be selected for each primary nurse. If it were on a bay or group of rooms basis, it would be no different from a patient allocation system. Their main concern was that they would be unable to observe dependent patients if their allocated patients were dispersed throughout the ward. Another concern was the patient with whom the primary nurse had difficulty in relating. This can add to ward stress if not resolved and may culminate in 'distressed' nurses. Historically nurses were not allowed to express discontent in the ward environment without being made to feel guilty at their 'inability to cope'. After a fruitful discussion it was agreed that nurses experiencing difficulties in communicating with patients should bring this to the ward sister's attention. This is important because unresolved conflict in a ward environment can quickly lead to a divided and unhappy staff.

The meeting also focused on how primary nurses would be prepared for their new role. At this point I had not fully prepared a teaching package for this purpose, as I was still awaiting a decision on whether to try out the new system. I was mandated to work on this point and prepare it for the next agreed meeting.

At the next meeting the staff agreed to a trial period of 3 months, to start 3 months hence, once the ward teaching programme had been established and general ward management affairs had been explained and understood by the primary nurses. There was still doubt evident among the ward staff, but they agreed that if this system could be made to work it would benefit both patients and staff. The enrolled nurses varied in enthusiasm but did not dismiss the changes out of hand, agreeing to the 3-month trial.

During the discussion period the medical staff were approached and the unit consultant was initially somewhat bemused by the proposal for change. When primary nursing was explained, one doctor expressed fears about the confusion in relating to more nurses on a day-to-day basis instead of channelling all information through the ward sister. Nevertheless, the consultant was willing to participate in the trial, provided it was not detrimental to patient care or the efficiency of the unit.

Finally it was decided that after the 3-month trial we would evaluate the effectiveness of the changes and plan the future direction of the ward. All members of the ward team would participate in the evaluation, and the decisions would be democratic and positive.

THE FIRST MONTHS

The unit primary nursing programme began by selecting four staff as primary nurses. The primary nurses selected were three new staff nurse appointments and a staff nurse working on the unit before the upgrading. Each primary nurse was to work with an associate nurse, who was either a permanent enrolled nurse or a course nurse (RGN or EN) (see figure 8.1).

Selection of the staff to a primary nurse was made by the ward sister and primary nurse after discussion with the associate nurses. This was democratic and amiable as the majority of staff wished to try this system. There were fears about the primary nurse's workload so we encouraged each nurse to experiment with her own workload which she herself would critically evaluate. Primary nursing day 1 followed a public holiday so the unit was not busy. This was deliberate to give time to the primary nurses to establish their roles, to explain their new approach to care to their primary patients and to re-evaluate the care plans for individual patients and to reassess the nursing intervention required. It was hoped that by improving systematic care documentation there would be continuity of care throughout the 24 hour shift and that nursing care evaluation would, as a result, improve.

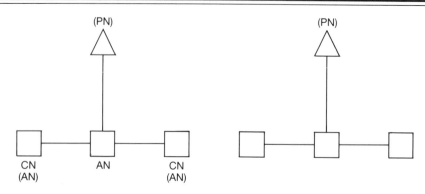

Fig. 8.1 Diagrammatic representation of primary nursing on the continuing care unit: PN, primary nurse; AN, associate nurse; CN, course nurse (EN or RGN).

Before the transition period the ward staff had created a unit teaching programme and invited others from the multidisciplinary team to participate in informal teaching sessions. This proved successful, giving the ward staff a greater understanding of the various roles and expectations of individual practitioners such as, for example, the occupational therapists. This was aimed at preventing problems of professional jealousy and role overlap.

It was essential to give primary nurses the confidence to discuss changes in care with other disciplines. The ward sister and myself had previously discussed the importance of confidence among the primary nurses and the need to provide a supportive environment until they became comfortable in their role. As this new role is stressful we felt that further responsibilities, such as participating in teaching and assessing course nurses, could be added to the remit of the primary nurses only when they felt ready. Alongside added responsibility for patient care came the commitment to relative participation in care, and patient and relative education. Given the unit philosophy for care the implementation of this ideal is potentially stressful because of the various levels of understanding required to help patients and relatives.

Discussions were made regarding formal and informal support systems for the staff. They decided that a more formal support group was unnecessary and they preferred an informal system whereby individuals could discuss problems with each other, the ward sisters or myself. This system was open to change at any time if the staff so wished. Recently, we have been looking at other systems of support, and change is likely in the unit although no final decision has been made (see chapter 13).

The transition was relatively trouble free, despite some concern about the diminished role of the sister as overall co-ordinator of nursing care. The sisters' role obviously changed. The main problem appeared to be the temptation to answer questions and deal with practical problems occurring on the unit without referring to the appropriate primary nurse. This habit was difficult to break. The sisters' role was to provide both management and specialist advice in circumstances that the primary nurse or associate nurse had not met, and to aid direction in their subsequent actions. The ward sisters work opposite shifts so there is usually a sister working an early shift when help and advice may be necessary.

The sisters will also act as associate nurses and provide nursing care if appropriate. They will also advise other associate nurses regarding change in care in the absence of the primary nurse. This decision, however, can be overruled by the primary nurse on her return should she think it inappropriate.

The enrolled nurses did not find this associate nurse role too demeaning, and those established in the specialty still felt able to contribute towards care planning. Course nurses obviously liked the continuity of care and the fact that working with primary nurses enabled them to have a 'mentor'. Casual comments from patients, who enjoyed contact with the same nurses, were favourable. They felt that nursing staff better understood their problems and that communication had consequently improved. Relatives began to ask for the primary or associate nurse by name and felt more comfortable discussing their intimate feelings and anxieties with a nurse who was no longer a stranger.

At the introduction of primary nursing the ward had two permanent night staff with the remainder of the night establishment maintained by internal rotation. This was a problem in implementing primary nursing as primary nurses also had to take their turn of night duty. This involved eight nights on and six nights off duty. Choosing a flexible system to suit our environment, it was decided that when primary nurses were rostered to nights the ward sister would caretake for the primary nurse during the day and that both would participate equally in evaluating care. As a result, critics may argue that a true primary nursing system is not being practised, but the primary nurse on night duty still has the opportunity to review changes in patient care and discuss future management with day duty staff at report time. The present primary nurse system is not ideal, but we have to work within the restraints of hospital internal rotation and this appeared to be the most effective compromise.

The course nurses employed as associate nurses were not left to take decisions beyond their experience, because in the absence of a primary nurse they could refer to the ward sister. There was also an opportunity to liaise with their primary nurse at report time. Report time consisted of a patient problem-orientated format and this report took place in the ward office with all the staff present.

The experience available to course nurses is extensive, enabling them to develop better communication skills and knowledge on pain and symptom control. To facilitate learning, the nurse needs both support and guidance in this often stressful specialty. Primary nursing offers an excellent learning environment in which the primary nurse sets the educational goals (sometimes in conjunction with the ward sister) and education is offered at a pace that suits the learner. Learner performance is evaluated by continuous assessment and formulation of course nurse ward reports, which now become the responsibility of the primary nurse. During the interim report the ward objectives are discussed. Realistic goal setting is very important from the outset, as unrealistic unachieved goals lead to frustration and stress.

During the first 3-months the night staff expressed frustration about acting as associate nurses. They felt excluded from the ward and there was negative communication between themselves and the primary nurses. This situation could quickly have led to division between day and night staff. The problem lay in the emphasis primary nurses were putting on specific nursing instructions in such a way that the night staff felt that there was no opportunity to use their initiative. The problems were two-fold: over-enthusiasm on the part of one or two primary nurses and their feeling that they needed to prove themselves in this role. In two specific situations the night staff found the nurses' authoritarian attitude unacceptable. This was exacerbated by ambiguous documentation of nursing intervention, which was found to conflict with the verbal report of patient care.

The ward sisters conversed with all parties concerned, attempting to redefine their priorities and roles. The situation required immediate clarification and positive reinforcement to avoid further conflict. A repetition of this situation occurred on one or two other occasions, again due to poor communication and role ambiguity. These difficulties were discussed at ward meetings where emotional stress was shared and dissipated. Gradually, trust and confidence overcame these disputes and a balance was restored. The fact that the primary nurse and night staff had night duty allocations together gave them the opportunity to clarify points and view each other's working style, and this seemed the most satisfactory approach to solving this conflict.

The 3-month trial passed quickly and at our evaluation meeting it was decided to continue with primary nursing as it appeared to suit our ward environment and specialty. The medical consultant expressed pleasant surprise at the quality of information imparted by primary nurses, and the ingenuity shown in the delivery of nursing care, but the best indication of the success of the trial in his view was the general satisfaction expressed by patients and their relatives.

THE ONGOING PROCESS

I will now briefly describe the continuing process of implementing and maintaining primary nursing and our subsequent modifications of the system.

As months passed, it became apparent that all the staff were motivated to explore different aspects of pain and symptom control. This was indicated by their undertaking various projects and studying various teaching packages, including a guide to using different products in wound care and a 'teaching box' on subjects pertinent to the specialty. One exciting project was a 'resource room', to which all the ward staff contributed relevant articles relating to nursing, management, research and education. Any member of staff was free to refer to the articles and add to the collection. We also keep a small library of books and the room is used for private study. The teaching programme on the ward continued to develop in both seminar and lecture form.

The clinical competence of the course nurse members was assessed by the primary nurses. It was gratifying to see their confidence grow in every case. Their enthusiasm was rewarded by the opportunity to undertake study days on relevant professional development courses. Enrolled nurses and night staff were also encouraged to participate in furthering their educational development. This enthusiasm was also notable in clinical practice, where the management of the clinical workload improved and use of research-based practice was tried and evaluated.

It was important to encourage the staff as their individual backgrounds varied and also because from our position the ward sisters and myself could sometimes perceive progress when the other staff could not. I made a point of introducing individual performance reviews so that both primary nurses and associate nurses were able to discuss their developmental needs and build on their skills.

From the practice of individualised care, the nursing process developed. The nursing process documentation has undergone revision at the Royal Marsden Hospital and the format used today is used throughout the hospital. Nursing in continuing care has in the past been based on a medical model of care. There is still a tendency for nurses to identify patients' medical problems as opposed to their nursing problems. However nurses have made a conscious effort to become nursing problem-orientated and to document nursing intervention in a systematic, individually planned format, thereby improving delivery and evaluation of nursing care. Primary nurses became responsible for this delivery of care and the documentation became a valuable tool in evaluating care and in teaching. Not everyone found nursing care plans easy, especially in defining goals for patients with varying prognoses. Help was available from the ward sisters and from the patients themselves to define limitations. This continues to be problematic for some nurses, but quality assurance studies, using Monitor, showed an improvement in the evaluation of care. As communication is so important we endeavour to describe problems in the patients' own language, especially when attempting to understand a patient's pain. If a common language is used between nurse and patient it assists in the evaluation of care (Manthey, 1980). Verbal communication has also improved, whereby theoretical reports are being replaced by problem-orientated reports. A recent change in the format of ward report has taken place so that the midday report is now given by the primary or associate nurse at the patient's bedside, thus including the patient in his own care. Care plans are kept at the bedside and improvement has been noted in vocabulary, both oral and written.

This system both underlies and reinforces the unit's philosophy to provide 'family-centred care'. The primary nurse is the pivot in providing information for patient and family to prepare themselves for changing roles at home and for the difficult time leading up to a patient's death.

The unit functions in a multidisciplinary framework of care. As the primary nurse communicates with all disciplines in this team her consistency in co-ordinating the individual patient's care and as a communication source is vital, so that staff, patients, and relatives can achieve continuity in their care.

The role of the unit has changed somewhat over the years as pain and symptom control have improved, and many patients have the opportunity to return home. Although desirable, home care is not without problems for both patients and families, and a degree of unit rehabilitation is usually required. Living with any disability (regardless of the prognosis) requires adaptation and education for the whole family. The primary nurse's responsibility is to collaborate with other members of the multidisciplinary team. Any social, physical or emotional deficits that will impede progress, must be assessed by the primary nurse and referred where appropriate (see figure 8.2).

Primary nurses do maintain contact with some of their patients and relatives and we encourage patients to ring the unit to speak to their primary nurse if problems

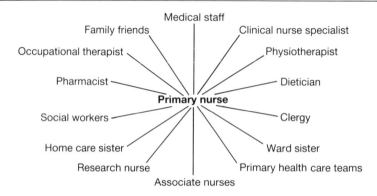

Fig. 8.2 Channels of communication within the multidisciplinary team.

arise. Occasionally, the primary nurse may go on a home visit with the home care sister to see her patient and this adds to the nurse's understanding of problems that can occur in the home. This new perception of situations adds to the nurse's knowledge and sensitivity when organising future services between hospital and community.

Research is an integral part of the unit's work. There is a wealth of knowledge on the effectiveness of drugs, especially on symptom alleviation and on drug delivery. The unit staff includes a research sister who participates in collecting and disseminating the information required to conduct research trials. Primary nurses have a responsibility to monitor standards in research protocols and any adverse drug side-effects. They participate in studies to provide valuable current data, and some primary nurses have themselves studied subjects pertaining to the unit's work.

THE FUTURE

The unit settled down and experienced a long period of stability when all the permanent staff were content and enjoying their work. Their individual career patterns emerged and three staff nurses left the unit to pursue new nursing roles. This caused an unsettled period with the introduction of new staff nurses and our second generation of primary nurses was born! They themselves decided when they felt it was appropriate to take on the primary nurse role, but our mistake was to make this transition period too general and not related to nurses' individual needs. This added to nurses' stress by not sufficiently preparing them for this role. Presently, we are making a checklist to cover essential information for staff to be able to take management and clinical responsibility so that all new primary nurses have constant information, and we are looking towards individualised development programmes. This list is being compiled by permanent staff on the ward who are all too aware of the shortcomings in the previous system!

As the unit is committed to primary nursing we will continue to strive towards improving standards of care for our patients. However, to move forward requires flexibility and critical evaluation, and therefore we expect to continue to learn and modify this approach to care.

In conclusion, nurses must be critical about the effect of change on their nursing practice and there is no more honest way than to listen to our colleagues. So I shall finish with comments from two nurses who have experienced the change:

- Initially I felt threatened by my new role as a facilitator, but the team had to establish and define new identities and realise that overlapping of one another's roles could be achieved and enjoyed. I could not envisage returning to the more traditional role of charge nurse, as I had previously worked. (Charge Nurse)

- Primary nursing has provided me with the openings to develop my 'professionalism' by providing avenues for individual accountability and initiative I'd never discovered before, despite supposedly having been 'trained' to that end. (Primary Nurse)

External demands and changes within the education system for nurses in the UK have implications for the practice of nursing. The future is uncertain, but it is important not to become complacent in our role, but to use ingenuity and further flexibility in practice to attain a standard of nursing that is acceptable to individual units. Primary nursing may be a way of continuing that change and providing that challenge to look at our practice, evaluate its effectiveness and plan for the future.

Medical developments are not isolated from nursing practice, and as we have to cope with new directions and procedures we must remain systematic, professional and ever aware of our individual development.

9

Meeting the Needs of People with Acquired Immune Deficiency Syndrome

Ann Taylor

When in early 1981 the first case of Acquired Immune Deficiency syndrome (AIDS) was diagnosed in the United States, few people could have anticipated the devastating effects that this disease was going to have on society, nor its implications for health care professionals. By Christmas 1981, when the first case of AIDS was seen in the UK, over 300 cases of AIDS had been diagnosed in the USA (Pratt, 1988). The number of new cases is now thought to be doubling every 13–14 months. UK figures for October 1990 show 3884 cases of AIDS and 2131 deaths (CDR Report). The World Health Organisation has reported 383 021 cases world wide in August 1990 (WHO September 1990). They also estimate that by the year 2000, 10 million children will be infected.

At present the majority of people with AIDS are from groups in society who may already be misunderstood, stigmatised and disadvantaged, such as homosexuals, intravenous drug abusers, and bisexuals. It is, however, important to note that figures announced for the third quarter of 1990 show that the number of cases of AIDS acquired heterosexually has almost doubled in the past 12 months, compared with an increase of 89% among intravenous drug users and 40% among homosexual and bisexual men (Delamothe 1990).

AIDS is a multisystem, grossly disfiguring disease which affects both the body and the mind, and one that places tremendous stress on those involved with, or caring for, individuals suffering from the disease. There should be little that is different about caring for people with AIDS as, like all patients, they have specific needs which must be met. They have the same right to the highest quality of care that it is possible to provide. In practice, however, nursing people with AIDS is different. Not only are its effects devastating, but it affects people in a young age group, many of whom may have watched their friends die of AIDS. The average age of those affected is 20–49 years. The majority of cases are those in the 30–39 age group. Many do not take to the sick role passively, but will question what is being done, and why, and go through 'life's last great adventure' with tremendous courage and dignity.

To meet this challenge, health care professionals must address many issues which have for too long been neglected or ignored. People with AIDS, like any individual with a terminal illness, experience tremendous feelings of loss, for example loss of:

- Control over one's life
- Control of one's body because of disfiguring conditions
- Control of one's mind because of neurological involvement
- Ability to care for oneself, both physically and financially
- Security – financial and emotional
- One's family and friends

Thus AIDS has been described as presenting the greatest challenge that the nursing profession has ever known (Snee, 1988). It requires the nurse to be flexible and adaptable, and to be brave enough to confront issues previously swept under the carpet.

MILDMAY MISSION HOSPITAL

Mildmay Mission Hospital is a Christian charitable hospital situated in the East End of London. It was founded as a medical mission in 1866 by Mildmay deaconesses to care for victims of the cholera epidemic which had broken out at that time. Closed in 1982 as part of the NHS reorganisation, Mildmay reopened in 1985 as an independent hospital serving the local community. Mathieson, a 24-bed ward, was opened first. It aims to provide respite, convalescent and long-term care for young people who are chronically sick.

In February 1988, Elizabeth Ward was opened as the first stage of a continuing care unit, providing respite, convalescent and terminal care for people with AIDS. A further eight beds on Tankerville Ward was opened in 1989.

The views of people with AIDS were sought when planning Elizabeth Ward. The overall aim was to create as home-like an environment as possible. The ward (figure 9.1) comprises nine single rooms, each with *en suite* Clos-o-Mat (an automatic WC combining flushing, warm water and hot air drying functions in one unit), but all sharing a large shower room, an assisted Arjo Bath (the height of which can be raised or lowered to a convenient height), sluice room, clinical room, and a communal sitting/dining area. A rooftop conservatory is planned for the future.

Figure 9.2 shows the hospital management structure.

ELIZABETH WARD

Staffing ratios are high, at 1:1.5 patients. There are several reasons why this is so:

- Part of the philosophy of the unit involves staff being able to spend as much time with a patient or his relatives as they need.
- Patients and relatives may require a great deal of counselling.

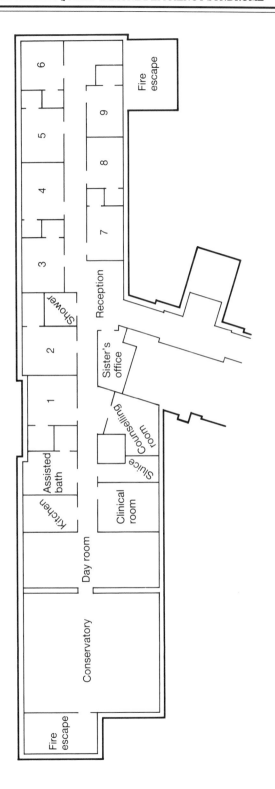

Fig. 9.1 Layout of the ward.

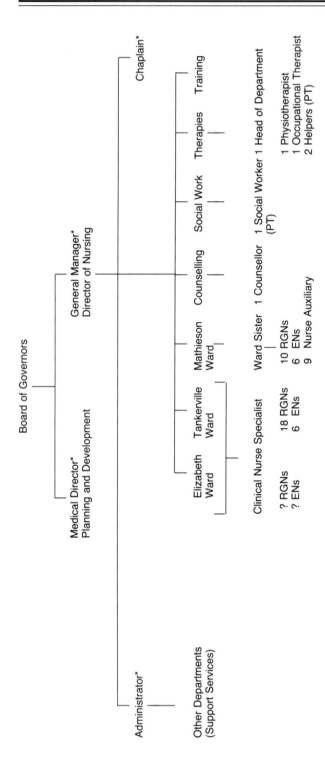

Fig. 9.2 Management structure of Mildmay Mission Hospital: *Senior Management Team; PT, part time.

- Many patients require highly dependent nursing care.
- Stress levels among staff working with people with AIDS has been found to be high. Adequate staff may help to reduce stress.
- It is difficult to supervise patients in single rooms.

It was decided that the nursing structure should be as flat as possible, to shorten lines of communication, and to encourage teamwork and the development of all members of staff. There is a clinical nurse specialist (CNS) responsible for management of the unit and co-ordinating the multidisciplinary team, whose line manager is the director of nursing.

Other members of the multidisciplinary team include a doctor, counsellor, part-time social worker, occupational therapist, physiotherapist, pastor and house-keeper.

PHILOSOPHY OF CARE

Mildmay was the first hospice for people with AIDS in Europe, and therefore there was no established model of care when the unit was set up. However, there may be no one model of care that is entirely suitable, as the disease is constantly changing and there are too many variables relating to it. Thus any philosophy adopted has to be flexible and adaptable.

Loss of control seems to be involved in every other type of loss individuals experience. It was therefore decided that the emphasis of care should be placed on allowing people to control their situation as much as possible by involving them in decisions regarding their care (self-directed care) and helping them to undertake their own care (self-care). To achieve this, the individual needs to have the necessary knowledge and space in which to make choices, and feel safe and secure in his environment.

When thinking or talking about AIDS, one automatically thinks of a terminal disease, but for many people admitted to our unit there is still a great deal of living to do. The emphasis within the unit is therefore on living, not on dying. Care is planned to try to make each day special. Some people return home, but for the rest the unit is not just somewhere where people die, but where they can live their last days as fully as possible.

WHY PRIMARY NURSING?

There were several reasons why primary nursing was chosen:

- It allows nursing staff greater autonomy as the unit is primarily a nursing unit. The nurse becomes accountable first of all to her patient and then to her manager, so areas of accountability are clear and can be readily exercised. This may improve standards of care and evaluation of practice.
- It appeared to fit the philosophy of the unit as it provides continuity of care and helps develop relationships by allowing patients and carers to get to know one

another. Each patient has a specific nurse, or nurses, with whom he can identify and work in partnership, so creating an environment suitable for making choices.

- It allows flexibility.
- It is viewed as being a professional style of nursing practice.
- It was felt that the unit should be innovative in its approach to its nursing practice.

Recruitment of staff for the unit began in November/December 1987. I was appointed as CNS, and was in post by 1 December, and the remainder of staff started to arrive at the beginning of January 1988. The time between January and the opening on 23 February was used for the induction of staff.

IMPLEMENTING PRIMARY NURSING

Only one of the nurses was familiar with and had worked using primary nursing before. A study day was arranged to look at the philosophy of primary nursing and to compare it with other methods of care delivery. This was followed up by informal discussions between staff and encouragement for individuals to do as much background reading as possible.

It was decided to have three primary nurses, each with a maximum case load of three patients. The first three primary nurses were chosen because of their previous experience of nursing people with AIDS. With a full establishment of 24 staff there would be seven associate nurses working with each primary nurse. Associate nurses were RGNs and ENs. The primary nurse would rotate to night duty, but would not be on 24-hour call. It was felt that the high stress levels involved with this area of care made it important that staff got away from work completely on their days off. However, if staff wished to be informed regarding patients' conditions while off duty, this would be supported. When the primary nurse went onto night duty, the case load was to be taken over by an identified associate nurse.

It was considered important that patients referred to the unit should be able to meet staff before being admitted. For many people the acute ward where they receive treatment is seen as a place of great security and a move to another unit can be difficult. It was thought that it might help, therefore, if the primary nurse visited the patient when he was referred, to assess his suitability for admission. Whenever possible the primary nurse would be on duty when the patient was admitted, to welcome him and commence an initial assessment. If the patient were discharged home, the primary nurse would remain the key nurse, and liaise with the district nurse. If there were any problems or difficulties, the primary nurse could visit the patient to maintain links, as necessary.

New patients are allocated to a primary nurse by the CNS, who takes the workload and the nurse's specific skills and expertise into consideration.

At first it was suggested that the role of primary nurse should be rotated among all the nurses. It was felt at the time that this would work, as the majority of the nurses had a great deal of experience, although not in the area of AIDS, and were capable of being primary nurses. This would have had the advantage of reducing the stress and workload of individuals as the primary nurse's role was perhaps more stressful and demanding than that of the associate nurse. It would also have broadened the development of all staff.

However, in practice, rotation was found to be impossible as it took quite a while for staff to adjust to the role of primary nurse and constant changes were unsettling for the unit. It was felt that perhaps it was better to develop the associate nurse's role to the full.

When the ward opened, the team comprised two primary nurses and four associate nurses. The aim to fill the ward slowly and to increase the nursing establishment gradually. Each primary nurse had one patient. By May there were three primary nurses. One of the original primary nurses had left, and two nurses involved in the unit from the beginning now acted as primary nurses. Each primary nurse has a case load of two to three patients. In practice the actual case load per shift was not greater than three. However, on occasions when a primary nurse and one of her associate nurses were on duty together, that primary nurse would act as an associate nurse for another primary nurse. As far as was possible, all shifts (internal rotation to night duty was in operation) had a nurse from each of the three groups on duty.

PROBLEM SOLVING

Staff meetings were held every month as a forum for staff to air any problems, difficulties and suggestions they had regarding their work on the unit. It was difficult initially both for staff to be open and honest about how they felt things were progressing, and for me as the manager to absorb criticism without having positive feedback with which to balance it. With time the meetings became more open and constructive, allowing adaptations to be made to the system.

The implementation of change is always difficult as it creates insecurity, and the problems on Elizabeth Ward were increased by it being a new unit, within a new specialty. In addition, Orem's self-care model of nursing was being implemented and there was continuous evaluation of nursing practices on the ward.

The problems outlined below were identified over a period of several months and are in no particular order.

COMMUNICATION

One advantage of primary nursing is claimed by Manthey (1980) to be improved communication within the ward, due to communication occurring directly from one person to another. It was found, however, that communication on the unit between nurses and other members of the team, regarding individual patients' care and general policy changes, was very poor. Messages and changes did not seem to be passed on. In an attempt to overcome this problem it was decided that the primary nurse, as far as possible, should attend all multidisciplinary meetings. (These important meetings are held every Monday, and it is here that plans are formulated, evaluated and reviewed.) This further reinforces the primary nurse's role as co-ordinator of care. To do this, the primary nurse no longer rotated to night duty. This appeared to improve communications, but it put an increased burden on the associate nurses as many worked one week in four on night duty. It is hoped that, once the system becomes more established, it may again be possible to rotate the primary nurse onto night duty.

SHIFT CO-ORDINATOR

The question of one person on each shift being designated as a co-ordinator, and whether or not this person should be a primary nurse, was discussed at length. It was felt that if the co-ordinator was a primary nurse, rather than an associate nurse, a hierarchy would be built into the system. Although it was important that specific tasks, such as ordering drugs, were done at certain times each day, overall, on a nine bed unit, the volume of work was not considered sufficient to necessitate a co-ordinator. Instead specific jobs were decided among staff at the beginning of each shift. The need for a shift co-ordinator is under constant review.

Nurses were encouraged to use a ward diary. A communication book was introduced, where changes in ward policy were recorded. Staff were encouraged to check this regularly, to keep up to date with ward changes.

PRIMARY NURSING AS PERCEIVED BY OTHER MEMBERS OF THE MULTIDISCIPLINARY TEAM

Initially, although every effort was made to ensure that other members of the multidisciplinary team were aware of the philosophy of primary nursing and our philosophy of care, it was difficult for them to see any advantages in using this approach to organising nursing, especially as communication between them and the nurses appeared to be poor. The team members were used to a more traditional system of care, and many missed the person-in-charge, be she the ward sister or senior staff nurse. They initially found it difficult to go to the nurse looking after the patient. They would often approach me as the CNS, as I was frequently on the ward and was seen as being in charge. It took a little while and a lot of encouragement to get the team to look at the wipe-off board outside the office to see which nurse was looking after which patient. This now appears to be working and is accepted as the norm. Communication does now appear to have improved and information is often more accurate when it is obtained and passed on first-hand.

On balance, once the team members became used to the system, they liked it and felt it offered an advantage over traditional systems in that problems were now discussed with the nurse who know most about the patient.

STRESS AND THE NURSE–PATIENT RELATIONSHIP

Anxiety had been expressed before implementation that primary nursing could cause increased stress within the nurse–patient relationship. One senior nurse in a well established hospice, with whom the implementation of primary nursing was discussed, felt that this form of nursing was totally inappropriate because of the possible increase in stress it might cause. Menzies (1960c) suggests that nurses will often both 'routinise' clinical care and concern themselves more frequently with administration, as a defence system, so protecting themselves from the stress arising from involvement and closeness with patients. There was uncertainty as to the effect of creating a situation in which those protections are removed and emphasis is placed on creating a close nurse–patient relationship, especially in a hospice where there is daily contact with death and dying.

It had been envisaged that the patient turnover rate on the unit would be high. Initially this proved not to be so. To date there have been patients who died soon after admission, but many patients were on the unit for months. (The average length of stay at the time of writing is 55.5 days.) There are several reasons why this may have been so:

- It is much more difficult to establish an accurate prognosis for a person suffering with AIDS than for a person with terminal cancer.
- Dementia is now being seen in an increasing number of patients. These highly dependent patients are said to have a prognosis of around 6–8 months.
- Some referrals were inappropriate, while other patients, ill on admission to the unit, improved after being there for several weeks. One can only speculate that nursing played a key therapeutic role. In both cases, however, ward staff were slow to realise the need to start planning for discharge early. Added to this the severe lack of suitable accommodation, such as half-way houses and assisted hotels in London, created enormous difficulties with rehousing.

Because of the prolonged length of stay, the depth of the nurse–relative relationship increased. There was a tendency for nurses and patients to become possessive of their respective patients and nurses. When patients did die the feelings of grief and loss that many nurses experienced was great, thus increasing their feelings of stress. It can be debated that it was inevitable that this should happen within a small unit. However, such stress would not be unique to primary nursing, and may well occur using other methods of care delivery, as patients will often form bonds with those nurses, and vice versa, with whom they relate best.

In general, in discussion with patients it was found that they liked knowing who was going to be looking after them and this helped them feel secure. It particularly helped those patients with dementia to have some consistency in the nurses looking after them. However, this was stressful for the nurse. Conversely some patients did not relate well or did not like the nurses looking after them and found the partnership less than therapeutic. Careful intervention was required in such cases, firstly in counselling the nurses involved and then in discussing changing the primary nurse as necessary.

Clearly in this context there are positive and negative aspects to primary nursing.

Problems must be dealt with sensitively. Support for staff was obviously of primary importance.

STRESS AMONG STAFF

It was anticipated at the outset of the project that the rate of turnover among nurses caring for terminally ill people with AIDS would be high and perhaps at least as high as in any other area of terminal care. It was recognised that, unless the carers themselves were cared for, they would be unable to provide a high standard of care and develop good relationships with patients.

To provide a support system, a freelance counsellor was appointed who was not part of the management structure. All grades of staff can see her in complete confidence. A weekly support group facilitated by the staff counsellor was set up soon after the unit opened. Staff are encouraged to attend, with time off in lieu given to staff attending on their day off.

Other forms of support include the encouragement of peer support among staff, making sure that they all have adequate time away from the unit, and ensuring that staff feel cared for by nurses in management posts.

It was felt that report at handover should involve all the staff, so that everybody knew all the patients and felt that they had some involvement.

Familiarity often breeds contempt. A problem arose when a degree of manipulation by several patients was observed. This was particularly distressing for those nurses involved. These instances were discussed at both the weekly multidisciplinary meetings and the support group and a definite course of action was drawn up. This allowed the nurses the security of the support of the whole team and the patient the security of a consistent approach.

THE ASSOCIATE AND PRIMARY NURSE ROLES

The role of associate nurse is viewed as being suitable for enrolled nurses, part-time and newly qualified registered nurses, bank nurses and post-basic students. (Mildmay does not as yet have student nurses.)

As the unit establishment grew, nurses were appointed only to the associate nurse role and many were as experienced as the primary nurses, if not more so in some respects. Out of the 18 nurses now in post, only six are ENs. The associate nurse's role was to work closely with the primary nurse, their knowledge and experience being used to provide the best possible care for the patient. It was also her role to update care plans and implement care in the primary nurse's absence.

At about the six month stage, a major problem arose with staff morale. Although regular staff meetings were held and problems raised, these appeared only to be scratching the surface.

To understand the problems and defuse the situation, an extraordinary staff meeting was held. This meeting was well attended and, as expected, several other issues in addition to primary nursing were raised. As already mentioned, a new unit creates insecurity as staff are not working on a secure foundation but trying to create one.

The issues raised in relation to primary nursing were:

- Dissatisfaction with the associate nurse's role
- Primary nursing being viewed as a type of hierarchy
- A lack of understanding of the philosophy of primary nursing
- A general feeling by associate nurses of being undervalued

Obviously the one problem underpinning all these was lack of understanding of the philosophy of primary nursing itself. Although considerable time and effort had gone into preparing for the introduction of primary nursing, this had not been continued.

The number of nurses had doubled since the unit opened and a mentor system was, and still is, in operation. All new nurses are allocated to another nurse who has been on the unit for a period of time. It is the role of the mentor to ensure that the new nurse is familiar with ward policies and the unit philosophy, in addition to primary nursing itself. It was clear that understanding had become diluted during this process and instead of primary nursing developing the nurses' autonomy and accountability (to the patient), the associate nurses felt that they were not in a position to make decisions or contribute to care planning and evaluation. The primary nurse was viewed as being similar to a ward sister and responsibility was seen as residing with them, not the associate nurse. This view clearly also contributed to the problems with communications.

It was realised that it was of vital importance that ongoing education should take place. Plans were made to have regular workshops on primary nursing, which all new nurses had to attend as soon as possible after joining the staff.

It was obviously immediately impossible and unnecessary to change the staff skill mix, so it was important to adapt the associate nurse's role to meet the needs of the unit and help each associate nurse develop her own specialty and area of expertise and feelings of worth. To complement this, the primary nurse also needed help to develop her own role and identify the strengths of the associate nurses working with her and then, working with the CNS, to develop these strengths to their fullest potential.

Before the problem of poor staff morale developed, separate meetings had been held between the primary nurses and the CNS. These meetings were to provide additional support for the primary nurses, to help them to develop their role, and to identify problems within the unit as early as possible. These meetings were initially very valuable for the primary nurses. They have since been discontinued as it was felt that they caused division between the primary and associate nurses within the team.

THE WARD SISTER'S ROLE

By giving individual nurses greater autonomy and responsibility, the ward sister's role has been changed. No longer can she be the all-powerful, all-controlling person that she was in the past. Manthey (1980: 43) describes the new role as one of 'clinical leadership and continuous responsibility for the overall management of patient care'. She defined a clinical leader as being a teacher, a validator of decisions made by her staff, a resource person, and the quality control supervisor of the unit. Although many of these elements have always been present in the ward sister's role, if trained staff are given greater responsibility and autonomy, these must not be taken back by constant checking and interference.

This new role can be difficult and create insecurity for the sister. The CNS role was often similar to that of a ward sister under primary nursing, and it was difficult at times to stand back and allow junior nurses to make mistakes in the process of arriving at the right answer. It was also difficult initially to direct other members of the multidisciplinary team to the primary or associate nurse on duty, rather than discussing specific problems oneself. It was very easy for the CNS (or sister) to feel insecure owing to loss of control herself! On the other hand, standing back too much was just as bad – after all, the sister does have some responsibility for maintaining the overall standard of care on a unit. This balance has been difficult to achieve and is still not quite right.

OFF DUTY

Although the aim was to ensure that each shift was covered by at least one person from each group, this proved impossible to do consistently. However, this may also have been an advantage in that it allowed staff to look after patients other than their own. This was at times a welcome break if the case load of a group was particularly heavy, and provided more flexibility within the team.

CONCLUSION

It is now nearly a year since the unit opened and primary nursing was implemented. That year has certainly not been problem free! Although it may be considered an advantage to create change rather than have change imposed externally, this does not make change a painless process. Certainly the amount of change within the unit created an enormous degree of insecurity among the staff. Not only was the environment new, but the system of care delivery was also new, so there was little that was stable for staff to lean on!

A year is much too short a period to evaluate fully whether primary nursing is working, and therefore no firm conclusions can be drawn. However, to date, in general, staff are in favour of primary nursing and although very aware of its disadvantages they are also able to recognise its advantages, those being mainly improved continuity and co-ordination of care and deeper and more satisfying nurse–patient relationships.

Although it is true that in this situation the deepening of the nurse–patient relationship can place increased stress on the nurse working within this environment, it may well be that, because of the type of patient nursed in this unit, this would have happened regardless of the method of care delivery. Stress levels would appear to be just as high on other units caring for people with AIDS but not practising primary nursing. However, these are purely subjective observations and there is no control against which to measure them. The depth of satisfaction experienced by the nurses in being with and beside the patient may help to compensate for the stress experienced, provided there is adequate support.

The importance of ongoing education cannot be underestimated, not only to clarify the issues relating to primary nursing, but to help the nurse develop professionally and innovatively.

Clearly, although no system is by any means perfect, primary nursing has, in the short period of time it has been in operation, generally met with success in this environment. It is important to remember that the philosophy of primary nursing is to help improve standards of care and it should not be seen as a punitive or rigid coercive system of regulation. The basic philosophy, however, may need to be adapted slightly to meet the specific needs of different units. Implementing primary nursing is exciting, but it requires tremendous enthusiasm, energy and determination on the part of those initiating and sustaining it.

10

Close Enough to Touch –

Primary Nursing in a

Psychiatric Unit

Chris Hart

It might be thought that the practice of primary nursing in psychiatry would place all the emphasis on the individual. In some senses this is true but, as in so many other things, it is the strength of the collective, and of a collective approach, that allows the individual room to grow.

I am going to write about primary nursing in the psychiatric setting I know, on Ward Six at the Maudsley Hospital. An attempt will be made to look at some of the psychodynamic aspects of our work. These aspects marry closely with primary nursing and it would be artificial to separate the two. This chapter will be largely about the relationship between primary nurse and patient, engaged in a process of continual 'negotiation' and renegotiation', with the nurse involved in every aspect of the patient's treatment and care. This leads to a degree of closeness and intensity between them rarely experienced in any traditional task – or team-oriented setting.

In examining this relationship, and its difficulties and advantages, I shall be looking at the use of care plans, and the use of 'support' and supervision networks within a multidisciplinary team, as well as the nursing framework and the primary nurse's position in relation to those teams.

THE SETTING

Ward Six is a small and cramped 17-bedded general psychiatric unit. We take both admissions via the hospital's Emergency Clinic and referrals from other hospitals. Primary nursing on the ward was initiated and refined over a period of several years, with ideas being used and/or adapted from elsewhere. As this system of care grew, a structured timetable also developed, giving a necessary anchor to both nurses and patients, who could look at it at almost any time of the day to see what activity was due and where they should be. It was an essential component in an environment where it is easy to become over-involved with the problems of others and to overstretch oneself, losing perspective of what one's original objectives were and not evaluating what progress – or lack of it – has been made. As the methods of organising and delivering nursing care have become more sophisticated, the timetable has altered to reflect this.

Sue Ritter, a former charge nurse, performed the extremely important task of documenting the work she and her colleagues were doing. In so doing she not only stressed the need for precise documentation but also ensured its survival after their departure, allowing those who followed to continue its evolution.

Ward Six has been described by one former consultant, quite accurately, as 'always either in chaos or on the verge of chaos'. This chaos results from having a very disturbed group of people crammed together in an environment ill designed for psychiatric nursing. However, rather than try to suppress individual patient's, or their collective, disturbance, we attempt to use it, working our way through its confused labyrinths. It is in trying to understand what the disturbance is about that we attempt – and we believe we succeed in that attempt – to help the patients.

Within the framework, however, the Ward Six approach has been one of paying attention to basics. We do not allow ourselves to get carried away either with psychodynamic principles at the cost of pragmatic management of a general psychiatric ward or with primary nursing that is aimed at flowery, high-blown objectives that do nothing to improve the basic quality of life of a patient or to address problems that have been identified as interfering with this.

DOES IT WORK? THE ROLE OF THE PRIMARY NURSE

The fundamental question of whether or not primary nursing can work in a psychiatric setting has been raised by many who perceive the work as more amorphous and difficult to plan, implement and evaluate than general nursing. This argument is extended to care plans, often associated with primary nursing. I have heard many psychiatric nurses state that they believe care plans cannot be formulated for psychiatric patients because there is nothing tangible to work with, nothing 'practical' that can be written down. (For more on the use of care plans, see page 145.)

It has also been argued that there is less reason to allocate a primary nurse to someone with mental health problems because, although it is an advantage to have a nurse who gets to know all the health problems and personal needs of a patient on a general ward, this is not the case in psychiatry. Even if it were, the argument runs, it is just too difficult, especially with the treatment regimens of many consultant psychiatrists – and, of course, the appallingly low staffing levels that exist on far too many psychiatric wards.

I would propose that not only does it work, it actually stands as part of a powerful alternative to nursing practice which is sometimes associated with the 'medical model' of psychiatry. Here, treatment regimens of pills and electroconvulsive therapy can offer little or no role for nurses beyond providing custodial care or, as is more often the case, the pattern of meandering out into the dayroom and talking to the first patient who wanders into view, and then the next, while the patient approaches another nurse, perhaps presenting a totally different picture of his needs. Such an approach does not allow themes to be followed up or problems of a more insidious or occult nature to be clearly identified.

In giving the opportunity for a consistent approach, gathering information as the nurse works, moving coherently from one problem to the next, primary nursing puts nurses in a strong, responsible position and fundamentally alters the relationship between themselves and the other disciplines on the ward, 'giving the nurse the necessary authority and confidence to negotiate directly with them' (Ritter, 1984). It can also provide hard information in the perennial battle for improved staffing levels and shows clearly what nurses can do given the resources.

Although the expectations of nurses are different according to their experience and position, the genetic role of the primary nurse remains the same for anyone on the ward. Even student nurses (who are assigned one or two primary patients according to their stage of training) can find themselves being asked their opinion on medication or a patient's safety, providing and presenting the nursing report in ward rounds, liaising with outside agencies such as hostels, or helping patients try to express their worst fears and feelings; or doing far more fundamental work, like trying to get the same person out of bed day after day, to attend occupational therapy or to agree to a care plan. It is not unfair to say that, in this sense, the primary nurse occupies the pivotal role in a patient's care. 'Talk to the primary nurse first' is a familiar piece of advice on Ward Six, given to everyone from doctors to dieticians.

The primary nurse's work can be said to fall into three broad categories:

- The nurse and patient getting to know each other (which will coincide with immediate safety care if the patient is new to the ward).
- Getting involved in the 'nitty gritty' work, such as the difficulties that brought the patient into hospital, problems arising during his stay, and helping him identify aspects of himself and his life that he wants to look at and change.
- The leaving, or separating, stage.

THE NURSE–PATIENT RELATIONSHIP

Once the patient is on the ward, it is not uncommon to find other, apparently different, problems arising that become intrinsically linked with these processes. They often revolve around the relationship with the primary nurse – or, more accurately, become apparent because of that relationship. It is accepted on Ward Six that these difficulties in relationships and with emotions are at least as important as any acute symptomatology that can be quickly treated. They may be secondary to other phenomena or closely bound up with them, but it is felt to be as necessary to address these problems as any other for the patient's long-term rehabilitation and prognosis. It is at this level that the primary nurse comes into her own – and that she often faces the greatest challenge. Issues of dependency *versus* independence, of responsibility and control have to be confronted, not only by the patient but also by the nurse.

One of the features of primary nursing in psychiatry is that, once a problem becomes apparent, it is much harder to ignore than when no particular nurse, or a different one each day, is allocated to a patient's care – the pressure is on the nurse and the rest of the team to confront it or accept that it is beyond their capabilities or constraints to do so. It seems an obvious observation that if a patient does not, for whatever reason, feel able to work consistently with their problems, it is actually advantageous for him to take them to different nurses at different times, imbuing the carers with little hard evidence but a lot of confusing feelings about the nature of the problem and what to do about it. So if a primary nurse is going to address this process and provide the boundaries within which the patient can express himself, the skill of confronting with sensitivity – thus mobilizing the patient's resources rather than demolishing him – is a very necessary one to develop. It is widely used on Ward Six and involves questioning everything (although not necessarily expressing these questions aloud – it is as important to know when to shut up as when to speak out), not accepting a communication simply at face value, not tolerating unacceptable behaviour, not letting the patient pass total responsibility onto the nurse except in exceptional circumstances, and being able to say no when necessary. It means risking the hatred of a patient unused to such limit setting, who, as the closeness engendered by such contact with the nurse develops, becomes fearful of the ambivalent feelings of dependence and attachment aroused, realising that there is someone who might be able to *help*, who reacts in a different way to that which they're used to, offering understanding yet, while raising hopes, inevitably threatening them with the prospect of change. And the nurse is, of course, as capable of mistakes as anyone else – and consequently a disappointment.

NEGOTIATION

Integral to all of this is the process of negotiation between nurse and patient, immediately questioning the assumption that they work from a common starting point. The expectation is there from the outset that, no matter how unwell the patient, he will attempt to negotiate any meetings with his primary or associate nurse, making clear when, where and why he wants to meet. This would, in many cases, be related to the care plan all patients are expected to negotiate with their nurse. This immediately confronts anyone who has experience of nurses as being trained to jump when a patient asks and to be there when the patient demands. It means nurses being able to allow patients to retain uncomfortable feelings long enough for them to cope with themselves and start the process of making sense of why they are uncomfortable, nurses not responding immediately to cries for help and not saying the words that will smooth things over temporarily.

A meeting, in this context, becomes very important. Both patient and nurse know when it will begin and end, and what is to be discussed. By implication, the subject matter and subject – the patient – are important. They are important enough for a nurse to go to all this trouble to talk about and to them.

As the process of negotiation develops, so does the relationship. In its early stages, particularly with a disturbed patient, it seems to be weighted strongly in favour of the nurse, who is often in the position of having to say no to aspirations which appear to exceed a patient's capabilities. It confronts patients with their own responsibilities as well as their ability to plan ahead.

It can be easier for a patient to say that either it is beyond them or that they are well and more than capable of looking after themselves. Many castigate nurses for expecting them to negotiate everything they want to do in the day, arguing that this fosters dependence on the nurse, which, to an extent, it does. Yet negotiation develops far beyond this. As patients acknowledge the expectations and limits set out for them, and work within them, they have the chance to explore that experience safely and move on to talk about the limitations their illness puts upon them and to set about making practical changes. The unevenness in the relationship diminishes and, as patients they become more independent, they have more opportunity to be involved with what happens to them and take a role in deciding their treatment and care.

CARE PLANS AND DOCUMENTATION

This work places each nurse in a position to make unique observations, different from but complementary to – and as important as – those of medical staff. Therefore, the way it is recorded has to reflect this. On Ward Six negotiated objectives have to be written down, with the interventions that will be used to meet them before the nurse carries them out, with a full evaluation of what actually happens then. Also required is a weekly evaluation covering the various aspects of the nurse's contact with the patient from the patient's self-care to mood and behaviour, from social and family to abnormal thoughts/feelings; a self-evaluation would also be given to the patient to complete at the same time, and any other necessary observations, such as weight, are recorded weekly.

If the work the nurse undertakes with a patient is a journey into unknown territory, then their map is the care plan. The practice on Ward Six is to keep one care plan to one problem or need, identified by the patient. (We try to frame problems or needs in behavioural terms rather than looking at 'feelings' in isolation, or simply talking about 'things'.) This is then formally agreed by patient and nurse and an objective is set, to be achieved by a specific date. The patient and nurse each have a copy of the care plan and sign both. If the nurse is a student, the care plan is countersigned by an RMN.

SUPERVISION

Carrying this type of responsibility on one's own would, of course, not only be intolerable, it would also be dangerous, for both the nurse and the patient. This is where the careful balancing act between the individual and the collective is put into practice. With the primary nurse at the 'coal face', involved in one-to-one work with a patient, often so close up that she cannot 'see' clearly or achieve the necessary degree of objectivity, supervision of the nurse is essential.

On Ward Six we strive to provide five important levels of support. Firstly each primary nurse has two associates who work with her, to carry on individual work with the patient in the primary nurse's absence, who should follow the guidelines laid down by the primary nurse.

The role of associate nurse is very important. They should be part of a team, acting as support for the primary nurse and feeding them information about what happens when they are not around, following care plans, acting upon requests from the primary nurse, and ensuring continuity.

There is, however, always the possibility – often a reality – that the patient may consciously or unconsciously create a 'split' among the nursing team, with one nurse being the 'good object' while the others have to contain all the bad feelings of the patient. So it might be, for example, that the patient describes Nurse X as being better than Nurse Y, or more caring, or says that he cannot possibly 'get better' unless Nurse Z is meeting with him. He perhaps won't negotiate with one nurse, but consistently does so with another, saving all the 'valuable' information for her and leaving the 'unwanted' nurses feeling inadequate or resentful.

Nurses – and this is never confined solely to students or inexperienced staff – might find themselves feeling isolated from their colleagues, sharply disagreeing with others' opinions about patients and their symptoms. It may even be that anger felt towards the patient is directed at a primary nurse very closely identified with him. A team might easily be split in the classic 'special patient' scenario (Main, 1957).

In such cases we attempt to understand these problems as a team (what it's like to be 'at the sharp end', how/when/if the issue is going to be addressed, and by whom), aiming to provide not only support but also direction for future work with the patient. This may come from the trained nurses on the ward at the time or may involve staff from other disciplines in the management team (who may, indeed, be protagonists in the problem). This, of course, happens outside the primary nurse system and is very common on psychiatric wards, with one group of staff convinced that a patient is very ill while others think he isn't. The process surrounding the 'special patient' has been well documented (Main, 1957), but it is much easier to address in a ward practising primary nursing (where an individual nurse is purposely close to the patient) and which has an extensive support network for that nurse.

The management, or multidisciplinary, team aims to provide another layer of support in the form of a management round held each week to review the patient's progress – or lack of it – over the previous seven days and to decide what should be the aims of the next week and beyond, providing advice and supervision as necessary. The primary nurse should be attending these meetings regularly to offer a report of her contact with the patient and to be involved in any decisions made, even if this is 'only' to continue the present care.

Regular supervision, provided by the nurse's supervisor – always an RMN – often focuses on issues to do with a specific patient, or may refer to a patient in relation to the topic under discussion. The charge nurse or staff nurse working directly with the patient's consultant (and who attends all ward and management rounds, except in extraordinary circumstances) will give feedback from those meetings where the primary nurse is unable to be present or is afterwards unclear about any aspect of the work.

Finally, there is the 'on the spot' guidance of the planning and evaluation meetings, where a registered nurse will listen to what arrangements the nurse has negotiated with the patient, then listen to her plans for the shift, and offer whatever advice or guidance is felt necessary, such as at what level to pitch an intervention, what is appropriate in a particular context or setting, and whether to be confrontative, supportive, directive or simply to listen. Once the nurse has carried out those plans with the patient and the shift is drawing to a close, the nurse evaluates again under the direction of the registered nurse, how the planned activity has gone. As with the planning meetings, evaluations should constitute a collective activity, with all the nurses on the shift paying attention to each other and contributing.

MANAGING AND STRUCTURE

Ward management in this system is essential. Our experience is that the charge nurses cannot have primary patients. This has many advantages, not the least of which is that they can bring a greater degree of objectivity to the overall management of patients in ward and management rounds, taking on the role of nurse consultants in many senses, and acting as a resource person for other staff. However, direct and close contact is maintained with the patients through the ward's groups and charge nurses maintain an outpatient case load. Each charge nurse works with a particular consultant and by being present in all of his ward and management rounds she can develop a sense of continuity available to few other members of the team. It is also the job of the charge nurses to provide the strategic management of the ward, liaising with other disciplines and areas of the hospital, freeing the staff nurse to manage on a shift-by-shift basis. We have found that close contact between charge nurses and staff nurses leads to a sophistication of management that can only improve the delivery of care; also, regularly attending the meetings that other disciplines such as medical staff do means continual nursing involvement in the decision-making process

There has been work done on the anxieties faced by nurses in traditional ward settings, where elaborate social systems minimise the intimate contact with patients (Menzies, 1960d), but for primary nursing in psychiatry to work many of these must be, by necessity, stripped away. Those new to Ward Six encounter an intense and intimate culture that is often very confusing. The demands on their time and resources from the patients (and, sometimes, other staff) can be enormous.

To help nurses with this, contact is limited by the timetable, but the closeness between nurse and patient means that nurses are often left with powerful emotions after being with their patients. This can be a sense of confusion; of being 'stuck' and not knowing where to go next with a patient; or perhaps feeling very in touch with the patient's own pain and emotions and confusing them for one's own; even more seriously, it might be a far more pervasive sense of responsibility for a patient with suicidal ideas he does not seem to be in touch with, but with which the nurse most certainly is, feeling that the patient's life hinges on what she might do or say.

Nurses may feel weighed down by the responsibilities they are encumbered with and the expectations they feel the senior staff have of them.

It is therefore important that the trained staff aim to provide an environment in which the nurse feels safe to talk about her experience and identify her own feelings, the aim being to try to understand them and use that understanding in work with the patient. This is done by paying attention to self-awareness, which is encouraged at all levels on Ward Six, and nurses in evaluation meetings are asked to talk openly not only about the nuts and bolts of their work during the shift with the patients and each other, but also about their own perception of it. In doing so, we are asking them to share something of themselves with their colleagues, but only to a degree they are comfortable with and only about aspects that relate to their work.

Self-awareness on the part of the primary nurse can also help in understanding a patient in that the nurse is able to gain a sense of her experience with that person over a prolonged period, allowing her to measure the changes in a personal sense. This means knowing not only that she can now organise her day on a consistent basis, but also that she can negotiate and tolerate disagreement with someone very close to her. A very fraught relationship can blossom to one of great warmth and mutual respect and it is not uncommon to find a nurse, who said she couldn't stand working with a patient initially, becoming very fond of him. It of course bodes very well for those with mental health problems when they can enter into and sustain relationships, and this can be a very useful diagnostic tool.

A NUMBER OF PROBLEMS

A number of logistical problems arise from the ward being in a teaching hospital. One of these is that, because of the long-term nature of the care and treatment offered on the ward, students find themselves doing a lot of hard and draining work without seeing much movement from the patient, which may only come after several months and one or more changes of primary nurse.

Another lies in what has been described as one of the system's inherent 'faults'; it is nurse intensive. There must be enough nurses to fill the positions of primary and associate nurse for each patient. The system of allocating nurses to patients has evolved over the years and mirrored the ward's staffing levels; after profound struggles with the hospital's management, recent increases in the staffing levels have meant that each staff nurse now has two primary patients and three associate patients. This is an allocation that senior students can also be given, although it is more common for them to have just one primary patient. This enables the staff nurses to spend more time with their own patients and more time supervising their individual students. Junior Maudsley students and seconded students have one primary patient and up to four associate patients. Any ideas to leave them as associate nurses only have always been resisted, not least by the students themselves. As stated above, the ward's two charge nurses never have primary patients.

Primary nursing on Ward Six has developed to the degree where 'substitute' nurses are not allocated on a shift-by-shift basis to patients without a nurse on duty. When this is the case the patient has to negotiate with the nurse in charge of the shift and assistance is given for practical objectives (such as going to the hospital treasury to withdraw money) whenever possible, or a meeting might be arranged if thought necessary. Otherwise the patient is left to manage himself.

There have been times on Ward Six when patients have been without any associates, or perhaps a primary nurse, simply because of lack of staff. In the absence of someone who can caretake, there is a serious risk of important work being missed. This means those who are on the ward working harder (and this most often falls on the shoulders of the trained staff or nursing assistant) with everyone feeling they should be doing more and having to hold on to their anxiety about what a particular patient may or may not do without a nurse.

The level of demand on the registered nurses is such that they have little time (or energy) for development in the hospital by attending outside lectures or courses, but the recent increased staffing levels and some re-examination of the nurses' needs has led to the beginnings of a more formalised and structured programme of supervision for the staff nurses, by the charge nurses, and a personalised programme of development for each of them. The danger that a ward practising primary nursing – especially when it is isolated in this practice in the larger institution – will become introverted and inward looking has to be guarded against. This means, by necessity, getting off the ward to find out what others are doing, going on courses to enable the information and experience from them to be brought back onto the ward, and going outside to tell others what is going on in the primary nurse setting.

SEPARATING

The leaving, or separation, stage in the nurse–patient relationship is undoubtedly one of the hardest parts of the work. 'Leavings' occur in every nurse–patient setting. Primary nursing does not necessarily assist in resolving the difficulties that arise out of this phase, but certainly focuses them very sharply within the context of its intimate relationships, allowing for a 'working through' by the two individuals involved. On Ward Six leaving is an almost eternal topic in the groups, with someone always going or about to go, either patient or staff. The degree to which the leaving affects the ward is not always dependent on their length of stay or role, and can be as much about *how* they leave. As with so much else on the ward, there is the 'reality' of someone going, which one hopes is shared knowledge; but then there is the 'fantasy', which is more often unique to the individual. Leavings also awaken memories of previous separations, often traumatic experiences for patients, and it is then difficult for them to express the bewildering array of emotions they feel about important people in their lives going away, both 'positive' and 'negative', sometimes because they confuse such basic emotions as sadness or anger with mental illness. In such instances the staff try to help the patient by modelling modes of communication and limited self-disclosure, as well as listening carefully to what patients say to tease out a higher degree of understanding and clarity. For instance, it might be known that a student is going to be moving onto another ward, but this might not stop the patient from feeling that he is leaving because of something he has done or because the nurse cannot bear to work with him any longer. For those not used to the intimacy and intensity of working with individual patients over a long time, it can be difficult to acknowledge how important their departure is going to be. We always advise a 'leaving period' of at least two weeks, to allow the patient to work through the complexity of feelings aroused, and that this should be formalised through a care plan. Perhaps not surprisingly, it is not just the patients who procrastinate in this important area. Yet, if the work is going to be placed in perspective, if the patient is going to be helped to let go of the relationship and allow a new one to develop, an evaluation of what has happened in the nurse–patient relationship and of what it is like for two people to separate has to occur. This means facilitating the patient's expression of anger, disappointment, sadness, gratitude and, whatever else, loss.

CONCLUSION

Despite all of this – or perhaps because of it – primary nursing in a psychiatric setting can often be creative and fun. Being given the responsibility also means that nurses have the opportunity to bring in their own ideas in their work with the patient and to have their say in the making of decisions; what may, at times, seem a burden can also be liberating.

Also, the intensity of the relationship with the patient, while putting the nurse in the firing line of the psychological attacks, sadness and whatever other emotions and psychopathology the patient displays, heightens the rewards. As primary nurses, students often express a feeling of warmth and closeness towards the patient which they have rarely experienced in other forms of nursing and describe a deep sense of satisfaction at having been so closely involved in every aspect of the patient's care. But the relationship is far more important for patients. As they go through the hurdles of the relationship with their nurses, the relationship becomes a learning experience about relationships with other people, not just knowing nurses who give them tablets and serve up meals. For those previously handicapped in this area, it becomes a life-changing process. The skills and knowledge the nurse acquires towards this end and the benefit many patients derive from those skills are as strong an argument as anything else for the further development of primary nursing in psychiatry.

However, it cannot be stressed enough that primary nursing cannot function – or certainly not effectively – without the active support of the consultant medical staff. If the work, and evidence of that work, that a primary nurse brings to the senior medical staff is discounted and treatment plans are decided on the basis of a five-minute interview, it is not only a waste of time, it is the source of immense grief for the nursing staff and of utter confusion for the patient. With the fragile patient group implicit in psychiatric practice, this can be extremely dangerous. Similarly, the nursing management have to be prepared to translate sympathetic words into practical support whenever necessary. Although involving the individual focus of work, primary nursing is a team enterprise and as such is easily undermined, but it is a form of care that lends itself to systematic examination and a presentation of its advantages and disadvantages. Because of its nature and the challenges it throws up, in terms of both patient care and relationships with other disciplines – as well as other nurses who may not be practising it – primary nursing will never be easy, but will demand a high level of commitment and energy from all the nurses involved in its implementation, not just a zealous ward sister or charge nurse, or one or two individuals. Yet, as stated above, it is not only a system that may work in psychiatry; it is one that allows patients a system of individualised care and nurses the opportunity to be accountable for the care they provide and practise in a semi-autonomous manner.

ACKNOWLEDGEMENTS

Some individual nurses who have helped me to develop, and whose ideas have been represented, in part, here are Rita Bourke, Jamie Christison, Janette Goddard, Mrs King, Linda Langford, Katy Lewis, Peter May, Paula Morrison, Tricia Musa, Janet Rimmer, Sue Ritter, Beatrice Stevens, Thecla Wilkinson and Gary Winship. To them, my thanks.

11

Consensus – A Basis for Introducing Primary Nursing into an Acute Respirology Ward

Angela Heslop and Shelagh Sparrow

In this chapter we would like to describe how the organisation of nursing care has developed to its present form of a modified system of primary nursing on an acute medical ward in a London teaching hospital. The chapter is titled 'Consensus – a basis for introducing primary nursing' as we believe that it is through involving nursing staff in decisions about how care should be delivered that the modified primary nursing system we will be describing has emerged, and we wish to describe how we have adapted the theory to the needs of ward 5 West.

STRUCTURE – THE WARD WITHIN THE ORGANISATION

Before describing primary nursing on 5 West it is essential to discuss the ward structure, a key element that affects how and why developments take place. The word 'structure' is used to encompass the environment, the ward design, the people who work there, the patients we care for and the provisions of services. A ward is only a small part of an organisation and in consideration of this it is also necessary to contemplate areas in which change may be encouraged or impeded. It is only possible, within the boundaries of a chapter, to indicate briefly the role structure plays in developments.

Charing Cross Hospital is a 800-bed hospital which has been open since 1972. Being fairly modern it has the advantage of being spacious and having fairly modern equipment. Like all its wards, 5 West is of a race track design (see figure 11.1), which means that patient care areas are situated on three sides of a rectangle with a service area in between. A race track ward has advantages over the traditional Nightingale design, the main one being reduction of noise and an increase in privacy for the patient, but it means that the ward area is much larger and that immobile patients cannot see much activity. The hospital has a unique communication system whereby, if they require assistance, patients can call an operator who then locates the nearest nurse. The way nursing is managed on the ward does not necessitate the sickest patients to be nursed being nearest to the

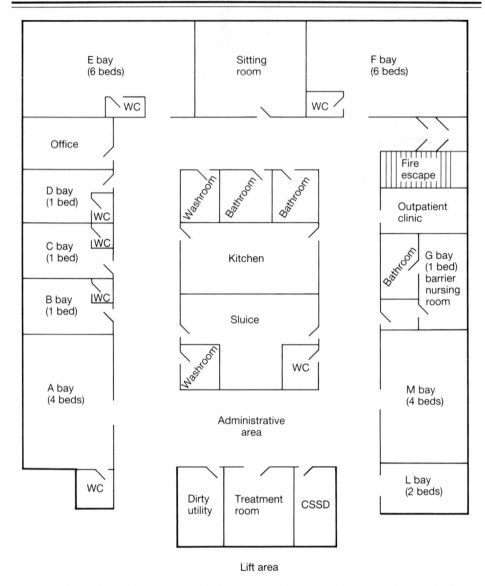

Fig. 11.1 Plan of 5 West. M and L bays constitute the Clinical Investigation Unit.

nursing station, but the provisions of a cardiac monitoring system in wards A and B does mean that on occasion patients may have to be moved from one part of the ward to another – an issue which will be discussed later in the chapter.

Charing Cross is composed of a 15-floor tower block served by 12 lifts, five of which are for the provision of services, removal of waste and transportation of patients. Despite this number of lifts it takes time for personnel and supplies to travel from one part of the building to another. Because of this structure the hospital also lacks the central corridor, common to many of its older counterparts, in which people could meet and cross-fertilization of ideas could take place.

The day-to-day management of a large teaching hospital is an enormous task. The hospital site is comparatively small and all equipment and supplies are provided from elsewhere. There are a large number of personnel employed who have no contact with patients but are only concerned with the day-to-day running of the organisation. This can lead to misunderstanding and conflict of organisation goals.

Charing Cross is situated between the residential areas of Hammersmith and Fulham, where there is a large mixture of young and elderly people with a mixture of financial resources. Many people live in environments which are far from conducive to good health and which can encourage respiratory disease. Ward 5 West has 26 beds and caters for male and female patients. Six beds are funded via a research grant and patients are admitted here short term for clinical investigations. These patients require routine observations, and educational and supportive care, and their care is divided between the other three ward management units, which will be discussed below.

Many of the patients cared for on the ward are suffering from respiratory diseases. Chronic lung disease is a disabling condition which restricts the lifestyle of the individual greatly. Patients often require hospital treatment for recurrent chest infections, and the hospital could provide a much better physical and emotional environment to the patient who has poor housing conditions or who is confined to his home by his need for continuous oxygen therapy.

The ward is part of a professorial unit and so has a predominance of medical staff, many of whom are doing research and spend only short periods of time in the clinical area. The three consultants spend 8 months of the year on the ward and 4 months in the outpatients clinic. Each has a senior registrar and registrar attached to him; two have a senior house officer and a house officer who changes every 3 months. Medical staff who have a belief in the therapeutic potential of nursing and who are open to change are essential if developments in nursing care are to take place. The power of the consultant and the predominance of the medical model can prevent a patient-centred care system for developing. As ward developments have occurred, medical staff have become increasingly supportive of the ideas expressed.

The ward has a large multidisciplinary team including physiotherapist, pharmacist, social worker and dietician, and their understanding of primary nursing is also crucial to ward developments.

The ward nursing team consists of two sisters (the authors) who work in a job-sharing capacity. Job-sharing ward sisters are rare and this was the first example in the country (Lathlean, 1987). Both sisters have other jobs within the hospital. Angela is employed as a respiratory health worker and as such she visits patients with breathing difficulties in the community; she concentrates on health education and ensuring safe discharge (Heslop and Bagnall, 1988). Shelagh is employed as a nurse researcher and is currently setting up a peer review system which will look at quality and standards. Both the sisters' other jobs are complementary to their ward work, and sharing the sister role ensures that they have the support that this job so often lacks. The ward has an establishment for ten registered nurses and two enrolled nurses to cover 24-hour care, with internal rotation to night duty (see figure 11.2 for an example of the off-duty rota).

One enrolled nurse does permanent night duty and is also employed in the

Riverside Health Authority
Ward: 5 West   Duty Rota

Month: January Date: 1989	2	3	4	5	6	7	8	9	10	11
Name	M	T	W	TH	F	S	S	M	T	W
Angela (Sister)	E	L	R	R	R	D	D	E	E	E
Shelagh (Sister)	L	E		R	R	D	D	R	R	R
A–C										
Tina (Primary nurse)	No	No	D	D	L	E	L	E	L	E
Dawn (Primary nurse)	Do	BH	BH	E	E	E	D	Study leave		
Zoe (Associate nurse)	D	L	L	E	D	BH	BH	AL———————→		
StN Cathy 3/86	D	N——————————→						N	No———	
StN Penny 10/88	L	E	L	E	E	D	D	D	D	L
StN Emma 10/88	E	L	E	D	D	L	E	L	E	E
StN Ann 6/86	———									———
StN Claire 10/87	———									———
StN Jerry 10/88	———									———
D–E										
Rob (Primary nurse)	D	D	L	L	E	L	E	L	E	D
Caroline (Associate nurse)	———————————————							Orientation		
Sen Leila (Associate nurse)	L	E	E	L	E	D	D	N———		
Erica 1/86	N	No						D	D	L
Caroline 10/88	E	E	D	D	L	E	L	E	L	E
Andrew 10/87	———									———
Emma 10/88	———									———
Penny 10/88	———									———
Sue (Primary nurse)	AL——————————→				D	D	D	D	L
Geraldine (Associate nurse)	N———————————→						No———→		
Elizabeth (Associate nurse)	E	SD	SD	SD	BH	D	D	L	E	D
Amanda 3/86	E	E	D	D	L	E	E	E	L	E
Jerry 10/88	D	D	L	L	E	L	E	E	D	D
Erica 1/86	———									———
Carole 10/88	———									———
Bank Nurse Carol		7.30–12.30						7.30–12.30		
Sen Lyn	No							N		
	5/3	5/3	4/4	3/3	5/3	4/3	4/2	5/3	4/3	5/3

Fig. 11.2 A typical off-duty rota: E, 7.30 a.m.–3.30 p.m.; L, 1.30–9.30 p.m.; N, 9.00 p.m.–8 a.m.; NO, nights off; AL, annual leave; SD, study day; D, day off; BH, bank holiday; R, research job; StN, student nurse.

Charing Cross Hospital

12	13	14	15	16	17	18	19	20	21	22	23	24	25	26	27	28	29
TH	F	S	S	M	T	W	TH	F	S	S	M	T	W	TH	F	S	S
R	D	D	L	R	R	R	E	SD	D	D	R	E	E	R	R	D	D
R	D	L	E	E	E	E	R	D	D	D	R	R	L	E	R	D	D
L	SD	D	D	N →							No →						
	→	D	D	Study leave →					D	D	E	L	E	E	E	D	D
	→	D	D	D	D	L	E	L	E	L	D	E	SD	SD	D	L	E
			→														
E	L	E	L														
L	E	D	D														
				L	L	E	L	E	D	D	D	D	L	E	E	E	L
				D	D	L	E	E	L	E	L	E	D	D	L	E	L
				E	D	D	L	E	E	E	E	L	E	L	E	D	D
D	E	E	L	E	L	E	L	E	D	D	A	L				D	D
L	E	D	D	L	E	E	D	D	L	E	E	L	E	E	E	D	D
			→	No →							L	E	D	D	L	E	L
E	L	E	E														
E	E	D	D														
				E	L	E	E	D	D	L	L	E	D	D	L	E	E
				D	D	L	E	E	E	L	E	D	D	L	E	L	E
				E	E	D	D	L	E	E	D	D	L	E	E	L	E
E	L	L	E	L	E	D	D	L	E	L	E	L	E	E	E	D	D
			→	L	E	E	D	D	L	E	L	E	E	L	E	D	D
D	L	E	L	E	L	E	L	E	D	D	D	D	L	E	L	E	L
E	E	D	D														
L	E	L	E														
				E	E	D	D	L	E	L	E	L	E	D	D	L	E
				D	D	L	E	E	L	E	E	D	D	L	E	E	L
		7.30–12.30									7.30–12.30						
				No							N						
5/4	6/4	5/3	4/4	7/4	6/4	7/4	6/4	7/4	6/4	6/5	7/4	6/5	6/4	7/4	9/4	6/4	6/4

adjacent sleep laboratory. The other enrolled nurse works as an associate nurse and her knowledge of the hospital and her ability to care are an important feature of the ward. The ward, like so many others in London, is subject to staff shortages and often less than full establishment is in employment. Comprehensive documentation and patient allocation ensure that continuity of care is facilitated if employment of bank or agency nurses is necessary.

Learner nurses are allocated to the ward for a period of 8–12 weeks. There are always four nurses on their very first allocation, two nurses in their second year of training and one or two third-year students. The hospital nursing management has a hierarchical structure with a clinical nurse manager, a clinical service manager and a director of nursing and inpatient services, and they have allowed the development of nursing care to take place and are supportive of future developments.

MOULDING THEORY TO DEVELOP CARE

Primary nursing and ways in which it can be implemented have been discussed earlier in this book. The development of primary nursing on 5 West has taken place vicariously and the concepts have been taken and adapted to the needs of the patient population, the environment and the nursing staff. We would suggest that it would not have been practical to have interpreted the theory in an idealised way and that each ward and each unit will develop primary nursing in a unique way.

It is suggested that a primary nurse has the autonomy to plan care for her patients and the authority to initiate that plan of care, and is accountable for her actions and the plan of care for a named group of patients. It is doubtful that nurses are prepared to accept that level of accountability. The concepts of authority and autonomy are also poorly understood and in a teaching hospital which has a dominant medical model and a rigid hierarchy they are not part of the dominant culture.

The system in operation on 5 West is referred to as modified primary nursing, and these modifications will be discussed below.

Angela Heslop became a ward sister having taken part in a research project which investigated psychotherapeutic interactions with breathless patients (Rosser *et al.*, 1983). Through the structural design of the project, Angela was valued and supported as a nurse and she felt that this enabled her to care for patients more effectively. Support and structure that aid the development of the individual have been key elements in the ward's development. The word 'structure' is used here in a slightly different way to encompass the framework of care. Over the years this framework has widened from concentrating on individual care through changing from a medical model to a nursing model framework to primary nursing. These developments have all occurred through a consensus reached by the qualified nursing staff who, through being valued and supported as individuals, have been committed to improving the delivery of patient care.

The word 'consensus' is used to indicate a majority agreement in the decision-making process. Consensus is difficult to reach in an environment where staff are changing or are away for long periods on nights off or on holiday. People who do not agree to the change are encouraged to express their doubts and are listened to by the other staff, and adaptations are made if necessary.

Shelagh Sparrow has not been a ward sister as long as Angela and she was previously a primary nurse in a Burford Community Hospital for 2½ years. Whilst at Burford visitors suggested to Shelagh that primary nursing could not be developed in an acute hospital where patient turnover was high and medicine and management imposed more restrictions. Part of Shelagh's role is to utilise the experience she gained at Burford to help develop the role of the registered nurses on 5 West.

DECENTRALISED MANAGEMENT

So how does this system of modified primary nursing work? What does it mean? In the remaining part of the chapter we will attempt to answer these questions and discuss their implications for the nurse–patient relationship and for learning.

Ward 5 West is divided into three management units plus the clinical investigation unit, and all the ward's activities are decentralised to these areas. Each area has three of four qualified nurses allocated to it, two of whom take on primary responsibility for a group of patients (usually six or seven). The other nurses and the learners act as associate nurses. Discussion between primary and associate nurses is encouraged.

Associate nurse roles are taken on by qualified nurses who do not wish to be primary nurses, or by nurses who are newly qualified. Any structure needs to be flexible to respond to emergency situations and staffing shortages. An associate nurse may need to take on the responsibility of a primary nurse, but she will be supported by colleagues and established guidelines. Since many nurses have developed within a hierarchical form of organisation it is difficult for nurses not to think of primary nurses being in a hierarchical position to associate nurses, but gradually the hierarchy in the ward is being flattened.

Student nurses are allocated to each area for two weeks at a time to aid learning, and every three months the staff working in each unit changes to enable student nurses to have the opportunity to work closely with other people and to work in other units, each of which cares for patients with different types of problems.

The role of the ward sister will be discussed later, but is educative, supportive and facilitative rather than managerial.

Apart from medicine administration, meal times and rest periods, patient care is delivered according to the needs of the individual patient. When medications are administered, at least one nurse working in that unit dispenses the drugs so that there is somebody present who has an in-depth knowledge of the patient. At the beginning of each shift the nurses working in each area examine the patient's care plan and assess what nursing interventions are necessary to aid goal achievement. Ideally, these discussions should take place at the bedside but tripartite discussions are difficult and nurses are often not sufficiently prepared with the requisite communication skills. Instead these discussions are used as learning opportunities in which students are encouraged to relate to the patient's physical, psychological and social needs.

Late shift staff receive details of all patients when they come on duty, but these details are centred around the main problem for that patient that day, and subjective comments that have no value are discouraged. This handover is performed to relieve students of the anxiety that they need to know about every patient, and they are encouraged to value quality information about a small group of patients rather than relatively basic knowledge about every one.

With the decentralisation of day-to-day management that occurs with primary nursing, the role of the ward sister or nurse 'in charge' alters dramatically. There is always a person acting solely to co-ordinate events such as fire or cardiac arrest, although the nurse is encouraged to have global knowledge of every patient. Other ward management activities are also decentralised and each registered nurse is encouraged to have responsibility for a specific area from ensuring that there is enough coffee to drink to ordering the supplies.

Medical and paramedical staff are educated about the care delivery system when they come to the ward and each are encouraged to go to the registered nurse in each area to discuss patient care. Nurses have had to find the relevant doctor for years, but doctors are used to communicating only with the sister or senior nurse on duty. Occasionally doctors express dissatisfaction at having to seek out the appropriate nurse, but in time they appreciate that, having found her, they are given quality information and medical prescriptions are heeded. Nurses do not attend consultants' rounds but are available to discuss patients and exchange information.

After each round the registrar discusses medical objectives with the registered nurse in each area, and these are clearly stated in the nursing document. Registrars appear to find this opportunity useful for clarification of what they are doing.

GROWTH OF THE NURSE–PATIENT RELATIONSHIP

● The uniqueness in nursing lies in 'being with' the patient. (Travelbee, (1971: 119)

● The single most important commitment at the present time is to ensure that qualified nurses nurse patients. It is illogical to do otherwise. It is whole point of professional training and ensuring professional competence and yet the majority of patients are nursed in the health service by the totally untrained or those in training. (Pembrey, 1984: 541–542)

The effect primary nursing has on the nurse–patient relationship is explored in detail in chapter 12. Primary nursing allows the registered nurse to 'be with' the patient for greater periods of time and the less experienced nurses may learn from more experienced colleagues. Through spending time with the patient, observing and communicating with him, the nurse has the opportunity to develop detailed knowledge about the patient and his family. Patients refer to the nurses caring for them by name and willingly discuss the suggestions that 'Sue' or 'Dawn' have made. As mentioned in the discussion about the ward structure, patients are sometimes moved to another part of the ward. This situation is avoided if possible but is sometimes necessary. Because of the layout of the ward it is physically difficult for a patient to keep the same primary nurse. This is an example of another way in which primary nursing is modified on 5 West. Good communication and clear documentation help to ensure that the patient's care is affected as little as possible by the move.

The removal of barriers operating within task-orientated modes of nursing, and the potentially increased likelihood of stressful situations occurring with primary nursing are considered in chapter 13. Accountability is a concept which is poorly understood (Lewis and Batey, 1982). It has been found that many nurses are unable to define the term or state to whom they are accountable, and so are unable or unwilling to accept the accountability inherent in primary nursing. Stress can arise through concern that the plan of care is inappropriate, that the nurse has acted as the patient's advocate with insufficient knowledge, or that the care plan will not be followed in the primary nurse's absence. To help avoid this stress (at the present time) is another reason why primary nursing has been modified on 5 West. By keeping the concept of a team in each management unit, primary nurses are encouraged to support each other in their work, being perceptive to other nurses' needs and offering assistance if appropriate. Stress, however, can also occur if conflict arises within the team.

Nurses are encouraged to discuss problems they have, whether these arise in working relationships or in disagreeing with a plan of care, rather than let the situation get out of hand. It often appears easier to avoid a situation rather than to confront it. It is part of the sister's role to be aware of potential conflict and act to disperse it. If a patient or his treatment is a cause for concern, the nurses are encouraged to discuss it, often with the multidisciplinary team. An example of this is a gentleman in severe heart failure whose family had been told he was dying. He was aware that his family was upset and was attempting to guess why, but the family was adamant that he should not be told. The nurses met with the registrar to discuss the situation and as a result permission was gained from the wife to inform her husband. The patient's anxiety was dispelled and in fact his condition stabilised so that he was able to be discharged home.

As a further measure to encourage nurses and doctors to be aware of situations that may create a sense of unity, a monthly evening meeting is held convened by a psychotherapist. At this meeting a patient who is causing some concern may be discussed or the topic may be less specific – for example, ward communication difficulties or how staff have been affected by a patient's death.

One question the nurses on 5 West are asked repeatedly about primary nursing is what happens if you do not get on with the patient. The possibility of the patient not getting on with the nurse is rarely considered. The identification of the 'unpopular patient' is a cause for concern. All too often this patient has been cared for by a different nurse every day and each nurse has been reluctant to do so because of the labelling of the patient and anticipated difficulties. In such circumstances the patient is discharged and the reason for his behaviour is not sought.

We do not expect every nurse and every patient to get on together, but encourage situations to be faced rather than ignored. One approach we have used is that of a patient contract in which a patient is offered specific acknowledgement for demonstrating behaviour which has been negotiated between the patient and the nurse. Contracts are used frequently in psychiatry but less so in general nursing and skill is needed to use them effectively and not punitively. Contracts have been used on 5 West and the labelling of patients avoided. For example, a patient who disliked bathing became annoyed when a nurse asked if he wanted a bath each day and commented on his hygiene level. After discussion with the patient it was decided he would bath every Friday and would not be asked in the interim. This information was put in the care plan.

5 West, like many wards, is a hectic environment in which it is difficult to find privacy, to be by oneself or to talk with other nurses or patients and relatives without being interrupted. In recognition of this the ward obtained use of a room in an adjacent corridor. This room was decorated and furnished in non-clinical style with the help of the League of Friends and is known as the Quiet Room. It has a variety of uses from a place where nurses talk to each other or with patients or sit alone, where relatives can be alone with patients, or where the recently bereaved can sit undisturbed. Despite its name it is also a place where emotions can be expressed in privacy. It has been described as a refuge in a storm, and plays a vital part in the functioning of the ward.

LEARNING: A SHARED RESPONSIBILITY

The need for education beyond registration is slowly becoming accepted and we would suggest that newly registered nurses do not have the skills or the knowledge to adopt the primary nurse role. The need to learn is a value central to the ward. Each nurse, from first ward student nurse to sister, is encouraged to take responsibility for her learning and to be aware of learning opportunities.

Learning is seen as a two-way process in which both the teacher and the student can gain from the situation, and registered nurses are encouraged to be perceptive to the views and reactions of student nurses as well as to those of colleagues.

Registered nurses are encouraged to reflect on the care they give and prescribe, and to take action where they find their skills, knowledge or attitudes need developing. The office has a number of books, a filing cabinet of articles, and noticeboards circulating information, current affairs, recent research and often a specific topic of interest related to the care of a patient on the ward. The registered nurses are encouraged to utilise the knowledge and experience of the ward sisters, who may be able to help to locate the information required and help in its interpretation to use. Utilisation of specialist nurses is also encouraged, as well as use of medical and paramedical staff. Registered nurses are actively encouraged to go on courses, study days and conferences. The ward itself held a conference about the development of primary nursing, and proceeds from this were used for purchase of books or for nurses to attend conferences. The hospital also has an active continuing education department and nurses are encouraged to attend where possible.

One nurse is responsible for ensuring that information about continuing educa-tion is up to date, and anyone who attends a course is encouraged to report back to a staff meeting and to make information available for other staff members.

Newly qualified nurses are encouraged to observe the skills and knowledge of their more experienced colleagues. They are given the opportunity to learn about the nursing management of a group of patients and then a management unit before being left as the senior nurse on duty. Consideration for colleagues is given high priority so that issues are dealt with as they occur; for example, a new box of syringes should be opened if you remove the last one, or you should arrange for a new light bulb to be replaced if you find one is broken. Joint responsibility for the environment is also stressed and the importance of having a pleasant environment in the office so that you can have a break or read in comparative comfort.

Learners are encouraged to take responsibility for their education while on the ward and to recognise learning situations other than the formal education programme which is repeated every 10 weeks. The planning round is central to the students' learning opportunities and they are encouraged to relate the care they will give to the patients' condition and treatment.

The students spend two weeks working in each area. The reason for this is to allow them to work closely with a group of patients and nurses but to gain experience on the different types of care that the ward offers. While working with learners the registered nurses are encouraged to give them regular feedback and to document this, stating clearly the learner's progress, what she manages well and areas for improvement. The registered nurse who works with the student next is then able to continue this feedback. The registered nurses used the ward objectives as a basis for discussion with a learner (Sigsworth and Heslop, 1988).

Learners at different stages of training respond differently to the learning opportunities offered. First ward student nurses respond well to the flattened hierarchy and willingly ask registered nurses for help, or challenge them on issues. Second-year and third-year nurses have more difficulty adapting to the ward. They are used to being used as pairs of hands rather than students and feel that their position in the student hierarchy is threatened. They are preoccupied with tasks and very concerned with the attainment of shifts as opposed to knowledge and attitudes. Careful explanation of the ward and the way in which it operates, and encouragement to express dissatisfaction, help them to settle in.

Learner meetings are held at regular intervals, which encourages the learner group to inform the registered nurses of the positive and negative aspects of their experience on the ward.

CONCLUSION

Writing this chapter has been a useful exercise, both in analysing what has been achieved and in planning future developments. We often compare introducing change in the ward environment with mountaineering. When climbing a mountain, so often what you perceive as the summit turns out to be just a lower peak and there is still a long climb ahead. However, at the peak it is possible to stand back and survey the land from a clearer perspective than that gained on the ground, and this creates a sense of achievement which spurs you on to the next step. Likewise, with each achievement on the ward, another horizon appears but, before continuing towards it, it is important to span what has been done and to celebrate success.

Mountaineering needs group collaboration. A climb cannot be commenced until much thinking, talking and planning has been carried out and tasks, responsibilities and anxieties shared; the same is true of any development in nursing. Group collaboration may lengthen proceedings but the benefits outweigh this. Mountaineers often encounter treacherous conditions and unforeseen problems. Likewise nurses have to manage themselves, nurse sick and distressed patients 24 hours a day 365 days a year, and communicate with a large multidisciplinary team and other hospital personnel as well as with anxious relatives, and all these factors can impede change.

The ward we have described is not an ideal example of primary nursing and we doubt if we will ever reach the ideal or if we wish to. It is, however, a dynamic environment which is slowly developing a primary nurse framework. The people working in the ward are the key to the success of developments but they are a transient population in the main, and change of personnel also reduces the speed of change. However, as people leave, they go on to develop what they perceive as the good aspects of the ward, and new people bring new ideas and fresh enthusiasm. Each student nurse, doctor, paramedic, patient and visitor may have an important contribution to make about the ward. Negative as well as positive reactions are valuable as they encourage us to analyse and defend our actions.

As we write we are discussing ways of developing the primary and associate nurse roles and investigating issues such as accountability and quality assurance further. Plans are in progress to abolish the drug round and introduce individualised patient drug administration in which patient education will be given a high profile from the day of admission. However, we are also experiencing for the first time a shortage of registered nurses as the popularity of working in London continues to wane. This period is impeding developments but is turning out to be fruitful, enabling consolidation of the existing nursing teams and organisation of the ward.

We hope that this chapter has provided you with food for thought. We did not set out to provide any answers, but hopefully will help you answer some of the questions you have about introducing primary nursing into the acute medical ward situation.

PART 3

The Implications of Primary

Nursing

12

Primary Nursing – Implications for the Patient

Steven Ersser and Elizabeth Tutton

It is a great challenge to nurses to create a method of organising nursing work which provides the optimum benefit to patients and nurses. As each new development in nursing emerges we are challenged not only to consider whether it will be to the patient's satisfaction but also to reflect on the fundamental question of its practicality and the implications it has for the patient's welfare.

Discussions of accountability in nursing tend to refer to the need for nurses to account for particular actions. Little discussion is evident on the importance of nurses accounting for the way nursing is organised. However, nurses will face problems if they rely on a review of the literature to provide them with the answers. Despite voluminous writing on primary nursing it is perhaps surprising that there has been little study of the implications of primary nursing for the patient. Furthermore, the existing research literature is often narrow in scope, lacks adequate working definitions of the specific components of practice involved and is inadequate in the rigour of both the research design and the methods used (see chapter 17).

Here an attempt is made to provide a critical analysis of selected research literature concerned with the relationship between primary nursing and the quality of care the patient receives. This is followed by an attempt to explore the relationship between the aspects of a nursing situation claimed to be of therapeutic potential and the organisational features of primary nursing, an area of which we know little. This chapter therefore focuses on the most significant indicator of the quality of nursing, the effect nursing may have on patient outcome and how this relates to a method of organising nursing.

THE EFFECT OF PRIMARY NURSING ON THE QUALITY OF PATIENT CARE: A SELECTED RESEARCH REVIEW

Quality is defined as 'degree of excellence' by the *Pocket Oxford Dictionary* (Fowler and Fowler, 1969). Various methods have been used to measure the quality of nursing care. These measures include asking the patients if they are satisfied with their care and measuring what the nurse does or says she does. Many studies have tried to ascertain the effect primary nursing has on the quality of nursing care. All of these are hampered by the lack of definition of the method nurses used to organise their care (whether primary nursing or not) and the problems of assessing the effect of this method on the quality of nursing. However, to begin to explore the relationship between primary nursing and the quality of nursing care, 13 research studies are reviewed here. They are chosen on the basis that they compare primary nursing with team nursing in hospital environments. A brief critique of the studies will be provided together with a description of the quality assessment tool used to aid critique. This is followed by a review to establish the extent to which the studies support or negate the following two hypotheses:

- Primary nursing increases patient satisfaction with care.
- Primary nursing improves the quality of nursing care.

Critique of Studies

Most of the research evidence we have so far concerning primary nursing in hospitals and its effect on the quality of nursing care is American in origin. Only two of the studies are British (Reed, 1986; Pearson et al., 1988).

The choice of study design is mainly experimental, utilising post-testing with a control group, or pretesting and post-testing using the subjects themselves as their own controls. All the studies choose to compare primary nursing with team nursing as methods of organising nursing care.

Most of the studies are flawed in that they did not standardise the nursing competencies in their control and experimental groups. For instance, Felton (1975) included nurses with one master's degree, five baccalaureate degrees and five diplomas in the primary nursing group, but only one baccalaureate degree nurse in the team nursing group. In consequence the nursing competencies were higher for the primary nursing unit, as were the measurements of the quality of nursing care. Shukla (1981) tackles this issue by attempting to equalise nurses' competencies before measuring the quality of nursing care. The results of the study indicate that the competence of nursing staff might have more effect on the type of nursing care received than the organisation of nursing. A later study by Shukla (1983) attempted to equalise nursing competencies, in addition to staff levels and workloads, and found no significant differences in the quality of nursing care. The studies will now be considered within the context of the two hypotheses.

Primary Nursing Increases Patient Satisfaction with Care

Research in this area generally utilised patient satisfaction questionnaires. Many of these were author designed and showed little evidence of reliability or validity testing. An exception to this is the Risser patient satisfaction scale used in two of the studies (Mayer, 1982; Ventura et al., 1982). Daeffler (1975) utilised an omissions-in-care tool and Pearson et al. (1988a) a patient service checklist.

Author Designed Questionnaire

Sellick (1983) devised his own patient satisfaction tool and administered it to patients on the day of discharge. Patients nursed by primary nurses as opposed to team nurses perceived the nurses to have greater understanding of their patients, to show more concern and to communicate more with their families, to be more likely to give information, to contribute positively to the experience of hospitalisation and to give greater consideration to discharge planning. In a survey of patients after discharge Ciske (1974) found that they believed that primary nurses took more initiative than team nurses in providing opportunities for patients to talk about complaints and problems. Carey (1979) interviewed a random sample of patients on the day of discharge and showed that primary-nursed patients were more able than team-nursed patients to name their medications. Though not statistically significant, primary-nursed patients were more satisfied with the information they received about the nature of their illness and about their tests and treatments. They also had more confidence in their physicians and nursing staff and in their own ability to help themselves. However, more team-nursed patients knew the names of their medical problems and were clear about their food and activity regimens. A higher percentage said they obtained complete relief from their medical problems. Carey also performed a telephone follow-up of the same patients 4 months later. All the primary-nursed patients, compared with 90% of team-nursed patients, said their treatment plans were clear. More primary-nursed patients said they followed their medication plans, although no figures were given in the text. Of primary-nursed patients, 42% said they received complete relief from presenting symptoms, compared with 23% under team nursing. This opposes the results in the discharge interview and therefore questions the validity of the study. Descriptive results from Laforme (1982), giving no quantifiable or comparison material, found that primary-nursed patients perceived their care as more personalised (although the author infers that patients' responses reflected an increase in patient communication with primary nurses) and all said primary nurses treated them as individuals.

Other researchers have not found any differences between methods of organising care and patient satisfaction and have found opposing results. Roberts (1980) demonstrated that patients felt that they had more continuity of care and that their care was more individualised with primary nursing than with team nursing. However, overall scoring showed the patients to be equally satisfied with primary and team nursing. Giovanetti (1980) found patient satisfaction to be slightly higher with team nursing, although satisfaction responses were high in both units.

Risser Patient Satisfaction Scale

The Risser questionnaire contains 25 items subdivided into three areas covering the technical–professional area, interpersonal education relationships and interpersonal trusting relationships. Response to the questionnaire is made on a five-point likert scale from agreement to disagreement (Risser, 1975). A well designed study by Ventura et al. (1982) used the questionnaire and found no significant difference in patient satisfaction between primary and team nursing. Mayer (1982) utilised the same scale to measure satisfaction in patients who could and could not identify their nurse by name. Mayer found that patients who knew the name of their nurse demonstrated significantly more satisfaction by their response to six statements. Patients who did not know the name of their nurse demonstrated more satisfaction by their response to only one statement.

The study was limited by the fact that the author was unable to assess in depth the variations in the different methods of organising nursing care. Valid comparisons between the elements of primary nursing and patient satisfaction cannot therefore be made.

Omissions Checklist

Patients' perceptions of care have also been measured using an omissions checklist, which is intended to measure feelings of inadequacies in the nursing service. Daeffler (1975) used this tool in a comparison study with team nursing and discovered that primary nursing had significantly fewer omissions in one of the seven categories – dietary needs. Team nursing had significantly more omissions in three categories – rest and relaxation, dietary needs, and contact with the nurse.

Patient Service Checklist

Pearson *et al.* (1988a) utilised a patient service checklist devised by Hall *et al.* (1975) and used extensively in studies evaluating the Loeb Centre in New York. The checklist consists of a list of 46 statements to which the patient can answer true, not true, or not applicable, for instance:

- The radio or TV was noisy.
- The nurse was usually in a hurry.

The results of the study demonstrated that the patients nursed by primary nurses had significantly higher scores than those in the control group. In response to an open-ended question from questionnaire data 73.6% of the primary-nursed patients had no complaints compared with 41.6% in the control group.

Conclusion

In conclusion there is some evidence to support a hypothesis that patients nursed using primary nursing systems are more satisfied than those using team nursing. However, the evidence can only be considered as good as the tool used to obtain it, and most of the tools had not been assessed for reliability or validity. It is interesting that a better designed study using a tool that had shown some validity and reliability (Ventura *et al.*, 1982) showed no difference in patient satisfaction. Ventura argues that patients are unwilling to express negative feelings while they may still need the care of the staff. Marram van Servellen (1980) indicates that we do not know what satisfies patients; it could be clean sheets, medications on time and hot meals, which they could get with any system of care. She also raises the questions of self-fulfilling prophecy; would satisfaction be higher if primary nurses educated their patients to expect individualised care?

Studies relating to the second hypothesis will now be considered.

Primary Nursing Improves the Quality of Nursing Care Patients Receive

The measurement of the quality of nursing care is extremely complex. Most authors try to use a variety of methods to cover as many aspects as possible. The methods used in these studies are as follows:

1. Direct observation of nursing actions or competencies:
   - Quality of patient care scale (Qualpacs)
   - Rush/Medicus quality measuring methodology
   - Slater nursing performance rating scale
2. Direct observation of nursing time spent with the patient
3. Nurses' and physicians' perceptions of quality
4. Auditing of nursing records
   Phaneuf's nursing audit
5. Performance indicators

To provide a deeper understanding of the methods, a brief synopsis of the four main tools will be presented.

Quality of Patient Care Scale (Qualpacs)

The Qualpacs scale was developed from the Slater nursing performance rating scale at Wayne State University by Wandelt and Ager (1974). It aims to measure the process of nursing by direct non-participant observation and with reference to nursing care plans. The scale is composed of 68 activities organised under six headings. Each of the items is written as a statement and the observer judges the extent to which she agrees with the statement on a scale of 1 to 5. Normally two observers will observe one or a group of patients for 2 hours and will compare their results to reduce observer bias. It is assumed that the quality of care received by the randomly chosen patients will reflect the general level of care provided by the ward (Wiles, 1988). Fox and Ventura (1984) demonstrate that Qualpacs is reliable and shows some evidence of validity.

Rush/Medicus Quality Measuring Methodology

This tool was developed by nurses from the University of Rush–Presbyterian–St. Luke's Medical Centre and statisticians from Medicus Systems Corporation. It is based on the nursing process and has 250 criteria, in two parts, which are then grouped into six classes of objectives and further subdivided into subobjectives. Not all the criteria are applicable to all patients. Four dependency groups are identified: self, partial, complete and intensive care. These groups are used to determine which criteria are appropriate. The tool may be used in many specialties and claims to be valid and reliable (Jacquerye, 1984).

Slater Nursing Performance Rating Scale

The Slater scale (Wandelt and Stewart, 1975) covers the same six areas as Qualpacs but has 84 activities. The focus of attention in this scale is on the nurse and she is rated from best through average to poorest nurse. The tool takes approximately 2.5 hours to complete and may also be used retrospectively. The authors argue that the tool has displayed evidence of validity and reliability.

Phaneuf's Nursing Audit

Phaneuf's nursing audit is a retrospective method of assessing the quality of nursing care as reflected in the patient's records. It is entirely based on the assumption that the care given is identical to the care that is written down. Phaneuf (1976) based the tool on seven functions of nursing that tend to reflect a medical model of nursing.

The tool has 50 items identified from the seven functions, and each has to be answered with a yes, no or uncertain response. The final score reflects the quality of the care planned on a five-point scale: unsafe, poor, incomplete, good and excellent. Studies to ascertain the reliability and validity of this tool are inconclusive and further studies are needed (Manfredi, 1986). The results of the research may be considered by returning to the five main methods identified.

Direct Observation of Nursing Actions or Competencies

Several studies indicated higher Qualpacs scores in primary nursing than in team nursing. Felton (1975) demonstrated a significant increase in Qualpacs scores in primary nursing situations. The results of Eichhorn and Fevert (1979) indicated increases in mean scores following the implementation of primary nursing, with significant increases in the medical and burns patient groups. In a case study by Reed (1986) a higher score of 4.35 out of 5 was obtained by primary nursing compared with 3.98 in team nursing. None of these studies considered the nurses' level of competency. Shukla (1981), realising the correlation between high Slater competency scores and the quality of care, equalised the nursing competencies on two units. The results demonstrated that primary nurses still scored higher in five out of six Qualpacs subscales, but only one was significantly higher. In a follow-up study in 1983 comparing three methods of organising nursing and equalising nursing competencies, staff level and workload, Shukla found no significant differences.

The Rush/Medicus quality measuring methodology was used by Martin and Stewart (1983). They found that primary nurses scored significantly higher in formulating care plans, attending to non-physical needs of patients and evaluating patients' responses to care. Culpepper *et al.* (1986) performed a large retrospective study using an adapted form of the Rush/Medicus quality measuring methodology. They found significant improvements, all relating to the four primary nursing design elements: increased patient teaching, patient orientation or admission, respect for privacy and civil rights, and extension of social courtesy.

Direct Observation of Nursing Time Spent with the Patient

Two studies considered the amount of time nurses spent with patients. Shukla (1983) found no differences between primary and team nursing. In contrast

Giovanetti (1980) found a significant difference in that team nurses were spending more time during the day shift on direct care than primary nurses were.

Nurses' and Physicians' Perceptions of Quality

Shukla's (1983) was the only study to ask nurses and physicians their perceptions of care, and it found no significant differences, although in one subscale physicians perceived team nurses as doing better planning and discharge preparation than primary nurses.

Auditing of Nursing Records

Several studies utilised Phaneuf's nursing audit. Felton (1975) found significantly higher audit scores in primary-nursed as opposed to team-nursed patients and primary nursing had correspondingly higher Slater nursing competency scores. Reed (1986) found primary-nursed patients to be in the excellent category and team-nursed patients in the incomplete category. A large study by Pearson *et al.* (1988a) showed the audit scores of primary-nursed patients to be significantly higher in each of the subscales and in the total overall score. Primary nurses also had a higher concurrent audit score in Giovanetti's (1980) study, where she used an unpublished concurrent nursing care review scale. None of these last three studies considered nurse competencies.

Performance Indicators

Objective data concerning the rate of infection demonstrated no difference between primary- and team-nursed patients. However, a clinical quality-of-care index performed by observing nurses setting up an intravenous infusion and rating their performance showed team nurses to be significantly better than primary nurses.

CONCLUSIONS

These studies raise some interesting issues. Is the competence of a nurse a more significant factor in determining the quality of care provided than the method of organising care? Furthermore, do nurses of greater ability migrate to units practising primary nursing? Primary nursing does not guarantee competent nursing practice (Ciske, 1980; Manthey, 1980). It may be that emphasis on developing the competence of individual nurses is of greater necessity than major changes in the organisation of nursing. In general, the studies are limited in their chosen method in both choice of design and use of tools. Kitson (1986) suggests that tools such as Qualpacs or Phaneuf's nursing audit are inherently subjective as they are designed from a professional consensus of the meaning of quality care. This limits their validity as measures of care. Kitson used a different approach and devised tools to assess the quality of care in terms of the degree to which nursing may be therapeutic, based on a conceptual nursing framework. The validity of this study, however, depends on the extent to which the conceptual framework is accepted. Therapeutic nursing care was perceived to be that which promoted independence, allowed patient participation, and treated the person as a unique individual. The results of the study indicated that high-quality nursing care was provided on wards where the sister had a high therapeutic nursing function score. It would seem, therefore, that the nurse's perception of her role and how she functions are important factors in the provision of a quality service. The therapeutic potential of primary nursing for the patient will now be explored further.

THE EFFECT OF PRIMARY NURSING ON PATIENT WELL-BEING

● There is a need to examine nursing and find out: What can nursing do as a therapeutic, educative process? (Peplau, 1952: 9)

So far in this chapter an examination has been made of a number of studies exploring the relationship between primary nursing and the quality of care through the use of existing quality assurance tools. One component of the measurement of the standard of care is to identify the effectiveness of nursing (Crow, 1981). Among the indicators of quality used in research on primary nursing there is little mention of outcome indicators that specifically reflect a change in the patient's health and how this may relate to the practice of primary nursing. This section specifically explores the issue of the potential effect that primary nursing may have on the well-being of patients.

Only a small number of studies have been located which claim to identify a relationship between primary nursing and patient welfare, and many of these have design weaknesses. For example, Jones (1975b) attempted to explore the effect primary nursing had on the welfare of renal transplant patients in an experimental study. From the literature it was argued that such patients were said to have a high incidence of psychological problems postoperatively which may be alleviated by nurses working directly with them and being present when patients needed to vent feelings. Despite statistically significant support for hypotheses showing an association between patients nursed under primary nursing (experimental group) and shorter mean length of stay and postoperative complications, there are various threats to the rigour of the study. The total sample size was very small. Reliability and validity tests were not conducted on the questionnaire and the behaviour measurement rating scale used. Furthermore, the limited details given about the data collection tools makes its difficult to evaluate their validity. Despite little attempt to define primary nursing operationally (as the experimental variable) and to measure its introduction, an adequate description was given of the organisational method to distinguish it from other methods.

The lack of studies examining the association between primary nursing and patient outcome may be attributed to the research difficulties involved, some of which are briefly referred to here and are explored further in chapter 17. Some of the complexity of the cause–effect relationships involved may be illustrated using an analytical framework loosely based on those used by Donabedian (1969) and Inman (1975). Such methods may be viewed as a type of structural factor (a feature of the context in which nursing is provided) which may influence the pattern of specific nursing activities (process) which, in turn, may influence patient outcome in various ways (see figure 12.1). For example, primary nursing may influence the pattern of nurse–patient communication on a ward, which may subsequently affect patient well-being. It may be seen from figure 12.1 that numerous structural factors surrounding a ward will shape the delivery of direct care (process) and thereby the patient outcome, making it difficult for the researcher to tease out the influence of primary nursing. This is illustrated by the studies of Shukla (1981, 1983), referred to earlier. These studies compared the effect of team and primary nursing on the quality of care provided and indicated that other structural factors, such as the competence of the nurse and staffing levels, may also have a significant impact.

Figure 12.1 indicates that it may be possible to explore the effect of primary nursing on the patient's well-being by considering two questions:

● What aspects of the nursing situations are therapeutic for patients in hospital (potentially therapeutic nursing activities)?
● In what ways does primary nursing enhance or compromise these aspects?

Aspects of Nursing that are Potentially Therapeutic in Effect

The origins of the terms 'nursing as a therapy' and 'therapeutic', used in a nursing context, are unclear; however, the nursing literature has made regular reference to this concept since the 1950s, with Peplau's notable statement in 1952. Nurses' use of the word 'therapeutic' may be based on assumptions and premises which are not explicit. There would appear to be a lack of shared meaning which hinders any attempt to study the area. The dictionary defines 'therapeutic' as 'of the healing art'; it is a derivation of the Greek *therapeutikos*, meaning to wait on (McIntosh, 1951). To explore the concept further, it is proposed that nursing which could be described as 'therapeutic in effect' could be said to comprise that behaviour of a nurse or group of nurses which has a positive effect on the well-being of patient or client. This will be used as a working definition.

The notion that nursing may be viewed as a therapy is not new. Nightingale (1859) recognised the '. . . extreme importance of nursing in determining the issue

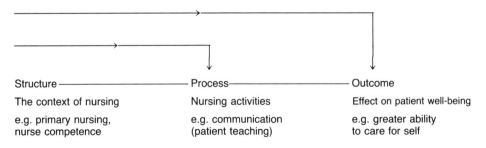

Structure ———————————— Process———————————— Outcome

The context of nursing   Nursing activities   Effect on patient well-being

e.g. primary nursing,   e.g. communication   e.g. greater ability
nurse competence   (patient teaching)   to care for self

Fig. 12.1 The relationship between primary nursing (structure), nursing activities (process) and patient outcome.

of disease'. More recent references to nursing having therapeutic potential have been accompanied in some cases by attempts to clarify the nature of nursing. For example, Peplau (1952: 5) said:

● . . . it can be easily seen that it [nursing] is an interpersonal process and often a therapeutic one.

Since the theoretical work of Peplau many nurses have explored this notion, including theorists such as Hall (1969) and Orem (1980), researchers (for example Kitson, 1984; Ersser, 1990) and clinical nurses such as Muetzel (1988). Reference has been made to the nurse's ability to use herself in a therapeutic manner in the term the 'therapeutic use of self' (Travelbee, 1971). However, there appears to be little understanding of the relationship between the therapeutic features of nursing that result from the personal qualities of the nurse and those consequences that arise from carrying out particular nursing activities. In the psychiatric nursing field, Mellow (1966) has also viewed nursing used as 'therapy' as a deliberate process. Pearson *et al.* (1988a) refer to the therapeutic effect experienced by patients admitted to a nursing unit; however, the nature of the therapy was not clearly defined.

The nursing literature abounds with descriptions of the activities of nurses which may enhance the health of patients. However, discussion of the therapeutic elements of nursing will be confined to those features of nursing which appear to bear some relationship to ward organisation and which illustrate some of the possible mechanisms involved.

Influence of Work Organisation on the Pattern of Nursing Care

As an organisational method, primary nursing is essentially a framework through which nurse and patient are brought together in a particular way. Primary nursing, like all approaches to organising nursing, may produce variations in areas of practice such as:

● Frequency, duration and consistency of contact any one nurse has with any one patient.
● Opportunities for information exchange and the types of communication channels existing between any one nurse, other staff, the patient and his relatives.
● The nurse(s) responsible and accountable for planning the nursing of any one patient and the degree to which this nurse (or these nurses) give direct nursing care.
● The number of nurses responsible and accountable for the quality of nursing the patient receives over a 24-hour period.
● The way in which nursing work is assigned to nurses over time.

These, in turn, may influence the effect the nurse has on the patient.

The consistency of contact between the nurse planning the care and the patient receiving it is highlighted as being particularly significant in terms of the opportunities created for the nurse to benefit or harm the patient. (Examples will be given later.) Whenever on duty a primary nurse will tend to nurse the same group of patients, who are her responsibility. The off-duty rota may not ensure that the patient is nursed by a consistent set of associate nurses. However, primary nursing often allows the off-duty rota to be organised so that each patient is nursed by a smaller group of nurses than is usually possible with other methods of organisation. It is on this basis therefore that primary nursing provides scope for greater consistency of contact between the nurse planning care and the patient.

Hegyvary (1977: 192) said that as the size of the work group increases (as is likely with team nursing) the average amount of interaction with the patient by any individual nurse is liable to decrease. Therefore one would expect greater nurse–patient interaction with primary nursing. However, the research available does not support this fact. Shukla (1983) observed no differences in the amount of direct care given to patients between team and primary methods. Furthermore, Giovanetti (1980) found that contact time was less with primary nursing to a significant degree. Neither study appeared to have any significant design faults. However, despite the possibility that the total nursing contact time may be less with primary nursing it would seem plausible that the patient is likely to have contact *with any individual nurse* (primary) on a more consistent basis when compared with other methods of organisation. This may create more opportunity for nursing that has a therapeutic effect as well as that which has an adverse effect on the patient, depending on the competence of the nurse and other surrounding circumstances.

It may also be conjectured that those internalised values and beliefs which may accompany the uptake of primary nursing (for example the value of providing care that meets the needs of individuals) could also influence nurse–patient interaction and its consequences. As described in chapter 1, if in practice primary nursing is viewed not only as a method of work organisation but also as a working philosophy, embodying a set of values about nursing work, then developing this system may involve changes in the ward culture which affect the delivery of care and in turn the patient's welfare. However, it could be said that in practice nurses may adjust only to the organisational changes and not to the attitudinal changes that primary nursing involves. Furthermore, beliefs about the type of nursing it is desirable to provide, such as that which meets the needs of individual patients, may be sufficiently broad as to be shared by nurses using any patient-orientated work method.

Because of the complexity of this area of study and the significant gaps in knowledge, two aspects of nursing that have therapeutic potential will be used to illustrate the possible ways in which such factors may be influenced by the practice of primary nursing. These are:

● The nature of nurse–patient/staff communication.
● The social environment created by nurses and their orientation to their work.

Potential Effect of Primary Nursing on Nurse–Patient/Staff Communication

Effective communication between the nurse and patient is recognised as a very important feature of nursing because of the significant need patients have for information (Wilson-Barnett, 1977; Hockey, 1984; Moores and Thompson, 1986) and the potential for it to serve therapeutic benefit (see Macleod-Clarke, 1984, for an overview of this area).

Various writers have argued that primary nursing can improve the continuity of care (see introduction to this chapter) to a higher degree than is often possible with other organisational methods. The method of assigning nurses to patients creates opportunities for more consistent interaction between the primary nurse and the patient. Effective nurse–patient and nurse–staff communication is dependent on the consistency of interaction. This can be illustrated with reference to care planning, patient teaching and discharge planning, which require nurses to convey accurate information to the patient in a planned, consistent manner.

Primary Nursing and Care Planning

The value of the care plan is, in part, dependent on the value of the information on which it is based. Therefore, it is important that the nurse who is responsible for planning care has regular opportunity to get to know the patient and to assess initial and changing needs and to observe his response to the nursing planned. Having consistent contact with the patient, the primary nurse has the opportunity to develop the trust needed to work co-operatively. Furthermore, primary nursing provides the scope for information, such as the negotiation of rehabilitation goals, to be communicated directly between the primary nurse, the patient and other staff planning his care.

Patients have reported that primary nursing provides an opportunity to develop greater insight into a patient's individual needs (Kratz, 1979[b]). This is supported by some evidence of improved identification of nutritional need with this system (Coates, 1985: 88).

Consistent contact with the patient also provides the primary nurse with greater scope for effective evaluation because she is both a planner and a provider of nursing and so has regular opportunity to try out specific interventions and adapt them as necessary over time for each individual. Hausmann *et al.* (1976) report that primary nursing may enhance the effectiveness of the nursing process.

Despite the potential care planning benefits offered by primary nursing, it is the effective use of this opportunity that would seem to be important. Drawing in the evidence of the importance of the influence of a nurse's competence on patient outcome cited earlier, there is no guarantee that such opportunities will be used more effectively in a primary nursing situation compared with any other system.

Primary Nursing, Patient Teaching and Care Co-ordination

Effective patient teaching requires the nurse to provide relevant information based on a careful assessment of need and delivered in a consistent and systematic way. This has been illustrated with patients requiring rehabilitation (Wilson-Barnett, 1983) and is supported by studies such as those by Kirovac and Fortin (1976). Again, at each stage of patient teaching from assessment to evaluation, the primary nurse is potentially advantaged by her consistent contact with the patient and also her scope for direct communication.

The co-ordination of care has been described as a key function of nursing (Wilson-Barnett, 1984). The success of nursing and treatment in meeting health needs will rely heavily on the nurse's ability to co-ordinate care efficiently. Primary nursing is ideally suited to ensuring effective co-operation of care (Hegyvary, 1982). These opportunities arise because the primary nurse is in a position to develop a greater knowledge of a smaller number of patients and again to engage in direct communication with all those involved in a patient's care. This would also suggest that practices which rely heavily on careful co-ordination, such as discharge planning, may improve under this system.

Discharge planning is often problematic because nursing decisions are not communicated effectively (Skeet, 1983). Mountain's (1984) small-scale study exemplifies the problems that arise when the perceived needs of discharged patients are not adequately identified by nurses. Opportunities to improve communication, care planning and co-ordination may help to avoid these difficulties. Furthermore, there would be no uncertainty as to which nurse was responsible for discharge planning, with the primary nurse being accountable at least for those aspects of planning which are concerned with nursing needs (Manthey, 1980: 34; Ciske, 1974).

Social Environment Created by Nurses and their Orientation to their Work

The social group that surrounds the patient has long been thought to influence his welfare (Peplau, 1952). Nightingale's (1859) writing reflected a belief in the importance that the ward environment may have on the well-being of patients. More recently, Revans (1964) identified a significant relationship between ward atmosphere (including staff morale) and patient recovery, in terms of the patient's length of stay. The behaviour of people within social treatment environments and their effect on the inhabitants has become a subject of research (Moos, 1974).

It would seem from such work that the social environment of a ward, created by the interaction between staff, patients and visitors, may have some bearing on the welfare of patients. The method of organising nursing adopted by each ward is likely to influence the nature of this environment, through its effect on the pattern of interaction, and possibly through nurses' expression of the beliefs and values associated with each method of their work.

In general nursing, two major studies have explored the consequences of the different forms of nursing organisation and orientation for the patient. Miller (1985 b&c) compared the dependency of patients who were admitted to wards of either patient or task orientation. At the onset patients were judged to be of comparable dependency in each ward type. However, she found that those who had been on the patient-orientated wards for more than one month were less dependent and the proportion of discharges to deaths was higher in the patient-orientated wards compared with the task-orientated setting. Although many patients are not in hospital for this length of time, this study is indicative of both the therapeutic and iatrogenic potential resulting from the social organisation of ward nursing.

Kitson (1984) examined nursing's therapeutic function in the care of hospitalised elderly patients. This study pointed to the existence of a relationship between the way nursing was organised and orientated (on the basis of task or patient), and aspects of care which were deemed therapeutic. Nursing identified as therapeutic included the nurse demonstrating a capacity to enhance the ability of patients to care for themselves, and the existence of positive attitudes to the elderly. Wards having a patient orientation displayed greater evidence of practice deemed therapeutic than those having a task orientation. Although both of these aspects of nursing could legitimately be described as therapeutic, the validity of Kitson's therapeutic indicators does rest on the extent to which one accepts her conceptual framework on which it is based (Kitson, 1986: 162).

These studies point to the benefits that patient-orientated nursing may provide. Primary nursing is designed to enable nurses to provide highly individual nursing (Marram *et al.*, 1974). Therefore Miller's and Kitson's studies indicate that the primary nursing system may help to create the conditions under which patients become more independent more than systems using a task-orientated approach. However, there is no certainty that specific patient-centred approaches to organisation, such as patient allocation or team nursing, are any less effective in enhancing patient independence. It may be useful to repeat Miller's research design by comparing patient outcome for wards practising primary nursing with those adopting other patient-centred methods.

Despite the opportunities that primary nursing may provide to enhance the therapeutic potential of particular nursing activities, consideration needs to be given to the ways in which this system may have a compromising effect on patient well-being.

Could Primary Nursing Compromise Therapeutic Interaction?

It cannot be assumed that primary nursing will foster practice which is therapeutic in effect. From the preceding line of argument it is logical that the consistency of contact between the primary nurse and patient could in fact create greater opportunities for the incompetent nurse to do harm.

Robinson (1988) has warned that access to nursing expertise may be more restrictive with primary nursing because the primary nurses in any one unit are likely to have variable expertise. To some extent this may be true because they would often work opposite shifts to other primary nurses. However, the primary nurse does not work in isolation and has opportunity to liaise with associate nurses and other primary nurses, all of whom could operate in a consultative capacity. Primary nurses need to draw on the range of experience and expertise of their associate nurses by actively encouraging them to contribute ideas to the development of the nursing plan, while continuing to uphold their own responsibility for the care plan. Our own experience of this practice has been positive. The patient's restricted access to the group of nurses on a unit may also be problematic with primary nursing if patient and nurse are insufficienty matched as personalities and the nurse fails to recognise this or chooses to do nothing about it.

THE DIFFICULTY OF IDENTIFYING THE IMPLICATIONS OF PRIMARY NURSING FOR PATIENTS

Exploring the implications of primary nursing for the patient is a very difficult undertaking and so this chapter can achieve little more than raise some issues. An attempt has been made to highlight the conceptual and methodological problems and complexities facing the researcher. In particular, the researcher is challenged to develop valid and reliable tools to describe adequately the wide range of methods of nursing organisation and various patient outcomes. To complement the research endeavour, a reasoned approach to exploring the possible consequences of changing the pattern of nurse–patient interaction for the patient is advocated.

In chapter 1 the concepts that underpin the different methods of work organisation were described as being on a continuum. It was argued that when identifying the nature of the method used on a specific clinical unit it is of greater value to place emphasis on identifying the presence and development of those features of the actual method, such as the degree of continuity of care, which are believed to benefit patients, rather than on whether a specific type of method is in use, such as primary nursing. The assumption is that the development of such factors of the organisation as the level of accountability for nursing, continuity of care and direct communication channels may help to create the conditions in which nurses may benefit patients. Future research studies need to explore how these concepts are expressed in the behaviour of the nurses on a ward and then to examine the consequences of these behavioural patterns for the welfare of patients.

13

Primary Nursing –
Implications for the Nurse

Jan Dewing

Nurses are subject to the influence of changes in the organisation at ward level and within the wider health system within which they work. Some of these changes will have an effect on the nurse's welfare. Organising and delivering care through a system of primary nursing, where a more traditional system has been in practice, necessitates changes in nursing and demands change from nurses as individuals, not just as nurses but in deeper, personal ways. This chapter focuses specifically on those nurses working in a primary nursing system.

The consequences for nurses arising from working within a primary nursing system may be different from the stresses previously associated with nursing. If the nursing environment and the resources within it, including nurses, are managed effectively and with sensitivity, the consequences of working in a primary nursing system need not be negative for nurses. All too often it seems that the management of the health care system itself is given priority over the people. The study of primary nursing should not be confined to how care is organised differently but should also examine more closely the consequences to nurses and clients. A general theme of this chapter is that the *people* should be given priority when changes are made in the organisation of nurses' work.

WHY FOCUS ON THE NEEDS OF NURSES?

It may well be questioned as to why nurses are focusing increasingly on their own welfare. Seemingly, nurses have always coped in the past. Their own welfare was not considered to be an important factor; nurses have apparently just got on with the job (Faulkner and Macguire, 1988). Perhaps this has not really been the case but nurses have not vocalised their own needs until recently. Rogers and Salvage (1988) argue that the continued failure of nursing to face up to preventable problems associated with working in nursing is responsible for the high levels of stress and illness among nurses. They argue that stress can arise from three possible sources, societal, employer-induced and professional. Nurses are generally exposed to one or more of these sources at some time during their careers. Within nursing, unsociable hours, poor facilities and uncaring senior staff all take their toll on the welfare of nurses (Salvage, 1985).

Centrality of the Nurse–Client Relationship

One of the central issues concerning stress in primary nursing relates to its potential impact on the conception and development of the nurse–client relationship. The risk of stress developing in nurses who work in a primary/nursing system is possibly greater. This is because of the personal nature of nurse–client relationships and other factors, such as the amount of time spent in contact with clients and the intensity of personal involvement of the nurse. In primary nursing, nurses are being asked to develop relationships that involve emotional closeness and personal involvement. Such relationships are often new experiences for many nurses, who may find difficulties in coming to terms with new working practices. This new closeness with clients may mean that some nurses experience different types of stress from those they may have anticipated. Nurses may not have prepared themselves in any way for such changes and may be surprised to find how they are reacting and coping.

Continuing professional developments within nursing are giving nurses greater opportunities to examine their attitudes to practice; for example, communication skills and assertiveness workshops. Many recent developments in nursing concern those areas of practice directly associated with delivery of care. Such developments often have wide-ranging effects on nurses at different levels of the organisation. These may vary from asking nurses to change their hours of working, to asking them to re-examine their attitudes or working practices. Often the effect that new working practices may have on nurses is overlooked to the expense of the welfare of nurses. Many educational experiences, such as study days, neglect to give nurses the opportunities to discuss the implications for themselves and their working practices. Knowing that change will directly benefit client care is reassuring for nurses but at the same time can put them under great pressure to change regardless of the personal cost to nurses in terms of time, energy and stress.

The Needs of Nurses

Nursing currently promotes the use of nursing models to serve as conceptual guides to nursing (Aggleton and Chalmers, 1986). Nursing models encompass sets of beliefs and values about people. Nurses who ascribe to the belief and values of nursing models should also be prepared to apply those same philosophies to themselves and other nurses. Nursing models are not just about patients or illness; they are about people and about health, in which case they can be easily utilised on a wider basis to include nurses. Maslow's hierarchy of needs (Maslow, 1954) is often referred to when focusing on individual clients' needs. Higher levels of needs, such as self-esteem, can usually be met only when more basic needs, such as physiological needs, have been met. This framework can also be applied to nurses. Rogers (1970) states that individuals require the following to achieve a state of health:

- A balance of ingoing and outgoing energy
- A continuously evolving direction to life
- A sense of predictability and organisation to the pattern of life

● The ability to conceptualise, think, relate and experience sensations and feelings that promote the development of self-esteem and self-satisfaction

Many nurses will be able to relate these factors contributing to health to themselves. It will be argued, later in the chapter, that the needs of nurses should be assessed, planned for, met and evaluated in ways similar to those employed by nurses caring for clients. As Salvage (1985) states, nurses should not presume to care for others unless they care for themselves first. An environment that is intended to be healing and therapeutic for clients should not be a potential source of danger for the staff who work within it.

It is important to value the needs of nurses as individuals in society and the value of nursing as a resource in health care. Because nurses are involved in health care, essentially a 'giving' service, does not imply that their own health needs should take second place. The statement 'who cares for the carers' is becoming too familiar amongst nurses (Tschudin, 1985b). The obvious answer to this is that nurses should actively care for themselves and each other. There is, perhaps, a need to turn such rhetoric into action so that carers will come to experience working in a caring environment and being cared for themselves – as individuals.

STRESS IN NURSING

Flint (1986) states that nurses are working in an emotional minefield, where their every action and word is noted by clients, colleagues and peers. Individual nurses are offered little protection against the demands of caring for people. New approaches to care, such as primary nursing, may highlight the position of the individual nurse rather than the nursing team. In this way individual nurses are readily identifiable by clients and colleagues for their actions. Traditionally, nurses obtained some sense of protection from feeling they were part of a homogeneous group of workers. Despite the greater emphasis placed on the nurse's individual responsibility and accountability within primary nursing, these concepts may still appear to be new for many nurses facing them for the first time (see chapter 4). In particular, the stress of translating the concepts into day-to-day practice may prove an additional burden for nurses in the primary nursing setting.

No matter how nursing care is organised, nurses today are facing more stresses associated with the nature of their work (Mitchell, 1988). There are many references to support the presence, nature and effects of stress in nursing (Bond, 1982). Stress in nursing arises from three broad areas: the environment, the system in which nurses work, and the daily contact nurses have with clients (Tschudin, 1985a). Salvage (1985) describes nurses as being in the difficult situation of delivering intimate personal care on a 24-hour basis and, in addition to this, having to make ends meet in the face of 'efficiency savings, cuts and resource realloca-tions'.

Defence from Stress in Traditional Nursing Systems

Traditionally, nurses have been protected from the stresses of caring for people by working in and developing a task allocation system (see chapter 1) that allowed them to remain personally distant and anonymous in relation to clients. This system operated as defence mechanisms against the stresses or anxieties that invariably arose from working in a caring relationship (Menzies, 1960c), some features of which are still being practised by nurses today (Melia, 1987).

The traditional method of organising nursing appears to have served as a relatively successful avoidance and defence system against stress. It would seem that nurses allowed stress to develop and tried to fend it off by avoiding the sources of stress. However, if the system had scored as a positive coping strategy there would not have been the degree of stress or stress-related problems which now appear to be present in nursing. Defence systems surrounding task allocation may have offered a degree of protection for nurses against the stresses associated with caring, but they did little for clients.

Task allocation enabled many hierarchical nursing practices to flourish, such as the delegation of work according to status and the belief that sister's judgement was always right and unquestionable. Many nurses still feel unable to question decisions made by senior nurses, even if they do not understand or agree with them (Pearson and Vaughan, 1986). This system has also led to the majority of qualified nurses spending the least amount of time delivering care. For example, Pembrey's (1980) study found that ward sisters spent less than 1% of their working day engaged in delivering care.

Positive Coping Strategies in Primary Nursing

Primary nursing requires nurses to alter their practices in such a way as to make them more exposed to the stresses associated with caring for people. Traditional defensive systems that encourage personal detachment from clients are not entirely appropriate in primary nursing. Individual nurses must acknowledge the presence and possible effects of stress and be prepared to learn and develop positive coping strategies both personally and with other nurses to enable them to cope effectively with stress. The strategy of each nurse will be individual. Also, nurses in each clinical area will develop strategies that are suitable for their own needs. There is the risk that if nurses do not act to develop positive coping strategies the traditional systems of organising care will be replaced by those which may both exert stress and fail to assist nurses to cope with the stresses inherent in nursing generally.

Potential Stresses in Primary Nursing

Primary nursing may support the development of relationships between nurse and client which are potentially therapeutic (Muetzel, 1988). To work in this way with clients, nurses are required to develop their nursing skills in learning to relate to clients in more personal, effective and caring ways. Muetzel (1988) argues that this can only be achieved when relationships have value and meaning for those concerned. For nurses this implies personal involvement. Bond (1986) states that, through socialisation processes in nursing, nurses have been taught that any form of personal involvement is viewed as negative and to be avoided. For professional carers to work effectively and in sensitive ways they need to give something of themselves (Flint, 1986). Again, this implies involvement for nurses. Flint speaks of nurses being 'cherished' by each other and the organisation.

Primary nursing, as a philosophy of care, is no guarantee in itself that nurses will be supported and cared for in humanistic ways (Salvage, 1985). Manthey (1980) argues that primary nursing is only a system through which care is organised. The most valuable assets to this or any system are nurses. Shukla and Turner (1984) and Shukla (1982) have shown that the competencies of nurses are likely to have a greater influence on quality of care than the way in which care is organised. Many of the skills nurses regularly use can be useful in nurturing relationships with peers and colleagues. If primary nursing is to be successful for nurses as well as clients, it will be necessary to incorporate supportive strategies for nurses as a part of normal practice.

Shukla (1982) argues that the success of primary nursing is partly dependent on effective support systems, for both nurses and the environment. The demands primary nursing makes on nurses to change their practices may prove stressful for some nurses. The difficulties associated with introducing primary nursing, either for an individual or for a group of nurses, may initially make it appear to be a more stressful way of working for many nurses. Support systems to cope with stress need to be developed as primary nursing is being introduced and not as an afterthought. These systems need to be in place to deal with problems as they arise and not brought into operation to cope with crises.

Relationships formed by nurses in primary nursing may be more intense and perhaps of a different nature to more traditional nurse–client relationships because of the case method and the greater consistency of contact with clients.

Stresses for Primary Nurses

Primary nurses and clients become the central figures in primary nursing. To some extent all other nurses may perceive themselves to become a supporting cast; this is an issue that will be dealt with further on in this section. Primary nurses may have to contend with the demand placed on them to develop close and, perhaps, more intimate relationships with clients, in the belief that this will help them to be more effective nurses.

Nurses have not always received the educational preparation to provide them with the knowledge and skills required to achieve this new type of relationship (see chapter 3). Adequate preparation for the role of primary nurse will place staff in a far stronger position to be able to understand what is being required of them and to cope with any associated stresses. Too often nurses are put in the position of taking on the role of primary nurse without educational preparation. Lack of preparation can mean that nurses never achieve their maximum potential, as well as making life more difficult for themselves and for clients. Because of the importance of the nurses' competence to the success of primary nursing, a structural change in the organisation of nursing should be accompanied by staff development so that nursing skills are improved (Shukla, 1981).

The knowledge and skills required from primary nurses to achieve potentially therapeutic relationships may appear to some nurses to be of an advanced level or perhaps of a different nature from those they have previously sought to acquire. If nurses are to use themselves in therapeutic ways they need to develop their self-awareness so that their personal concerns do not interfere with their relationships in ways that are harmful to clients (Hall, 1964). Given the intensity of nurse–client relationships with primary nursing, nurses need to acquire more 'people-orientated' skills, such as communication skills, assertiveness and counselling skills. Such skills contribute to the development of the nurse's self-awareness. Sparrow (1986) argues that there is a clearly defined responsibility of one nurse who is accountable for the care given to clients during their hospital stay that makes primary nursing different to other forms of nursing. Punton (1985) found that for some nurses this may be a source of stress. They may feel inhibited in making decisions on their own. Positive recognition from peers and colleagues can ease the load of accountability (Holmes, 1987). Primary nurses have the added demands placed on them of having to account for written care plans and perhaps for verbal ones too; they cannot be anonymous care givers and planners. Primary nurses must clearly identify themselves to clients and sign their name to care plans (Holmes, 1987).

Individual accountability can be highlighted by the ways in which primary nurses work, seemingly isolating them from colleagues and peers inside and outside clinical areas which may be a further source of stress. Traditionally, nurses have been used to working in pairs or in teams. Primary nurses often work on their own. Incorporating more flexible working hours and break times can have the effect of further isolating nurses. The high visibility of primary nurses to clients, relatives, and medical and paramedical staff can make additional demands on primary nurses. Primary nurses must have a high level of visibility to others, especially to clients, but not to a level that becomes harmful for the nurses.

Most nurses require some point during a busy day when they can have a few minutes to themselves, perhaps to think about a problem or simply to relax after a stressful incident. This may be incorporated into an official break or it may be needed during working hours. Primary nurses should not be expected to maintain high levels of visibility to all people at all times. The added responsibility of being a direct channel of communication can, in some ways, be balanced against the fact that primary nurses are not powerless to act. In more traditional systems nurses may find coping as a direct channel of information difficult because they have to act in the way sister would in the same or similar situation. This may not always be the way they know or believe to be the way they would want to act. Having to deal with a larger patient group and often having unclear authority, in practice the nurse in charge of the ward within the traditional system of organisation may experience significant demands. Manthey and Kramer (1970) observe that different levels of competencies between primary nurses become clearly visible. This may prove to be a difficult situation for inexperienced primary nurses or for those who are lacking in knowledge and skills. It does serve to illustrate the point that learning and development need to be ongoing. The styles of primary nurses within one ward team will differ. They may lead primary nurses to compare themselves with others and the ways in which others work. It may be a useful exercise if the primary nurses come to value each other's style of working and the contribution each member makes to the ward team. The individuality of primary nurses is a vital component of what they take with them into their nurse–client relationship and needs to be nurtured. However, primary nurses can add to their stress by feeling that they are competing with each other to be the best primary nurse.

Outside clinical areas, primary nurses may not always have highly developed social support networks of peers and relatives. Nursing colleagues may not be familiar with the stresses associated with primary nursing. Often partners or friends, however caring or well meaning, simply do not understand the pressures in nursing. Not all nurses have supportive families or partners to return home to after work. It is often the case that where nurses do have families they go home to continue in a caring role (Oakley, 1981). Nursing has a responsibility to attend to its own 'walking wounded'. Nurses suffering from the effects of stress in nursing should be cared for by nursing.

Clients may provide the major source of job satisfaction for primary nurses. To balance the stresses against the rewards it is important that primary nurses are aware of their successes, as so often nurses notice only where they have failed and not where they have succeeded. Experienced primary nurses are able to identify how much of an outcome to attribute to their care. When this happens primary nurses may find that there are actually more successes than failures.

Pearson (1988a) argues that the collegiate relationships established in primary nursing make it less stressful than more traditional and hierarchically based forms of nursing. Primary nursing may promote the development of collegiate-type relationships between nurses if they have the knowledge and skills to be able to work effectively in this way. Where the system is found to be more stressful, nurses should examine the wider areas of their practice, such as management issues and the leadership of the senior nurse and their own abilities as individuals and as a team to cope with the effects of stress.

Stresses for Associate Nurses

Associate nurses may be either registered or enrolled nurses. They may be newly qualified or clinically experienced nurses working either full-time or part-time. Associate nurses must be recognised as a valuable resource and an essential feature to primary nursing (Manthey, 1980; Sparrow, 1986; McMahon, 1988). However, in practice, their contribution may appear to be neglected. This often leads to associate nurses perceiving themselves as being devalued by nursing. The traditional hierarchical structure that nurses have allowed to develop can be damaging to the self-esteem of nurses. This may contribute to misconceptions about the lack of potential within the role. Associate nurses may perceive their role as not fully recognised by primary nurses.

The failure to acknowledge fully the work done by supporting workers is not a problem restricted to nursing. Primary nurses can do much to alter this misconception. Primary nurses often work as associates for other primary nurses, as do more senior nurses. It is possible to have registered nurses working as associate nurses alongside enrolled nurses, which can provide a good skill mix among the associate nurses. Burns (1988) feels that the experience of being an associate is vital preparation for a primary nursing role. The structural network in primary nursing in formal terms is less hierarchical. Informal hierarchies are very subtle; these may still develop within primary nursing and may exert considerable pressure on some nurses. Clinical regrading may have enhanced the effect of this informal hierarchy. For example, it is possible to find associate nurses on the same ward in differently graded posts.

Many associate nurses will go on to be primary nurses. If they have worked in a system that is caring and supportive to them, they are in a better position to treat their associate nurses in this way in the future. Associate nurses may feel they are powerless in following care plans written by primary nurses where they do not understand or agree with the plan. Sisters need to be aware of this potential problem and bring the nurses together to assist them in resolving their difficulties. Primary and associate nurses will be able to establish open discussions about these issues without associate nurses fearing reprisals from primary nurses or sisters. A useful way for primary nurses to communicate the value of associate nurses to these nurses is to show them respect. An important way to show respect is to listen to what someone has to say. Although the primary nurse is ultimately responsible for the overall direction of care, she would be unwise not to listen to the contribution of associate nurses, many of whom will have valuable and varied clinical experience.

Some associate nurses work part-time because of family commitments. They may feel that they have in some ways been forced into an associate nurse role simply because of the number of hours they work and not because of their level of knowledge or skills. In reality, this group of nurses may be some of the most clinically experienced nurses in the profession. Once these nurses start to work in primary nursing systems they can usually see that primary nurses almost always need to work full-time hours. Many primary nurses incorporate flexible working hours into their practice, which in most instances does not fit in with the demands of caring for children or other family members. Some associate nurses will need to acquire new knowledge in order to go on and practise as primary nurses in the future. They should not be prevented from educational development as part-time workers, in terms of either time or funding. Role preparation for the future should be encouraged at the present time. It is possible that some associate nurses, especially enrolled nurses, feel that they are being treated unfairly in primary nursing. Traditionally they may have performed the same jobs as many registered nurses, despite not being trained or financially rewarded in the same ways. Breaking with tradition, however appropriate, is still difficult for some nurses to accept and requires sensitive handling.

Stresses for Nursing Auxiliaries

The philosophy of primary nursing expresses the belief that clients have the right to have nursing care delivered by qualified nurses (Manthey, 1980). This leaves the position of nursing auxiliaries uncertain. In some areas the solution to this has been to alter the role of auxiliaries into generic care assistants (McMahon, 1988). Care assistants assist nurses with aspects of care requiring two persons and perform some non-nursing duties traditionally performed by qualified nurses, but do not perform any nursing duties on their own. Although nursing as a profession may be slowly moving in this direction, in reality there are large numbers of auxiliaries who still identify with a clinical role. Nursing auxiliaries may expect to perform certain aspects of nursing care either alongside qualified nurses or under the supervision of nurses. Many nursing auxiliaries resent the implied change in their role as they value contact with clients. Becoming a care assistant may also be associated with shorter working hours and many auxiliaries are not in a position to be able to afford to do this.

It can become difficult to balance the beliefs of primary nursing against the demands of managing staff in caring and supportive ways. Many nursing auxiliaries have very caring attitudes towards clients. Often they are persons who have wanted and for some reason been unable to train as nurses. Additionally many auxiliaries are more mature, with a lot of life experience which many younger nurses have not yet acquired. It is possible that role changes can be discussed with auxiliaries and changes agreed on. In these instances, it is also reasonable to expect that most auxiliaries would feel powerless to argue their case against qualified nurses. Primary nursing requires nurses to value individuals for their personal worth. This need not stop when it comes to auxiliaries; otherwise, nurses are really saying that personal worth decreases with status. There are ways in which nursing auxiliaries can be positively utilised in clinical areas, although this will differ from area to area. The position of auxiliaries has been further complicated by the emergence of the support worker (Rowden, 1989). Salvage (1988a) argues that it is still unclear what preparation and role they will undertake.

There is an argument for altering the role of the traditional auxiliary. If this is the road nursing is to take, change can be gradually introduced. This would result in temporary organisational difficulties for sisters and senior nurses but, if nurses really value working in ways that are caring and supportive, these difficulties can be overcome. Auxiliaries are not exempt from experiencing stresses associated with changes in role. The role of the auxiliary or the support worker needs to be examined in a wider context, as part of a means of providing the best combination of skills for clients (Salvage, 1988a). Although it is argued by some (e.g. Pearson, 1988a) that all clients deserve care by skilled qualified nurses, and many nurses would believe this to be the case, there are not as yet any solutions as to how to go about introducing this in the NHS without causing a severe manpower shortage.

Stresses for the Ward Sister/Staff Support Nurse

Details of the role changes to be undergone by ward sisters during the change to primary nursing have been outlined in chapter 4. The role of ward sister has been said to be vital to the development of clinical nursing (Pembrey, 1980). Ward sisters determine the style of nursing and the ward climate (Orton, 1981; Melia, 1987). Traditionally ward sisters have been the central figures in clinical areas, and all aspects of nursing have revolved around them. In primary nursing systems it is the primary nurses who assume much of this central role, at least where issues related to client care are concerned, and ward sisters may perceive themselves to be devalued or redundant in some ways. Manthey and Kramer (1970) find little difference between the roles of the sister and the primary nurse. The only difference they concede is that sisters are responsible for planning staff development. If primary nurses could assume greater self-responsibility for this and for many other areas that traditionally senior nurses have maintained in their control, there may not be a need for ward sisters. Organising staff development for all nurses in a clinical area is not to be devalued or underrated. Perhaps it is preferable that one person assumes responsibility for providing appropriate educational opportunities for nurses. The role of the ward sister may have become more sophisticated since Manthey and Kramer wrote their article. Keeping a group of primary nurses and other ward nurses functioning as a team requires skilful management. If primary nurses take on too many managerial tasks, eventually their contact with clients will diminish.

As a result of having less responsibility related to direct client care, sisters are now in the position of being able to develop many other aspects of their role, which in the past have often been neglected by sisters, such as teaching students, and counselling and talking to staff, as well as organising and developing ongoing educational programmes for nursing staff. It may be that ward sisters will find their role less stressful in primary nursing as the demands placed on them and their time become less intense.

The importance of the sister's role does not diminish with primary nursing. Successful role transition of ward sisters is vital to the success of primary nursing (Manthey, 1980). Sisters need to adapt and alter their practice to enable primary nurses to develop their own autonomy for practice. Sisters paying only lip service to allowing primary nurses to be autonomous in practice will not develop a successful primary nursing system. Sisters, like any other nurses, can experience stress associated with role transition. They may find themselves in a dual position. While being the ones to suggest change to primary nursing they may then find themselves in the position of having to undergo some of the greatest changes, and still be required to be a leader for the rest of the nursing team and support them through their role changes.

The role of ward sisters in providing staff support is perhaps the most important feature of their total role and probably the most underdeveloped by many sisters. Often it is seen as something that comes into operation when there are problems in clinical areas, but it is something that should be occurring continuously as a means of preventing the effects of stress to accumulate and to assist nurses to develop effective coping strategies. If ward sisters became known as staff support nurses it would assist them in defining the priorities of the role more clearly. The exact nature of what comprises staff support is more difficult to define. McMahon (1988) simply states that they provide advice and may use counselling skills to help nurses. Providing support that is of value for nurses is more complex than this. It begins with the attitude of ward sisters to their staff. Many sisters may feel they are supportive, but invariably the needs of the organisation become paramount, although this is not always the fault of sisters. They are managing situations with skills they have acquired often through trial and error or by the only way they have been taught. Too often sisters and senior nurses ascribe to commitment to caring for staff but when difficulties arise they continue to manage in traditional ways with very little thought for the needs of individuals.

The needs of all individuals cannot take priority at all times and there is the real problem of deciding where the dividing line falls. As was argued previously, nurses are individuals with needs. To some extent these needs must be planned for and met by similar processes to the way in which clients' needs are met. This increases demands on the ward sisters' time and skills. More human relationship skills are needed. Sisters who have not developed their own self-awareness and communication skills will find staff support more stressful than those who have developed these skills.

STAFF SUPPORT SYSTEMS

It should be clear that it is the responsibility of every nurse to attend to the effects of stress. Within the organisation sisters are better placed than some nurses in providing support systems for nurses. Outside the organisation each nurse can achieve as much as any sister in providing effective support systems. If nurses cannot take responsibility for directing their own needs, it can be questioned whether they are in the position to direct clients (Bond, 1986). Support systems should be equally balanced between those inside and outside the organisation. They are not meant to make nurses dependent on them or the organisation, but they should be enabling nurses to become more independent and self-confident practitioners. Bond (1986) is rightly suspicious of support systems that encourage dependence. McMahon (1988) does not specifically describe any staff support systems but points to staff councils, staff support groups and staff seminars as being channels of direct staff communication. Nurses must have confidence and trust in the systems provided. It is not uncommon for nurses to leave meetings without having said anything, taking away with them the same stresses they brought to the meeting. It could be argued that creating a caring and supportive environment extends further than providing formal structures. It extends from providing a physical environment that is complementary to nursing practice to providing the more formal means of staff support systems and to the attitudes of the sister and nurses towards themselves and each other.

Nurses need to work in environments that are comfortable. This is not to demand four-star hospitals, but simply to have the facilities that other professions take for granted. Too often nurses tolerate working conditions that are below standard, such as poor quality changing rooms, staff rooms that are far from comfortable, and small overcrowded offices. The effects the working environment can have on nurses is too often ignored (Rogers and Salvage, 1988). Faulty equipment can be taken away for repair, but it is not so easy when nurses are in this position (Tschudin, 1985b). Tschudin also notes that the resources allocated to staff support are given a low priroity. Some changes in the working environment can be planned and budgeted for by sisters and senior nurses. Nurses should, within reason, be their own press managers for larger-scale changes.

Positive Coping Strategies

Nurses can learn positive coping strategies to assist them in leading healthier lives both in and out of work. Nurses as individuals can adopt some relatively easy measures to ensure that they are fit and healthy to practice. Bond (1986) discusses the value of diet and exercise to physical health. Although nurses are well aware of the importance of diet and exercise they often allow themselves to adopt unhealthy routines because of pressures of work. Nurse educationalists can assist nurses by providing the knowledge they need to improve their interpersonal skills (Kagan, 1985; Faulkner, 1988). Counselling and communication skills can be learnt, as can assertiveness and self-awareness skills. These 'people skills' can be utilised by nurses personally and professionally. Nurses can also learn other skills such as massage and relaxation techniques, perhaps including the use of aromatherapy and music. Skills such as these can be used by nurses in self-help groups. Groups could be held in clinical areas at the end of the day, or during times that are identified as being particularly stressful. Clinical areas could link together to share these facilities and to teach skills to other nurses.

Bond (1986) thinks that nurses have hidden abilities that can be brought out through formal staff support groups. Nurses give each other support in numerous ways without the giver being aware of what she is doing or the receiver knowing she is receiving support. Educating nurses about giving and receiving support will often assist them in organising the skills they already possess and make them aware of what they are doing. By facilitating nurses to be responsible for their own support, groups can become independent peer groups, rather than being dependent on the skills of group leaders. Initially most nurses require the assistance of someone skilled in group work. Finding leaders can be difficult. Problems may also be experienced in finding time in which the group can meet. Receiving support is not always an easy process as some nurses may experience some personal difficulties related to group dynamics. They may have difficulties in talking openly and honestly, especially in front of more senior nurses. The reverse may hold equally true for senior nurses. There is no quick remedy to this problem. Nurses in staff support groups have to learn to trust each other and that confidentiality within the group will be maintained. Once established these groups can have several benefits. Peers can share problems, such as difficulties they are having in establishing relationships with clients of colleagues. Particular events that have proved to be stressful can be discussed and coping strategies can be developed for the future (Faulkner and Maguire, 1988). Support groups for specific purposes can be established in some areas, for example stopping smoking. Different groups of nurses from different or similar clinical areas can set up their own peer support groups.

CONCLUSION

Ultimately, the needs of nurses must be given priority over the needs of any nursing system, as it is the competencies of nurses that determine the success of any system.

Nurses need to learn how to cope effectively with the stresses associated with primary nursing to enable them to function as effective primary nurses. Coping with stress in primary nursing is not strictly just about coping; it is also about personal development. It is about enabling ourselves and others to achieve our potential. Stress in nursing must be dealt with by positive methods. To achieve this, effective support systems that will meet their needs must be developed by nurses. A great sense of self-satisfaction can be obtained from knowing that the environment in which nurses work and the way primary nursing assists them in delivering care have been managed in such a way that the personal growth and development of nurses becomes evident.

Introducing primary nursing into practice must include an awareness of the stresses associated with this system. There needs to be a firm commitment to providing effective support systems for nurses.

14

Managerial Implications of Primary Nursing

Heather Jane Sears and Shirley Williams

As a method of organising nursing, primary nursing is closely interlinked with management practice as illustrated in this chapter. The term 'management' covers a range of different roles and styles of practice. This chapter reflects the managerial implications for primary nursing explored from two different perspectives:

● A nurse manager with devolved general management responsibilities in a community hospital
● A director of nursing services for a hospital providing acute services

---

MANAGERIAL PRINCIPLES

Definitions of management are wide and varied. Heller (1972) suggests that management is 'achieving results from other people'. Kramer (1975) considers the key role of the manager to be that of arbiter between conflicting interests: 'management's task in general is not to widen conflicts but to strike a balance between divergent interests and constantly strive to harmonize them'.

It is perhaps more fruitful to consider some general principles from which most managerial practices derive. Four important features are considered:

● *Planning*   This encompasses setting objectives, forecasting, analysing problems and making decisions, to formulate policy.
● *Organising*   This involves determining what activities are necessary to achieve the objectives, classifying the work and assigning it to groups and individuals.
● *Motivating*   There is a need for the manager to inspire staff to contribute to the purposes of the organization. Drucker (1977) emphasises that motivation and communication are important ways of influencing people to work effectively.
● *Controlling*   There is a need for a manger to exert some control over work performed by checking performance against the plans made. The word 'measurement' has been used instead of 'control' (Drucker, 1977). This suggests a shift in emphasis from seeing that orders are obeyed to setting objectives and providing the yardsticks for self-control.

With the above four functions, some authors (e.g. Urwick, 1947; Brech, 1975) include co-ordinating. This would seem to be a too general term to be satisfactorily described as a feature of the manager's job; it rather involves all of the functions described. According to Calsune (1951: 24):

● The concept of co-ordination does not describe a particular set of operations but all operations which lead to a certain result.

Drucker (1977: 55) makes an important addition to the four functions by emphasising that management must involve the development of people. A manager:

● directs people or misdirects them, brings out what is in them or stifles them, strengthens their integrity or corrupts them, trains them to stand upright and strong or deforms them.

NURSING MANAGEMENT AND THE ORGANISATION OF WORK

The management of the organisation of nursing work is also shaped by the prevailing nursing ideology.

Traditional nursing management arrangements were developed in response to a task-orientated understanding of the nature of nursing work. Nursing work was believed to involve a series of predetermined tasks, derived typically from the patient's medical condition, often irrespective of his individual needs. While such a belief held sway, bureaucratic management arrangements were entirely appropriate.

Nursing work was organised, managed and supervised on a shift-by-shift basis. Nursing manpower was controlled centrally and staff were redeployed hospital-wide in response to shortages or increased workload on the assumption that any nurse was capable of carrying out any task anywhere. Nurses handed over their responsibility at the end of each shift, and since the ward sister worked only during the day it was considered necessary to have a supervisory sister during the night.

The role of the senior sister nurse manager was largely that of a controller of resources. By her very ownership of these resources, together with the authority which she had to award or deny them, she drastically curtailed the practising nurse's ability to function in anything other than a task-orientated short-term way.

Such management arrangements are clearly inappropriate for the support of professional nursing, where the decisions about each patient's unique need for nursing are determined, in the main, by one particular nurse. The primary nurse accepts professional accountability for the care of her patient from admission to discharge. Much of that care will be delivered by associate nurses working to her plan, and of course the primary nurse will discuss her patient's care and progress with her associate nurses, but that does not diminish her own 24-hour, 7-day week accountability.

Thus in primary nursing there ceases to be a need for a traditional managerial 'supervisor' who is not directly involved with the clinical activity on the ward other than as a nurse working in a consultative capacity. Indeed, any attempt by a nursing officer or clinical nurse manager to impose clinical managerial supervisory rounds will lead to conflict with the professional nurse. A 'top down', controlling management approach will at best be seen as interference and at worst will entirely inhibit the effectiveness of nursing. That is not to say that a service built on individual professional practice does not require management; far from it. It is our belief that it is important that nurses do not take as their role model the medical consultant, whose autonomous practice has caused major problems both for the individual patient and for the planning and delivery of the health service as a whole. The consultant's insistence that he must treat the patient before him in the best way that modern medicine has decreed, regardless of available overall resources, often results in 'other' patients being denied any access at all to his time or care. An even more fundamental issue is raised when we realise that the overall pattern of hospital health care provision is more often determined by the clinical specialist interests of the consultants in post than by the epidemiological needs of the local population.

It is perhaps desirable that autonomous primary nurses are managed in such a way that they are allowed to provide for patients' actual health needs which are amenable to nursing. We will now look at the managerial implications of primary nursing from the perspective of two different nurse managers.

PERSPECTIVE 1

This section, written by Heather Jane Sears, examines primary nursing from the point of view of a nurse manager with devolved general management responsibilities for maintaining primary nursing in a community hospital.

Context

The Hospital

Didcot Community Hospital is a 30-bedded unit in Oxfordshire. It has a 24-hour minor casualty, staffed from the existing ward establishment, and a busy outpatient department with clinics in every specialty.

The job of hospital manager at Didcot was created two years ago following the Griffiths Report (Griffiths, 1983). The previous posts of Nursing Officer and Administrator were combined, at the same time as the devolution of the hospital budgets, to ensure that the principles of general management would work at subunit level.

The Patients

Patients are admitted to the hospital in three different ways:

- Referral by general practitioner – patients who require 24-hour nursing care for a short period of time, plus some medical intervention
- Referral by district general hospital – usually elderly patients, after surgery or medical crisis, who require rehabilitation
- Referral by district nurse or health visitor – patients who require 24-hour nursing care for a short period of time, whose family needs respite from caring.

The Nurses

Primary nursing principles can be adapted to work within the confines of a cash limited service. All managers have to live within their resources and few units are fortunate enough to have the optimum ratio of professional staff to patients. The implementation and evolution of primary nursing takes time. Managerial decisions have to be made on various fronts; the size of case loads, the minimum number of nurses required on duty at any one time, consideration of the fluctuations in workload, skill mix and whether or not ancillary workers are available to relieve nurses of non-nursing tasks. At Didcot we now have a part-time ward clerk and volunteers who, for example, help make the beds, thereby increasing the time that nurses can spend with their patients.

Establishment and Skill Mix

One of my greatest reservations about introducing primary nursing was the relatively small size of our nursing establishment, along with the high ratio of unqualified staff. When we first began we had a very different structure than we have today (figure 14.1(a)).

There were three primary nurses, each responsible for a case load of ten patients, and linked to one of the GP surgeries. The idea was to orientate each group of GPs to 'their' primary nurse, and thus improve communication and co-operation.

From experience, we soon discovered that this system had two drawbacks. Firstly, one of the surgeries admitted more patients than the others, which led to an unbalanced workload, and cynicism from the doctors, who were yet to be convinced by our new system! Secondly, the primary nurses could not manage a case load of ten patients. After much discussion, we split the nurses into two groups, with case loads of seven or eight patients each, but found that this was still unsatisfactory (figure 14.1(b)). Our patients are all typically elderly and very dependent; coupled with this, the primary nurses also acted as associate nurses for their colleagues and staffed our minor casualty unit from the ward. Thus we developed our third structure (figure 14.1(c)). The case load of five patients was manageable and the nurses had more time for the psychological aspects of care. This structure has recently changed again (figure 14.1(d)) because of an increase in the number of trained staff.

A major managerial problem not anticipated when we increased the number of primary nurses was that of the Clinical Grading Review. Having increased the ratio of primary nurses, I had to state my case for sufficient F grades to reward them. It must be difficult for senior management, who are struggling to achieve parity across the region, to understand all the local idiosyncrasies that influence the primary

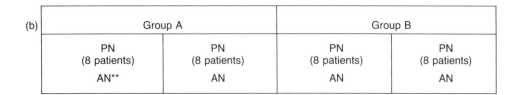

Fig. 14.1 The evolution of our primary nursing structure: PN, primary nurse; AN, associate
nurse; * ward sister; ** clinical practice development.

nursing structure. One would assume that, by directly comparing two community
hospitals of similar size, one would be able to standardise skill mix ratios, but this is
not necessarily the case. There are many variables, not least those caused by the
dynamic evolution of primary nursing (Table 14.1). A good example of case load
management, influenced by the gradual change in skill mix at Didcot, concerned
one of our primary nurses. Carole worked part time (27.5 hours) but wished to
increase her hours to 34 (the minimum we would expect for a primary nurse). The
problem was at the time we still had too many nursing auxiliaries; therefore we had
to wait for someone to leave (natural wastage) before we could change our skill mix
and transfer the hours to Carole. In the meantime, it was decided that she would
still take on a case load of four or five patients, but in view of her hours they would
all be long-stay patients. This enabled Carole to keep up to date with her care
plans, as the majority of the problems tended to be of a long-term nature. The
rationale behind our primary nurses working a minimum of 34 hours is that they are
then on duty for 5 days a week, thus improving continuity of care. This is essential
when the condition of acutely sick patients changes rapidly and decisions about
their appropriate care have to be made on a daily basis.

Table 14.1 The unit nursing establishment

Establishment	Proposed grade	Whole time equivalents
Hospital manager	I	1.00
CPD nurse	H	1.00
Day sister	G	1.00
Night sister	F	0.59
Primary nurse	F	4.60
Associate nurse	E	3.65
Nursing auxiliaries	A	10.90
		22.74

The Multidisciplinary Team

Medical staff are not resident, but are available for consultation by phone. We have a part-time occupational therapist who works for 15 hours a week and has an untrained helper. The Physiotherapy Department provides a full outpatient service, but unfortunately only 2 hours of in-patient physiotherapy a week. A chiropodist, dietician and speech therapist are available for consultation, although they are based in a neighbouring town. The hospital's social worker is based at Didcot, but works for only 18 hours per week and also has responsibility for three other local hospitals.

The Organisation of Primary Nursing: A Change in Routine

Alexander *et al.*, cited in Anderson and Choi (1980) believe that 'a clear definition of primary nursing must acknowledge the organisational context that fosters and reinforces the roles and activities assumed by primary nurse'. The interdependence of nursing activities on other departments needs to be considered when planning change. One example of this has involved allowing patients choice about the time they get up in the morning. The ritualistic 6 a.m. tea round is thankfully now a thing of the past and meal times are now negotiable. The 'morning rush' to bath patients has also been reduced, as patient choice of care has increased.

Staff Development

Much emphasis has been placed by necessity on the importance of facilitating appropriate educational opportunities for staff. Many others would agree, but do they honestly put that philosophy into practice? It is not always easy to find the time to organise teaching programmes or to find the resources to let staff off the ward, but it *can* be done. Indeed it must be, if we are to make a serious attempt to improve the quality of care.

Lack of financial resources is our biggest burden, and yet funding education is our greatest weapon against the recruitment and retention problems of today. If we are to promote primary nurses as managers, I believe we must ensure that clinical practice gives value for money.

The following approaches have been found helpful in raising money for staff development:

- Apply for extra training money from the health authority. It is their duty to provide some, however little that may be. I have found that the most successful approach is to invite senior managers to visit and see for themselves what has been achieved, to develop greater interest in primary nursing.
- Keep a 'back pocket' of money set aside from other funds. This helped to supplement the training budget when it ran out in the latter part of the financial year.
- Inform staff of the trust fund bursary schemes and scholarships that are available; information can be found in the nursing press.
- Establish a trust fund into which donations from visitors and perhaps businesses may be paid. These have to be properly administered according to treasurers' and national auditors' rules.
- Explain the financial situation to your staff, so that they come to realise that they may have to meet you half way. Pointing out the costs involved in paying for fees, books, time off and travel expenses may be helpful. The UKCC Code of Professional Conduct (UKCC, 1984) states that there is a need to ' . . . take every reasonable opportunity to maintain and improve professional knowledge and competence'. Above all it is important to be fair; some staff may demand more than others.
- Conduct a regular staff appraisal. (We endeavoured to complete our staff development and performance reviews every 6 months.) This enables us to have a basis on which to assess further training needs.

Maintaining Staff Support

As well as providing resources and encouragement for staff development, it is important to maintain primary nursing by the provision of adequate staff support. Stress may be derived from many sources (see chapter 13). Some of these are described below together with managerial attempts to tackle them.

'Bureaucratic Hassle'

The contact between the primary nurse and the staff of ancillary services such as the central sterilising supply department, pharmacy, catering and domestic services may expose them regularly to the distractions of bureaucratic red tape, adding to the frustrating struggle with priorities. The manager may help to reduce this kind of stress by handling these contacts more efficiently and by arranging an extra supply of linen, dealing with the works department, and ensuring that the necessary equipment is available and in working order. I have already mentioned the appropriate use of clerical staff, for filing and the phone, but we have also found that nursing time can be saved by extending their role to stocking up the ward supplies. Domestic staff, too, can be a great help, for example by making relatives tea or fetching flower vases.

The Anxieties of Peer Relationships

The primary nurse has 24-hour accountability for her group of patients throughout their hospital stay. The stress of this was found to be compounded because the primary nurse did not trust the nurses who cared for her patients in her absence. Effort has been made to use every opportunity to foster trusting relationships throughout the staff and promptly to resolve any misunderstanding or conflicts that could undermine mutual confidence.

Another area of stress related to peer relationships concerns the blatant disregard of care plans by some associate nurses. Often, the time and energy spent by a primary nurse in developing a plan seemed pointless, resulting in frustration and resentment. When conflicts like this arose, it was imperative that the nursing manager supported the primary nurse and clarified the role and responsibilities of each nurse once again. All staff needed to understand clearly the responsibilities of their own role and how it fitted in with those of the rest of the team.

The primary nurse provides total care for her patient and has in-depth knowledge of their current response to treatment. Frequently she steps into an advocacy role between the patient and his doctor. Conflicting concerns or threatened egos were found to be another source of stress. An attempt was made to help the nurses to work more effectively with doctors, by serving as a role model for communication skills and assertiveness.

As primary nurses developed and adjusted to their new degree of autonomy, their confidence grew. They no longer had to funnel all information through the traditional ward sister, but communicated directly with the doctors, who in turn had learnt to appreciate the nurses' greater understanding of the patient concerned.

Mutual trust and respect evolved into what has been described as 'interdependence and collaboration practice' by Coluccio and Maguire (1983).

Managing Priorities

An additional source of stress arose from the demands of managing priorities. At Didcot, the primary nurse acted as an associate nurse for several other patients. Naturally, more time and energy were devoted into caring for her own case load and as a result staff sometimes experienced guilt over their relative neglect of the patients for whom they were acting as associate nurse. This was found to be a sensitive issue, but one that I feel needs managerial input. It was found to be important that the nurse manager or ward co-ordinator ensured that all patients felt well cared for. By speaking to patients, the nurse manager can promptly assess the situation. Rarely did the patients who were being looked after by a primary nurse other than their own feel neglected, although obviously this is a pitfall to be aware of. More often than not, such neglect is only the perception of other members of the team, who apply peer pressure to the primary nurse concerned. We have found that by discussing such matters openly at staff meetings, or informally at coffee breaks, these difficulties can be avoided.

Another problem that affected not only primary nurses, but many in our hospital team, was the loyalty conflict between work and home. This was accentuated for women when their children were ill or they had problems with their childminder. Attempts have been made to provide flexible working hours. It was not always easy, but it was definitely worth the effort.

Isolation

Although there may have to be two primary nurses on duty together each day, they work independently of each other and have separate meal breaks to ensure ward cover.

Nurses are trained to work as part of a team, but primary nursing can isolate the nurse from her peers. By being aware of such a potential stress factor, one is already half way to avoiding it. As far as possible I tried to make myself available to chat to staff informally at coffee breaks, especially when I felt that small tensions were building up or a primary nurse had a particularly stressful situation to cope with. Many patients are admitted for terminal care and the nurses give a lot of themselves to the grieving relatives. I found that a series of such patients would have a temporarily adverse effect on morale, especially if the patients had been admitted for long-term care and the families involved were well known to the team.

Intense Patient Involvement

Primary nurses tended to invest much effort and skill in the care of their patients, which can leave them emotionally vulnerable. Patients' relatives sometimes demand a great deal, especially if the patient is critically ill and they need a lot of support. One primary nurse recently admitted to me that she felt 'completely drained by a family, as though they were leeches', sometimes feeling as if she had 'nothing left to give'. Overwhelming feelings of guilt, inadequacy and failure are unfortunately common (Holmes, 1987) and the nurse manager must be prepared not only to support her staff, but also to develop counselling skills. There is a need to watch continuously for signs of stress.

Arriving at work early in the morning provided an opportunity both to see the night staff and to discuss the patients with the primary nurses before the day began. Another way which we found helpful in getting to know one another was occasionally to meet socially outside the hospital.

The Associate Nurse

The potential stress facing primary nurses has been noted (Sparrow, 1986), but little reference has been made to the other essential member of the nursing team, the associate nurse. Support is also directed towards these nurses, who sometimes perceive their role as a difficult one to come to terms with. Many associate nurses have extensive background experience and expertise and it is vital that primary nurses and managers acknowledge this.

Despite the fact that role definition and responsibility was clearly defined before the current Clinical Grading Review, many problems have since arisen. Sometimes experienced associate nurses have felt downgraded and devalued because of the grading differentials. They may well wish to take on primary responsibility, but because of family commitments be able to work only part time. Part-time hours are often incompatible with the concept of continuity in primary nursing care. However, exception has been made in certain circumstances, taking into account different client groups. The example of Carole looking after a smaller case load of long-stay patients was referred to earlier. The manager also has responsibilities to foster understanding among staff. Pembrey (1988:1) has said:

● It is necessary that the primary nurse and associate nurse understand and respect each other's contribution and communicate effectively with each other.

Evaluation

Nurses have too often tried new ideas before really analysing them. From the managerial, consumer and professional perspective, we can no longer afford to do this. We have tried to measure the effectiveness of primary nursing at Didcot. We now have a team of eight nurses who have been trained in the use of quality assurance tools, including one primary nurse who is currently training to develop research skills. (Day release is given on alternate weeks, and some financial assistance is given with books, but she has put in equal efforts on her days off and pays for her own travel expenses.)

As a hospital manager, I find that evaluation is one of my main areas of concern. With so many other responsibilities I find it difficult to devote sufficient time to this essential activity. Evaluation involved reviewing our original objectives, to see if they had been met:

● Had the quality of nursing care improved? The results of the quality assurance tools Qualpac and Nursing Audit compared favourably with those obtained before the introduction of primary nursing.
● Had the professionalism and job satisfaction of the staff improved? Morale is high and a recent survey had pleasing results. There are other positive indications, such as recruitment patterns and absenteeism rates. We continue to be fully established, with a significant decrease in both staff turnover and days lost through sickness.
● Had each staff nurse's growth and development increased? Staff have been encouraged to adopt an area of clinical specialty, developing expertise which contributes to the development of practice and the in-service training programme. The nurses became more aware of their strengths and weaknesses, and as a result asked for the appropriate training.
● Had the patients' satisfaction increased? I agree with the consensus of staff opinion that it has, but have no evidence as yet to support that view. We are planning to use a patient satisfaction questionnaire, along with a form of structured interview, in the near future.
● There is a need to look at the cost of running our system of primary nursing and

compare it with other systems. Are we producing equal quality care for less money or better care for the same money? Data from the Körner Report (1982) may be of more use in the future.

● There is also the question of whether the primary nursing system has achieved stability. One sign that this has already happened is that nurses become frustrated when they cannot perform their primary nursing responsibilities. Another is that patients ask for 'their' nurse by name. But perhaps the most significant test is yet to come: when the change agent leaves, will primary nursing continue?

Staff Appraisal

Efforts have been made to ensure that our staff evaluation is continuous and consistent with the hospital's primary nursing philosophy. Self-awareness is an important part of professional practice and attempts are made to encourage nurses to evaluate themselves and to help set their own goals. Informal feedback from other members of the team helps to give insight into a nurse's capabilities, and peer review of both strengths and weaknesses has been encouraged. When evaluating staff, an attempt has been made to avoid focusing on personality characteristics, appearance and work habits; instead the focus has been on their nursing ability in areas such as assessment, planning, emotional support of patients, knowledge and application, skills, documentation and leadership.

The successful practice of primary nursing is heavily reliant on effective managerial practices. Managers are needed to provide the organisational facilities for the practice of primary nursing, in terms of resources, skill mix and allocation of appropriate case loads. Skills of facilitation and support and the ability to motivate are required to enable nurses to develop their own potential in order to provide high-quality care for patients. The implications for the nurse manager's role are vast. The stamina and enthusiasm required will soon fade unless the manager motivates her staff as Herzberg (1968: 22) has said:

● I can charge a man's battery, and then recharge it, and recharge it again. But it is only when he has his own generator that we can talk about motivation. He then needs no outside stimulation. He *wants* to do it.

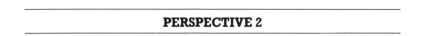

PERSPECTIVE 2

This section, written by Shirley Williams, examines primary nursing from the point of view of a director of nursing services for a hospital providing acute services.

Effect on Nurse Managers at Different Levels

The director of nursing services is responsible for creating the conditions for primary nursing through her work with nurse managers at all levels. Primary nursing requires a different style of management, which involves changes in the role of all nurse managers.

Sister/Charge Nurse

One of the most important elements of the sister's role is to lead her primary nurses in standard setting and in personally monitoring the standards of care on her ward. She must ensure that a system exists which protects patients from any possible aberrations on the part of a primary nurse. These must be challenged, and peer group reviews must take place.

For primary nursing to be successful, patient care management and resource management must rest at the same level in the organistion. Thus, as leader of her primary nurses, the ward sister must have authority over the nursing resources available for her ward.

The sister is responsible for informing the primary nurse of the resources available to support the nursing care of her case load. The primary nurse is then able to make an informed choice with the support of her ward sister, with regard to what care her patient must receive, in the event of a shortage of resources.

Night Sister

The role of the night sister has been radically altered with primary nursing. She moves from being a supervisor of tasks and deployer of staff, and becomes a source of professional support to associate nurses working at night. Associate nurses will need help in resolving unforeseen problems that arise, the most common being an acute staffing crisis caused by sickness. The night sister will need to negotiate help from a ward which is better staffed than the one with the problem, or in the event of the shortage being hospital-wide she will need to assist those nurses who are available to reassess their priorities. In addition, acute hospitals in particular need a site manager who can assume responsibility for overall co-ordination in the event of a fire or major disaster.

Nursing Officer

Supervisory rounds are clearly unnecessary since the primary nurse has 24-hour clinical accountability for the quality of care her patients receive. The ward sister is responsible, with the primary nurse, for measuring standards of care, developing the nurses and the efficient organisation of resources. Once each sister is responsible for ensuring effective deployment of manpower, the traditional role of the nurse 'on for the hospital' as being a redeployer of staff to fill gaps no longer exists.

Thus a tier of nurse management both on day duty and on night duty is freed from administration and supervision and becomes available both to support developing primary nurses and perhaps to undertake research and development work.

Director of Nursing Services

The management of a service in which responsibility for decision making has been devolved to the individual practitioner calls for considerably different skills from those needed by a bureaucratic administrator. The director of nursing services (DNS) is not only a change agent within nursing, but must also seek to bring about a cultural shift in the attitudes of the hospital management group as a whole.

In most instances, the DNS will be managing a developing service. Most wards will probably be somewhere along the continuum from task allocation to primary nursing.

To create a framework within which nursing throughout the hospital can move forward, the DNS will need to state clearly that she herself is committed to the concept and practice of primary nursing.

Devolving Responsibility

A sound knowledge of the principles of change management will be needed, as well as skills as a group leader.

During the developmental phase sisters will need the opportunity to clarify their own ideas and air their anxieties, and it helps if this experience takes place collectively so that a supportive environment is created. The skill with which the DNS facilitates this group's deliberations will have a crucial effect on the professional development within the nursing team. Once a strong supportive peer group of sisters exists, it is this group which must take on responsibility for agreeing hospital-wide nursing policies. This development must be overtly supported by the DNS and should be seen by her as a mark of her success in helping the sisters towards their professional goal.

A constructive peer group, with a clear organisational goal, will provide a source of support and encouragement for members who are experiencing difficulties, but at the same time it will ensure that any inappropriate behaviour on the part of one of its members is not allowed to sabotage the collective move forward. There is a considerable difference between a ward being supported in moving at its own pace, however slow that may be, and in allowing a ward to refuse to accept responsibility, the effect of which is that the more developed wards are penalised. For instance, either all ward sisters accept responsibility for staff deployment and for devising strategies for coping with short-term staffing crises, or there will be a problem between the wards which do accept that level of responsibility and those which do not. The latter may assume that staff from other wards will be redeployed to cope with their short-term problems. The DNS's role is to support this group through periods of stress and tension and to ensure that all members play their full part. She will need to ensure that an agreed record is kept of all policy decisions and she may need to remind the group from time to time of decisions which have been taken.

From Supervisor to Support Nurse

Many sisters have become deskilled in the art of resource management and this, coupled with the notion that management has nothing to do with clinical care, may mean that some sisters feel that 'I am responsible for the care of my patients, and 'they' are responsible for ensuring that I have the resources to deliver it'. This issue must be reviewed at a very early stage, for, unless the sister accepts responsibility for managing the resources available for her ward, clinical practice will be unable to develop. However, the DNS must not assume that the sisters' acceptance of responsibility necessarily indicates an ability to carry it out. The sisters will almost certainly need practical help in resource management, and in the development of quality assessment tools and workload assessment tools.

Hopefully, the nursing officers or clinical nurse managers will have skills in this area which the DNS can recognise and develop. The realisation that they are needed to support the sisters will help the displaced nursing officers to make the transition in their own role, from supervisor to support nurse.

In primary nursing, the DNS ceases to be the supervisor of the competencies with which procedures are executed, and takes on the much more demanding role of professional advisor to her nurses. The move from 'safe' procedures to individual decision making in a developing profession needs careful support and considered management.

The DNS will need to ensure that nurses recognise that they belong to a multidisciplinary team. It is important that primary nurses do not lose sight of the fact that nursing is one element of patient care and, in some instances, may not necessarily be the major element. Unilateral decision making is not possible, nor is it appropriate. For example, the issue of self-medication by patients is complex. The primary nurse may feel that an important part of her patient's therapy is for him to assume responsibility for his own drugs, but such a decision does not rest with the nurse alone and the legitimate views of the prescribing doctor and dispensing pharmacist must be considered. The DNS must ensure that the issue is thoroughly discussed with everyone involved, and a clear protocol must be agreed before any nursing change is introduced.

As primary nurses develop their relationship with their patients, they may take on the role of patient advocate. Although this is laudable in theory, nurses need great maturity and considerable knowledge of the rules governing their practice and that of other professionals if they are to avoid putting themselves at risk.

Nurses may also experience tension as a result of being both a professional and an employee if, for instance, the health authority that employs her decides to make a strategic shift in its health care priorities to the detriment, in her view, of the service the primary nurse is providing. For example, if the Health Authority decides to move away from providing long-term care for the elderly, this may be in fundamental conflict with the views of a primary nurse who is deeply committed to the concept of long-term care of the elderly within an NHS setting. Clearly, the primary nurse must voice her professional views and concerns, but at the end of the day she is an employee and, as such, her employer has expectations of her. The DNS will need to point out that the Authority will decide its priorities and the nurse will then be in the position of either accepting them or moving to a district whose priorities accord with her own.

The DNS has an important role in helping the primary nurses in their relationships with other disciplines, particularly in ensuring that she herself behaves in such a way as to educate others about the role of the primary nurse. The DNS may well have to intervene when other team members refuse to allow others to relate to her appropriately. Any interdisciplinary disagreement needs to be resolved by the primary nurse and the 'other' *with the support of* the DNS, not *by* the DNS on behalf of the primary nurse.

Effects of Primary Nursing on Members of Other Disciplines

Since there are many members of the nursing profession who have limited understanding of the developing understanding of the nature of nursing work, it is hardly surprising that the majority of those who are not nurses still think of nursing as being made up of tasks, undertaken in support of medical activity.

Members of other disciplines may regard the development of primary nursing as simply an attempt by nurses to extend their own sphere of control to the detriment of other professionals.

The devolution of authority and responsibility for decision making which comes with primary nursing can in itself cause problems for members of other disciplines. In a bureaucratic system there is one clear contact person, who both has authority to make agreements with others and is responsible for informing all nurses of changes in policies and in turn for ensuring that nursing practice accords with the agreed policies. In the past many nurses were willing to act as messengers for others, which of course made life relatively easy for the other people concerned. For instance, the duty nurse was often the recipient of all incoming telephone calls, and the loss of that role means that the switchboard operator now has to enquire which ward or department the caller needs and to contact them appropriately.

Allied Professions

The primary nurse's belief in holistic care may cause problems for the organisation of the physiotherapy and occupational therapy services. In the days of task allocation it was often the nurse's role to ensure that her patient was ready to receive his 'therapy' at the appropriate time. This therapy mainly took place between either 9.00 a.m. and 12.30 p.m. or 2.00 p.m. and 5.30 p.m. on Monday to Friday, and was usually scheduled at the convenience of the therapy department rather than in accordance with the patient's day. Since neither physiotherapy nor occupational therapy departments are designed to offer routine care outside office hours (although of course an 'on call' service is provided), the limits to the availability of their service imposes constraints on the primary nurse and tensions may ensue.

Support Services

The 'piece rate' approach to support services, in particular in such areas as cleaning and laundry, may mean that the objective of the manager of these services in respect to their ability to achieve 'efficiency savings' runs directly counter to the primary nurse's planning of her patient's day. The support services manager may wish to organise the cleaning of the ward floors sequentially, moving from one end of the hospital to the other. The nurses, on the other hand, will wish to have their ward floors cleaned at a time that suits the activities of their patients. The DNS will need to raise the issue with the support services manager; if, however, comparative costings show that the nurses' required cleaning pattern is more expensive than the sequential proposal, the matter will need to be taken to The Unit Executive. The DNS will need to argue her case in an attempt to persuade the Unit Executive to take a patient-centred rather than a finance-driven decision. However, it may be that to adopt the more costly option other cuts will have to be made. If this proves to be the case, the DNS will be forced to decide on the lesser of the two evils and will need to justify her decision to the nurses subsequently. Should the sequential option be decided on, the DNS must ensure that the Unit Executive is kept aware of the effects on patients of that pattern of cleaning.

Hospital Doctors

The move from task-orientated to patient-centred nursing practice is likely to have great effect on the primary nurse's relationship with her medical colleagues. The very individualised nature of the care which the primary nurse is planning may be incompatible in some ways with exclusively disease-determined treatment programmes. No longer does the care plan primarily state procedures to be undertaken, but instead it reflects the needs of the patient, taking into account the fact that he has undergone a specific medical or surgical treatment. Medical staff may feel that the primary nurse devalues medical activity because the high status accorded to activity in support of medicine in the task-orientated system may not necessarily be reflected in primary nursing. However, because paramedical activities are often of immediate consequence to the patient, medical staff may fear that the apparent devaluing of such activities by the primary nurse could result in their neglect, to the detriment of the patient. It is important for the DNS to ensure that the primary nurses recognise this anxiety in their medical colleagues. Also, there is a need to ensure that the nurses themselves acknowledge their legitimate role and responsibility in assisting with medical treatment and investigations.

The change in the role of the ward sister which comes about as a result of primary nursing may well be problematic for the medical staff because, in the past, the sister's prime role was to ensure that medical instructions were carried out to the letter. The sister was also the main nursing contact for the consultant at ward level and he felt confident that all he had to do was to leave instructions with her and they would be carried out. In fact, of course, this situation had changed long before the advent of primary nursing and the change had come about as a result of both the reduction of the sister's working week and the decreased length of stay of patients, so that it became possible for a patient to be admitted and discharged without even seeing the sister. The response of many consultants to this dilemma was interesting in that they demanded more than one sister. The primary nurse may not be seen by them as a suitable replacement for the sister. This may be partly due to there being more than one primary nurse caring for their patients, but is more probably because the role of the primary nurse bears little resemblance to that of the old sister, being patient centred rather than doctor centred.

Communications can be greatly improved if the sister ensures that nursing duty rotas are planned in such a way as to ensure that the appropriate primary nurses are on duty at the time of their consultants' medical rounds.

It is clearly important that medical staff know who is caring for their patients at any time and whether or not that nurse is in a primary or associate role. Doctors must know with whom to discuss their patients and to whom changes in treatment should be conveyed, and they must have confidence that appropriate prescriptions will be carried out. Once such basic trust has been established, the primary nurse–doctor relationship can shift towards being more of a partnership. The DNS has a vital role to play in the management of this fundamental change in relationships. She may have to be prepared to play the role of interpreter of doctors' real fears and prejudices to the nurses and vice versa.

The medical staff will almost certainly lack factual information about primary nursing, and the DNS will need to be prepared to run formal information-giving sessions with groups of consultants when appropriate. For instance, the medical staff may assume that the primary nurse is a staff nurse, the nursing equivalent of the houseman, and the DNS needs to spend time explaining to doctors both the knowledge base necessary to become a primary nurse and the level of account-ability that such nurses assume.

An equally important part of the DNS's role is to ensure that nurses appreciate the anxieties and difficulties that medical staff experience. It is essential that the sister shares information with her consultants about the stage of development her ward has reached. Many consultants relate to more than one ward (or even hospital) and can become very confused by the different organisational arrange-ments they meet.

Primary Nursing in the Era of General Management

The DNS needs to adopt an educative role in her Unit Executive with regard to primary nursing. Unit Executive members may have considerable difficulty in accepting the concept of primary nursing because it is almost certain that most of them will share the common perception that the NHS exists to support the medical care of patients. If the general manager perceives the medical consultants' exercise of their clinical freedom as being the source of most of his problems, he may view with alarm the increasing developments towards primary nursing, for he may see them as evidence of yet another group of staff exerting their professional influence and, consequently, fear the threat of this getting out of control. The DNS will need to convince the general manager that primary nursing is being undertaken as a rational way of improving patient care and not a means whereby nurses can indulge in professional aggrandisement. The general manager needs to understand the advantages that primary nursing brings.

Advantages of Primary Nursing: A Management Point of View

Resource Utilisation

Not only is the task-orientated method of organising nursing entirely discredited from a clinical point of view, but it is no longer managerially viable. Such an approach is simply not capable of responding to an increasing workload at a time of diminishing manpower, because the only response nurses working in such a system can offer is to attempt to perform an increasing number of tasks at an ever-accelerating pace. The carrying out of rote behaviour may in itself diminish mental effort, and thus the appropriateness or efficacy of the activity is never challenged.

There is often an automatic assumption that there is a whole series of tasks that need to be undertaken and the sole objective becomes the completion of them, a situation which may create a near infinite demand for nursing time.

Primary nursing, on the other hand, begins by assessing the unique nursing needs of each person and moves on to assess priorities and identify the appropriate actions that need to be taken. Thus it ensures that only those activities which each patient actually needs are undertaken. From a resource management point of view, the question moves from 'how quickly can we taken the temperature of all the patients in the ward?' to 'which patients' temperatures do we need to monitor and how frequently?'

With primary nursing there is a greater likelihood that nursing activity is carefully reflected upon, and thus expensive, wasteful, folklore-based practice and rote behaviour can be minimised if not eradicated. The devolution of authority and responsibility for decision making which comes with primary nursing means that each nurse's abilities are used to the full. Decision making, like any other skill, develops with practice, and the creative thinking and clinical innovation which is stifled by bureaucratic control is liberated by primary nursing and flourishes in an environment of professional practice, thereby increasing the total amount of available resources.

Developing Standards of Care

The primary nurse may feel more comfortable with qualitative rather than quantitative objectives for outcomes of care. However, this may be seen as idealistic and lacking in credibility by a general manager who has instructions to reduce a waiting list, and a conflict will result. If, however, nurses are prepared to accept that the general manager has finite cash and limited resources and to join with their medical colleagues in informing him how much work can be undertaken and to what standard within the resources available, they will have the opportunity of moving the service away from being led by medical demand and towards a more balanced service, catering for all patients' health care needs. The establishment of multidisciplinary resource management teams made up of the doctors and nurses responsible for the same group of patients has potential advantages both for the general manager and for nurses.

Workload agreements are invaluable to the nurse in her constant battle to provide a professionally acceptable standard of nursing care. A demand-led system generates unplanned peaks in workload which have the effect of arbitrarily depressing standards of care. Medical activities are often the patient's first need and consequently they are commonly undertaken to the exclusion of all others, with the effect that the nursing element of care is lost. Nurses are often aware of patients' unmet health needs, typically of a non-medical nature, but may receive little or no support from their medical colleagues when they seek to address the problem. Indeed, in the short term, nurses coping in such circumstances may actually receive praise from medical staff because the nursing procedures in support of medical activity are still being undertaken. However, if such a situation continues for any length of time, nurse–doctor relationships will become confrontational and nursing morale will collapse.

A multidisciplinary resource management situation, on the other hand, provides a forum for joint professional decision making and prioritisation by both doctors and nurses. As a result of working together, both develop a much deeper understanding of each other's working philosophy. Doctors begin to move from the 'rent-a-nurse' idea borne of task allocation and, instead, a constructive debate takes place about what standards can be achieved with the nursing hours available. The sister moves from being a mere responder to a medically created workload and becomes a proactive manager who is able to play a full part in agreeing care priorities.

Conclusion

Once acceptable standards of care have been agreed, it becomes possible to make statements about the number of nursing hours which are likely to be needed to care for a given group of patients. Thus establishment setting ceases to be a top down 'nurse per bed formula' exercise and becomes a statement of probable need for nursing which is derived bottom up from the care needs of patients. For the first time, general managers have a professional nursing group which is able to give them advice on resource requirements based on statements of care needs.

Finally, a deepening awareness of the managerial implications of primary nursing may help to create the conditions which foster improved standards of care.

15

Power and Communication Issues in Primary Nursing

Richard McMahon

INTRODUCTION: THE CONCEPT OF POWER

The innovation of primary nursing is of great significance for both the occupation and, in particular, for clinical nurses within it. As a system, primary nursing is not just concerned with altering lines of authority and enhancing autonomy for the practising nurse. It is also making a statement about the autonomy of the occupation as a whole. The underlying concept which explains these phenomena is that of power. The purpose of this chapter is to put primary nursing in perspective by examining the alterations in power relations that its implementation involves. This may seem highly abstract, but the ideas are simple and an understanding of primary nursing at this level can be crucial to its effective implementation in practice. It is through an appreciation of these issues that the nurse involved in primary nursing can gain an insight into the complexities of the communication patterns she sees around her.

The idea of 'power' is something about which we all feel we have some experience and understanding, yet we rarely consider the meaning of the word. The sociologist Weber defined power as:

● . . . the probability that one actor within a social relationship will be in a position to carry his own will despite resistance, regardless of the basis on which that probability rests. (Weber, 1947: 152)

This definition makes it clear that the exercising of power is an intentional, rather than an accidental, act. However, the wielding of power may, of course, create unintended effects around the power holder. People or organisations need not use power all the time, but we acknowledge that potentially they may do so; this is expressed when we say that they 'have' power. Also, the choice not to act can be as influential as the actual wielding of power. Power then is a simple concept, and it is one which is often used in relation to different occupations. For example, the so-called professions have power over their members and their clients as well as having influence at national and governmental levels. Within occupations, power is determined by such factors as the organisational level and the knowledge of its practitioners. Primary nursing raises issues in many of these areas and has implications for the modes of communication inside and outside the occupation. However, before these issues can be addressed, it is useful to examine the origins of primary nursing in terms of the frequently expressed goal of professionalisation.

THE RISE OF PRIMARY NURSING

The development of primary nursing is frequently seen as the culmination of a natural progression from task allocation through patient allocation and team nursing. The reason for this movement is often expressed in terms of the philosophical or conceptual values that primary nursing embodies, such as the intrinsic value of the nurse–patient relationship or the emphasis on consistent individualised care. However, a different interpretation is often put on those developments in nursing, namely that innovations such as the nursing process or primary nursing are steps towards, or characteristics of, the professionalisation of nursing. This claimed professionalisation is not merely a side-effect of these systems, but was a motivating force in their formulation and adoption. For example, Manthey in her textbook on primary nursing (1980) claims that the movement of the focus of nursing practice away from the home to the hospital resulted in the deprofessionalisation of the occupation. She states that:

● To regain the element of professionalism nursing once had it is necessary to create a *delivery* system that lives up to the expectations created by contemporary education and facilitates professional practice. That system is primary nursing. (Manthey, 1980: 12)

The spread of a new idea such as primary nursing is hastened by the support it gains from the leaders in nursing. For example, the Chief Nurse at the Department of Health, Anne Poole, revealed at the first national ward sisters' conference in Manchester in 1987 that it was her ambition for every in-patient to have a named nurse responsible for the patient's care alongside the medical consultant. Similarly influential bodies such as the Royal College of Nursing have organised conferences on the subject. Clearly support from this level does not come without careful examination of the political and interprofessional repercussions of the adoption of any new idea. How then might primary nursing fit into a strategy to professionalise nursing? To understand this, it is first necessary to consider the concept of a 'profession'.

OCCUPATIONS, PROFESSIONALISATION AND AUTONOMY

Sociology has provided a number of different ways of looking at professions and professionalisation. The most common of these is the 'trait' approach, in which it is assumed that certain occupations are typical 'professions'. It is then argued that common factors of these occupations can be identified and the traits or defining factors of professions in general isolated. Professionalisation can then be viewed as the process of acquiring these traits. Many lists of such factors have been drawn up by different academics; however, Millerson (1964) examined a large number of these and could not find one item that appeared on all of them. This absence of a finite list of attributes might suggest a considerable failure to agree by theorists. The trait approach has been criticised by Johnson (1972) for its assumption that some occupations may be unquestioningly labelled as professions, and that from those common factors can be isolated. Also the lack of a theoretical framework to link these concepts results in traits which are not mutually exclusive and which are sometimes derived one from the other. Regardless of these weaknesses, this is the framework most often used to judge whether nursing is a profession; and it is a judgement which nursing usually fails (e.g. Lembright, 1983; Chapman, 1977b).

A different way of considering the 'professions' is to adopt the approach used by Parsons (1957) when he described the medical profession. This way of looking at the professions has been called the 'functional' approach. Again, common characteristics are identified; however, in this case only those relating to professional *behaviour* and how this relates to either the client or to society are isolated. The kind of factor identified by Parsons was, for example, the fact that when doctors are examining a member of the opposite sex they concentrate on the process of making a diagnosis rather than any sexual purpose. Similarly, doctors are expected to work for the benefit of those with the greatest need regardless of their nationality or other characteristics (e.g. in a battle). However, such notions may be regarded as idealistic, because occupations such as medicine and law are not found in high concentration where greatest need exists, such as in the inner cities.

Having rejected the first two approaches, Johnson (1972) presented a third in which he redefined professionalism in terms of occupation control, which he relates to the producer–consumer relationship. He suggests that 'a profession is not, then, an occupation, but a means of controlling an occupation' (Johnson, 1972: 45). Johnson sees professional control occurring in a subgroup of those occupations in which the producer (e.g. the solicitor) determines the needs of the consumer (the client). He suggests that this occupational authority occurs only when there is considerable demand for the services of the occupation from a large, widespread population of consumers. The relationship is one of trust, based on a one-to-one relationship in which the consumer usually approaches the professional in the first instance, but which is terminated by the professional.

Autonomy is a concept that links the different ways of looking at the professions. It is a characteristic commonly identified under the trait approach and is crucial in the relationship between an occupation and both society and its client group in the functionalist approach. In Johnson's work, control of an occupation by its own members is a characteristic of the type of control that he describes as professional. Autonomy of occupations may be identified on two different levels (figure 15.1). At the macro level, the autonomy of the occupation may relate to independence from government (both in finance and governance) and also from other occupations. At the second, or micro, level it is the autonomy of the practitioner which is considered. This may relate to autonomy from bureaucratic control, other occupations and also from practitioners from the individual's own occupation. Therefore it could be argued that nursing must attain autonomy at both these levels if it is to fulfil the goal of professionalisation held by many in the occupation.

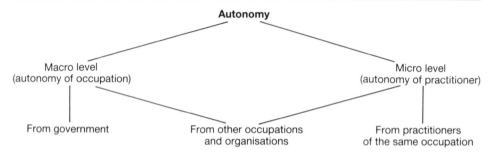

Fig. 15.1 Autonomy of occupations.

AUTONOMY IN NURSING

Autonomy in nursing has been defined as:

● freedom to make discretionary and binding decisions consistent with one's scope of practice and freedom to act on those decisions. (Batey and Lewis, 1982)

Although this definition was aimed at the individual practitioner, the definition may equally be applied to nursing as an occupation.

To attain autonomy at the macro level, nursing appears to have adopted a number of strategies. For example, the governing body of nursing, the UKCC, is making efforts to ensure that the occupation achieves many of the traits identified for professions. The UKCC is working for financial autonomy through the charging of periodic registration fees for all qualified nurses. It has issued a code of professional conduct, has taken responsibility for the disciplining of members of the occupation, and has attempted to upgrade education through Project 2000 (UKCC, 1986) – although Salvage (1988a) also questions whether professionalisation is the goal that this reform is leading to. However, nursing is not only working for autonomy at the macro level through self-governance. The development of 'nursing beds' in clinical nursing units (Pearson, 1983) is an attempt to demonstrate that nursing has a defined area of practice alongside, but separate from, medicine. Nursing beds are those to which patients are admitted by nurses under the care of nurses, rather than medical practitioners. In such a unit it is the nurse, not the doctor, who is accountable for the overall care of the patients, and as such represents a new provision within the health-care system in the UK (Pearson, 1988a).

Batey and Lewis (1982) suggests that autonomy for the individual (the micro level) is attained firstly through the willingness of the nurse to accept the autonomy and consequential accountability, and secondly through the organisational struc-ture in which she finds herself. It is at this point that the full implications of primary nursing can be appreciated. Primary nursing presents a radical lateral management structure which facilitates the exercising of individual autonomy by qualified nurses in the ward setting, which markedly contrasts with the traditional ward hierarchy and the divided hierarchy provided by team nursing.

POWER AND THE WARD MANAGEMENT STRUCTURE

Hierarchies such as those found on many wards demonstrate characteristics of hierarchies found in industry and most bureaucracies. Power is vested in the person at the top of the hierarchy who can influence the behaviour of all those below him or her. It most wards this is the ward sister who, although she is the centre of knowledge and communication on the ward (Pembrey, 1980), is necessarily remote from direct patient care. However, she controls the care patients receive by issuing orders which are passed down the hierarchy to the care givers. Where those care givers are the untrained or learners, they cannot function without clear guidance from above. Equally, the decision maker at the top needs data to fulfil her role, so information is passed up from the direct care givers to the nurse in charge.

Primary nursing presents a structure in which the care planner and principal care giver are the same person. The previous hierarchy must be dismantled and replaced with the new structure, as it would seem that attempts to superimpose one on top of the other leads to compromise of the underlying principles. It could be argued that the need for a nurse in overall charge of clinical care (e.g. the ward sister) is not a necessity in primary nursing, and in some areas the structure has been implemented without one (e.g. the Oxford Nursing Development Unit; Pearson, 1988a). Under primary nursing, knowledge and authority (that is, the legitimate exercising of power) is centred on the person who knows the patient best, that is, the primary nurse. That nurse has autonomy over the nursing care for her patients and is accountable for the quality of care that they receive.

The difference in the power relations in reality when wards adopting different management structures are compared has been highlighted by McMahon (1987), who suggested that in hierarchical wards power is vested not in an individual but in a *position* within the organisation, with little regard to who occupies that position at any time. Therefore great importance is placed on the ward sister, or whoever is in charge of the ward at any given time (traditionally that person holds the ward keys). Under primary nursing the position or qualifications held become of lesser importance. Instead, *individuals* become the centre of knowledge and hence the centre of power for those whom they nurse. Enquiries are passed on to the nurse who *knows* the patient, with the perceived rank of that individual within the organisation being of lesser consideration. Of course, accountability of primary nurses is on a 24-hours, 7-days-a-week basis, and so it may be that the off-duty primary nurse is contacted rather than any of the nurses on the ward making a major decision.

This chapter started by identifying professionalisation as one of the frequently expressed reasons for adopting primary nursing. Others are the 'philosophical' reasons relating to beliefs in the nurse–patient relationship or the nature of professional practice. However, nursing is not unique in moving to a lateral management structure, and a third reason may be identified by examining industry. Burns and Stalker (1966) looked at different companies in the electronics industry. They noticed two broad categories or types of management evident in those companies. The first was a hierarchical or mechanistic structure, which seemed to be most appropriate for those companies working in relatively stable conditions.

The second was a lateral or organic structure which was characterised by knowledge being spread through the organisation, with individuals being given the authority to act in their own area, yet working with an appreciation of the objectives of the organisation as a whole. This system seemed to be more suitable for environments characterised by unpredictability and change. It may be that this situation can be extrapolated to the development of lateral ward management structures in nursing.

For example, under task allocation and the more sedate throughput and technology in the 1950s and 1960s, routine and predictability seemed to be the goal and the norm of practice. However, with the advent of the nursing process and patient autonomy, along with the rise of high-technology medicine, there is a need for a system that can respond to constant change and unplanned occurrences. Primary nursing may be such a system.

THE PRIMARY NURSE AND OTHER HEALTH CARE PROFESSIONALS

Medicine has developed increasing influence throughout the health care arena over many years, including taking on responsibility for areas previously outside its influence, such as obstetric care. By keeping an esoteric body of knowledge and restricting access to registration as a medical practitioner, medicine has increased its power and control, for which it has been severely criticised (e.g. Illich, 1977). Friedson (1970) described this professional dominance in detail and suggested that at that time medicine was the only autonomous occupation in health care as it controlled the practice of all the others. Elsewhere he suggests that the paramedical disciplines must define or gain control of a discrete area of practice if they are to attain autonomy.

As nursing has developed and started to produce nurses with a clear concept of nursing and its boundaries, the potential for conflict with those who do not expect, understand or recognise these perspectives is heightened. For example, the doctor who recommends a type of dressing to be applied to a wound in the belief that this is his responsibility may be greeted with indignation from the nurse who believes that wound care is principally a nursing issue. The advent of primary nursing may help to strengthen the knowledge base of the nurse, and potentially increases the likelihood of conflict if the situation is mismanaged. Whereas with the hierarchical ward management system it was only the ward sister who was considered to have even the smallest right to challenge the doctor, under primary nursing the individual nurse can communicate on a care giver-to-care giver basis, with the nurse having expert knowledge of all her own patients. McMahon (1989) has suggested that, particularly in care of the elderly, the nurse can take on an advocacy role, because as primary nurse she will frequently know the patient, his family and his home environment more intimately than the doctor and hence be able to challenge decisions regarding the patient (such as discharge date) with the doctor from a position of strength (see chapter 1).

Conflict is rarely productive and can produce a backlash that results in a worse starting point than before. To prevent this, nurses must work hard to promote understanding and trust between the health care occupations. Nurses must earn respect by showing that their opinions are not based on whim or anecdotal evidence but on research or a sound theoretical knowledge base. Doctors may argue that nurses have no authority to make decisions in health care. Nurses need to show that they are willing to be accountable for those areas in which they wish to be the principal decision makers, and primary nursing makes that accountability clear. Finally, in an area where the turnover of staff in all disciplines is relatively slow, multidisciplinary seminars have been shown to be effective in helping different workers to identify their roles and how they interface with each other (Pearson *et al.*, 1985).

The use of group work benefits the relationship between nurses and other paramedical workers as well as those in medicine. Relations with these workers are also facilitated by the care giver-to-care giver relationship that primary nursing provides. Occasionally, other paramedical groups fail to acknowledge nurses as significant contributors to the therapeutic and decision-making process involved in a patient's care. This is probably a result of the medical model from which many of them are taught and the almost total lack of nursing input to their education (the reverse of nurse education, which has often welcomed contributions from physiotherapists, etc.). However, the lack of awareness of nursing that these workers may experience in their training is frequently reinforced on the ward, where even minor problems relating to the patients' care are automatically referred to the relevant paramedical worker. This would seem to be more prevalent on traditionally managed wards where the accountability for dealing with patients' problems is not vested in an individual direct care giver. There is some evidence (McMahon, 1987) that, on wards which have implemented primary nursing, nurses are more willing to identify patients' problems as ones which nurses can help to solve, and consequently deal with them without automatic recourse to the practitioner of a different occupation. However, this could be misleading in that nurses who choose to work on primary nursing wards may at this stage be those who already have a clear concept of nursing.

PRIMARY NURSING AND INTRAPROFESSIONAL COMMUNICATION

Primary nursing is not merely a cosmetic change to the nursing service on a ward in which nurses' job titles are changed. Instead it involves the taking on of completely new roles which demand different responsibilities and working practices. For example, Manthey (1973) states that the role of the senior nurse on a ward implementing primary nursing is ' . . . the factor most critical to the success of primary nursing'. Where that senior nurse was previously the ward sister, a particular effort must be made to prevent slippage into previous power relations. Primary nursing involves the devolving of knowledge and authority (and hence power and decision making) to the primary nurses (staff nurses). To some sisters this means 'letting go of the reins' of the ward and admitting to visitors and other health care workers that she is no longer the expert on all the patients on the ward. The ex-ward sister must trust her primary nurses and support them in their new role. That trust needs to be manifest, such as in allowing nurses space to make decisions, and, if necessary, to make mistakes. Clearly the senior nurse can easily trust only those in whom she has confidence, and nurses without the necessary knowledge, skills and values should not be asked to take on the accountability of a primary nursing post.

Although primary nurses are accountable for the quality of care for their own patients, the senior nurse on wards that retain such a post remains accountable for the overall quality of care on the ward. The way that this nurse may assure quality is not by controlling the care delivered to patients, as this is no longer her role. Instead, she can examine the practice and the care plans of her primary nurses and, rather than demanding that they fall in line with her own preferences, she can ask her primary nurses to give an account of the rationale behind the care given or prescribed. Where the nurse cannot give an adequate explanation based on theory or research (taking into consideration the gaps in both of these) the senior nurse may justifiably express concern regarding the care the patient is receiving. However, where the primary nurse can give an adequate account, the senior nurse should allow the primary nurse to continue unhindered, even if the nurse has chosen an intervention which the senior nurse mistrusts. The senior nurse does, however, have a responsibility to share her experiences or beliefs about the intervention to give the primary nurse the maximum amount of information on which to base her decision. As Zander (1985) pointed out, the emphasis in quality assurance under primary nursing moves away from the old model under which care is judged by the way in which it is performed. It is replaced by an emphasis on the outcome of that care. So where a patient's problem fails to respond to a specific nursing intervention, the individual responsible for that patient's care – the primary nurse – can be asked to explain her reasoning for continuing with that intervention. This should not be done in an accusing way; instead, it should be handled in a supportive atmosphere in which the individual nurse is helped to overcome a stubborn clinical problem by her colleagues.

Achieving an atmosphere which is non-threatening and supportive is essential to the successful development of primary nursing. Nurses must operate in a milieu that encourages the best care for patients and which facilitates innovation in nursing. This means allowing controlled risk-taking by primary nurses. Although there is now some guidance for nurses involved in this process (e.g. Carson, 1988), inevitably wrong decisions will occasionally be made. Where the nurse is in collaborative collegial relations with her peers it can be acknowledged that all practitioners make mistakes from time to time and a mistake can be used as a learning experience for all concerned. If, instead of this, the primary nurses watch each other and are quick to blame the nurse who makes a wrong decision or who takes a risk, creative practice will soon be stifled and nurses will make decisions based on how the care reflects on them personally, rather than on the best interests of the patient. Once again, it is up to the senior nurse to provide leadership in this and not to wield the power that she has as a result of her position in the organisation in a way characteristic of that which would be found in a hierarchical management structure.

The aim for the ward team would seem to be to achieve collegial communication networks and practices which are collaborative rather than divisive.

THE ELEMENTS OF COLLABORATIVE COLLEGIAL COMMUNICATION

The key to the successful implementation of primary nursing in practice is a genuine change from a hierarchical power structure to a lateral one in which individuals are not merely carrying out the orders of their superiors. Autonomy is, in one sense, power over oneself, and it is this freedom that may lead to increased job satisfaction for nurses (Reed, 1988). Communication within a lateral structure should not produce behaviour which is more typically found in the traditional management system. Nurses should not check up on each other in the way they often have in the past, and should not be ruling each other by dictat. Instead, the collegial communications should be collaborative. Nurses should consult one another and draw on colleagues' experience and expertise. Trust and a non-threatening atmosphere may well nurture creativity.

Beyer and Marshall (1981) identified eight elements of collegial communication, which might be found where the atmosphere is collaborative rather than divisive:

- Confidence and trust
- Mutual help
- Mutual support
- Friendliness and enjoyment
- Team efforts towards goal achievement
- Creativity
- Open communication
- Freedom from threat

In areas where primary nursing is claimed to be in practice, an absence of these elements may cause dissatisfaction and frustration among the nurses as the implicit value of the system comes into conflict with the reality of the situation.

Good collegial communications do not stop with the primary nurses. Relations between the primary and associate nurses, and with the untrained members of the team, can all embody the elements of collaborative relations. The creation of an elite of primary nurses is to deny the value of those in associate nurse roles and other members of the ward team who make a different contribution to the patients' care. It has already been suggested that autonomy can lead to heightened job satisfaction for nurses. McMahon (1987) showed that all grades of nurses on primary nursing wards can perceive collegial communication on their ward to be more collaborative than on hierarchically managed wards. It could be that this too may affect job satisfaction, and in its turn staff retention.

PRIMARY NURSING, POWER AND THE PATIENT

The final area in which power and control issues will be addressed will be in relation to the patient. The relationship between the nurse and the patient has in the past been one in which the nurse is in authority over the patient. (However, nurses were still subservient to the doctors, and Gamarnikow (1978) suggests that the way this was reinforced in schools of nursing resulted in a doctrine akin to the family; the doctor fulfilled a patriarchal role with the nurse cast as the mother and presumably the patient as the child.) However, the beliefs of theorists such as Hall (1969) are now gaining in popularity, resulting in support for a philosophy of partnership with the patient. This empowering of the patient to allow a degree of self-determination has been promoted alongside the development of primary nursing (Pearson, 1988a). Rather than keeping a complicated and inaccessible body of knowledge like the typical professions, nurses are being encouraged to share their knowledge actively with their clients in ways which can be easily understood. Although this may cast even greater doubt on the degree of professionalisation nursing can achieve at this time, it can be argued that by firstly empowering the patient and secondly acting as his advocate nurses have developed a new strategy for challenging the domination of the medical profession. It would seem that the general public are becoming less tolerant of a medical establishment which is becoming increasingly technologically advanced and dehumanising (see chapter 1). A nursing occupation which takes on the role of the people's friend is potentially a powerful force in the health-care arena of the future.

CONCLUSION

This chapter has raised discussions ranging over a wide area. It has attempted to show that primary nursing is of significance to the occupation as a whole as well as to nurses and patients at ward level.

The concepts of power and communication are linked; alterations in the latter are influenced by the former, and any move to primary nursing must involve genuine changes towards a laterally devolved power base. When operating correctly, primary nursing results in new relationships among nurses as well as with their patients and other disciplines. The acquisition of power is often viewed pejoratively, but in reality this is not necessarily so. The move to primary nursing is about acquiring and sharing power; I believe that in this case it is for a constructive purpose that will benefit patients and nurses alike.

16

Educational Implications

of Primary Nursing

Sarah Burns

This chapter seeks to outline the broad topics under discussion in nursing education today and to apply them to the issues raised by primary nursing. The chapter will also discuss the educational implications in relation to the following: the learning environment, current RGN learners, mentors to RGN learners, nurse teachers and ward sisters (see also chapter 3).

CURRENT TOPICS IN NURSING EDUCATION

The UKCC report *Project 2000* (UKCC, 1986) as its recommendations progress, now with Government support, is potentially one of the most radical innovations for nursing seen in the last 40 years (Clarke, 1986). The recommendations held with the *Project 2000* report could change dramatically the face of nursing education. It is relevant therefore to examine some of the proposals as they affect primary nursing.

One of the basic tenets in the report is that future nurse education must seek to prepare nurses who can and will respond to a changing society's demands. Nursing will have to respond to demographic changes, which include both a reduced birth rate resulting in fewer young adults coming into the employment market, and the increasing longevity of the population in general (*Project 2000*, Chapter 2). Nurses are often unwilling to change and find difficulty in undergoing change (see chapter 2). The antics of Sister Plume in the *Nursing Times* bear witness to reluctance among many nurses to consider innovations openly. The recommendation from *Project 2000* involves equipping the future nurse not only with the ability to be part of change but also with the personal willingness to participate. The amount of change described by recent innovators of primary nursing bears testament to the impact and depth of change required to move forward with primary nursing (Binnie, 1987).

The emphasis on the role of the 'registered practitioner' and 'specialist practitioner' referred to in the report encourages professional responsibility and accountability. These issues must be explored with all nurses and especially with potential primary nurses. It is our experience that some nurses have difficulty conceptualising professional practice for their own nursing practice and are equally inept in discussing this with other health care professionals, particularly the medical profession.

The common foundation programme of the proposed *Project 2000* curriculum is a planned programme which introduces the student to a range of settings and provides experiences within a variety of care groups. This will provide the potential primary nurse with an awareness of the contribution not only of other nurses but also of other professional workers.

The common foundation programme will reduce the heavy emphasis on general hospital nursing. Nurses will have a more rounded view of nursing activities in different care environments. This will be particularly helpful for primary nurses who need thorough knowledge of other nursing environments in order to facilitate referral to these nursing groups when most appropriate for their clients. Detailed knowledge of these care environments will not be required, but a working knowledge of the availability and suitability of these environments for the particular groups of patients will be.

The common foundation programme also provides an approach to a health care service founded in health, not illness, thus changing fundamentally the more traditional nurse training programmes. What may also come from this programme is a clear picture of what nurses themselves define nursing to be – a point which currently seems to hinder many nurses from professional progress.

By including in the proposals the notion of supernumerary status for students, the UKCC will allow a platform to develop whereby the decision-making process can be illuminated more easily for the student. Currently students find that decisions are made for them and they have little appreciation of how and why the decision was made. Removal of the apprentice role from training should allow the pressure of 'getting the work done' to be eased and allow the student with the primary/associate nurse to explore the decision-making process more openly. However, the inclusion of a 20% commitment to service needs (UKCC, 1987a) will allow the students to experience work responsibility and appreciate the demands of commitment and accountability for action within the team.

It is important to recognise that, although the issues raised here have come from *Project 2000*, other reports published over the last 20 years have also raised similar issues. For instance, the registered practitioner and specialist practitioner in the Brigg's Report (1972), the common foundation programme in the ENB Report (ENB, 1985) and Judge report (RCN, 1985).

NURSING EDUCATION RESEARCH

A second influence on educational thinking surrounding primary nursing is the increasing body of knowledge resulting from research into nurse education. The theory–practice gap has been identified in nursing for at least 20 years (Clarke, 1986; Miller, 1985a). Bendall's definitive study in 1975, *So you passed Nurse*, clearly demonstrated the problem. Alexander (1983) sought to facilitate the integration of theory and practice by implementing a programme of concurrent theory and directly relevant supervised practice of nursing. Her experimental study gave evidence that restructuring the basic curriculum to provide the concurrent experience would be advantageous. However, modifying the whole of a basic curriculum would require a major overhaul. Although many schools of nursing have approached this issue and are some way to implementing their new programmes, the underlying philosophy has not always changed, nor indeed can it while students provide such a large percentage of the workforce.

A second point is brought to light in Melia's study (1987), which is a qualitative study of the world of the student nurse from her perspective. The study pointed to a situation in which the majority of learning takes place in the clinical areas and in which the socialisation into the world of nursing, with the ethos of being there to get the work done, is extremely powerful. While aspects of this socialisation may be considered advantageous to nursing there are clearly some aspects that are detrimental to developing 'thinking' nurses. For example, one of the first issues that a new nurse sometimes has to ascertain is where she should have coffee breaks – in sister's office or the canteen? This issue takes precedence for some new students over, for example, identifying learning opportunities particular to that clinical area (Melia, 1987).

Further research conducted in the USA has been carried out to explore student learning in primary nursing and team nursing environments (Williams, 1981). While taking care not to generalise findings to the UK without due consideration for cultural and professional differences, it can be stated that the perception of students as to whom to go to for advice or assistance is an issue in a team nursing environment, while the enjoyment of following patients and their care through to investigations/treatment and discharge is highlighted in a primary nursing environment.

Bearing in mind the points raised thus far it is useful to clarify the principles of primary nursing and apply them to education.

APPLICATION OF PRIMARY NURSING PRINCIPLES TO THE FIELD OF EDUCATION

Moritz (1975) identifies five principles of primary nursing.

1. 24-Hour Responsibility

Educators exhort the value of total patient care and the use of a holistic approach to this care. However, students' ability to be fully responsible for patients' care is limited by their knowledge base, and this is particularly the case for more junior students. However, the opportunity to follow a group of patients from entering the care environment to discharge allows students to have a greater depth of knowledge of the individuals. Students can therefore become more responsible, especially when working with primary nurses who increasingly delegate care to the students, and encourage in the individual student an awareness of decision making and accountability in action. It is recognised that opportunities for working closely with students may be limited because of staffing levels. The quality of supervision and 'mentoring' has an effect. Where little or no preparation has been given to the qualified nurses for mentoring and where the staffing levels are so tight that it is difficult, if not impossible, for the qualified nurses either to supervise or discuss care with their students, the quality of mentoring will be compromised. Here is an opportunity for nurse educators in their clinical role to serve as role models for primary nurses. Lecturer practitioners, those holding joint appointments and clinical practice development nurses are all well placed to promote mentoring skills.

2. Case Method of Assignment

The case method of assignment allows primary and associate nurses greater depth of knowledge of their patients. However, this approach may inhibit the opportunity for a broader range of clinical problems in which the student may gain first-hand knowledge. The reduced exposure to a wide variety of clinical problems may affect the student's ability to complete the planned curriculum. In some respects this may be a problem, particularly with increasing specialisation in the medical field; opportunities may already be limited, and restriction to a case load may be too limiting for the students to gain experience of different illnesses. However, this may not be a problem when nursing curricula are based on principles which can and should be modified when applied to similar but different circumstances. If basic nurse education supports the ethos of bureaucracy and adherence to procedures and policies, students will feel disadvantaged as they will not encounter sufficiently diverse circumstances to feel adequately prepared. This may be a problem when students currently in training are gaining clinical experiences in varied traditional and professional nursing environments.

3. Care Giver-to-Care Giver Communication

An important part of this is the use of written care plans to communicate effectively all aspects of care. It would seem that we still have a long way to go before we can say that the nursing process is a well used tool in British nursing. The nursing process arrived in the UK from the USA in the mid to late 1970s (De la Cuesta, 1983; Ling, 1986; Dickinson, 1982). The General Nursing Council policy statement in 1977 indicated it was to be used in basic nurse education.

O'Brien et al. (1985) said that the introduction of the nursing process into practice lacked consideration of its underlying philosophy, structure and education. The results, known informally, of current efforts around the country to audit the clinical learning environments confirm the author's personal view that the implementation of the nursing process is not consistent. However, it has been observed informally that when team and primary nursing systems are introduced the quality of written care plans improves. In some areas, basic nurse education departments are exploring more thoroughly the use of the nursing process and have developed final examinations with a care plan component. However, in practice, students comment on the poor quality of care plans generally in use (Melia, 1987).

The awareness in a primary nursing environment of the value of care plans is increased, and what also becomes apparent is that the quality of verbal communication improves. Bed-to-bed handovers facilitate the inclusion of the patient in any evaluation, and also allow clearer exposition of any problems. The same group of patients are reviewed by the same group of nurses, which reduces the repetition of information and facilitates the retention of in-depth information for a smaller group of patients.

A further point for consideration is the poorly addressed area of counselling. Informally, nurses comment on their poorly developed skills in this area, and preparation for primary nursing should include remedial work in this area. The consistent contact of the primary nurse with the patient may make the patient's psychological needs more apparent, and some of these needs may be more amenable to counselling. Counselling should also be more clearly addressed in basic nurse education, but perhaps first we need nurse educators capable of effective teaching in this relatively new area.

4. Care Planner Being Care-Giver

The introduction of primary nursing focuses on changing the organisation of nursing work to allow the care planner to be the care giver, so in many respects this principle is well applied in practice. However, caution should be taken when students beginning to manage their own case load feel an almost tangible expectation from the ward staff that they should be able to carry out whatever is required as directed by the care plan – this is not necessarily so. In reality a student can be acting as an associate nurse, caring for a group of patients in a primary nurse's absence. While, in many instances, with appropriate information and supervision of practice the student is both able and willing, some students can feel pressure and expectation from the qualified nurses to continue to perform without the supervision they need. It is important for both mentors and other qualified members of the nursing team to recognise this as a potential problem.

5. Ward Sister as Role Model, Resource Person and Teacher

The principle of the ward sister acting as a role model, resource person and teacher can be applied to the nurse teacher. The ward sister and nurse teacher roles will be viewed here as within one post.

Moritz (1975) comments on the atmosphere of trust and support in risk-taking that the ward sister/nurse teacher should facilitate. The encouragement given to students to be self-directed in their learning should be matched by freedom to choose nursing care actions. Only by being consistent in our approach to nurse education – in the classroom and on the wards – will the end result be a nurse with effective decision-making ability.

There are major restrictions on allowing nurses to take risks. The biggest is nurses' general reluctance to move into unknown or uncharted territory.

Obedience to one's immediate superiors and the organisation has been and is encouraged at all levels. Deviance results in labels of troublemaker or rebel, matched with a strong covert and overt pressure to conform. There is a middle ground that should be strived for, namely that of greater independence, creativity and open mindedness. It is no coincidence that senior nurses have commented that they wish to employ 'nursing deviants' in a primary nursing environment (informal comment).

A number of writers have also commented on the ward sister's ability to 'let go the reins' of directing nursing care as being crucial to real implementation of primary nursing (Manthey, 1980; Hegyvary, 1977). Others have commented on the issue of the atmosphere and level of mutual trust and mutual regard for peers within the ward team (Burns, 1988). The open interest in and care of each other is new for many nurses. It is important that all members of the team work to develop an atmosphere in which individuals feel comfortable, disclosing their feelings without fear of ridicule or retribution (see chapter 13).

Current nursing programmes allow student nurses relatively short periods in any one clinical area. This rather militates against them being able to perceive the trust and encouragement to take risks as anything more than a warm and friendly environment in which to work. It should be borne in mind that only during the last two or three weeks of a placement are students beginning to feel confident enough to initiate nursing actions. It would seem therefore that for nurses to gain effective experience the amount of support and encouragement should be increased. It would seem very unlikely with current restrictions (e.g. EEC guidelines) on what must be included in training that the length of clinical placements can generally be increased. There is, however, room for examining the length of clinical placements in the latter part of training, particularly before final examinations.

EDUCATIONAL APPROACHES IN A PRIMARY NURSING ENVIRONMENT

Learning Theory

The learning theory which may underpin the educational approaches in a primary nursing environment is that described by Bruner (1966), Rogers (1983), Stenhouse (1975) and others whereby the student is the focus and the teacher takes on the role of facilitator and senior learner.

In preparing professionals for practice the notion of reflection on action is also gaining supporters. Zeichener (1981) draws on the work of Dewey (1933), who advocates open-mindedness, responsibility and wholeheartedness as prerequisites to reflective practice. This would seem particularly apposite for nursing. Work by Argyris and Schon (1974) on inculcating the ability to reflect on practice and apply lessons learnt to future situations has been described as appropriate to professional education. Previous work focusing on teaching and other non-health professions transfers well to the field of nursing. Strategies that may be employed to foster the skills of reflection include the use of a reflective diary, learning contracts between ward sister/nurse teacher and nurse, and counselling via job performance review interviews. Figure 16.1 illustrates how these strategies fit with the perceived learning needs potential primary nurses acknowledge (see chapter 3).

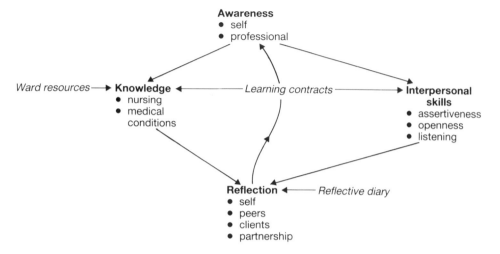

Fig. 16.1 Educational issues in primary nursing.

Learning Environment

In a primary nursing setting the learning environment is an important factor in the successful implementation and consolidation of learning. As has been described in chapter 3, the learning needs identified by the whole team, before implementation, can be huge and very diverse. Even when primary nursing has been introduced, the learning does not diminish because life-long learning is a necessity if the nurse is effectively to exercise her accountability.

It is important that the nursing team values education and that this is demons- trated in practice. There are three approaches available:

● Evident educational resources in the ward/department
● Learning contracts
● Access to in-house/independent continuing education courses and time out from duties for education

Educational Resources in the Ward/Department

The team should be committed to maintaining an up-to-date collection of articles and books relevant to the sphere of nursing. Often one finds out-of-date textbooks used merely as a back rest during handover. There are three problems identified in maintaining the quality of material: time, responsibility and money.

Time is difficult to identify in the sometimes rushed atmosphere and flat-out pace of work evident in many clinical areas. However, ward sisters have to be convinced of the value of maintaining this resource and of the need to plan in advance, so that staff nurses and students have time to use and add to the resources. If the management needs of the ward always take precedence over educational needs, the hidden message for all to receive is that education is less important.

The second problem with maintaining resources is whose *responsibility* it is to maintain them. It remains the ward sister's but with the wide range of pressing issues in her role it may be difficult for her to achieve this. However, primary nurses could identify areas of expertise and take responsibility for collecting relevant references in these areas. The administrative part, with regard to photocopying for example, can be delegated to someone other than a nurse, such as the ward helper. Another alternative may be to use some nursing hours to increase the ward clerk hours, or to invest in some part-time secretarial support.

The third problem is that of lack of *money* to buy books, subscribe to journals or photocopy articles. One approach is to ask the nurse training budget holder, normally the director of nurse education, for some money. As 70–80% of learning takes place in the clinical area, perhaps some direct finance for educational resources could be made available for the wards. A short-term solution might be to approach the ward team about spending a portion of donated money on books. Further possibilities include generating income from running study days or conferences. Subscriptions to journals can be expensive if one person is paying, but if the team jointly subscribes this may be more acceptable.

Access to Study Leave – In-house/Independent

Continuing education facilities nationwide vary from being woefully inadequate to excellent (Rogers, 1987). Access to courses and study days are hampered by service requirements. There is evidence to indicate that nurses attend study days in their own time and often pay fees out of their own pocket (informal comment from participants on visitors' days). Such high motivation to secure further information about practice or theory usually means that the staff return to their own unit and share the ideas with their colleagues. This in turn will positively affect the service they provide. However, managers do need to be challenged on their responsibility in this matter to try to secure funding and time out for study leave. Direct fund raising is one possibility. Enterprising units hold sales in hospitals – cakes, plants, etc. – and use the funds raised for study leave. The running of local study days on relevant issues of local expertise yourself, using companies to cover costs, should raise revenue from fees for the ward. Another approach may be to discuss with the ward budget holder the possibility of employing part-time staff during term time (which may suit mothers well) to replace the study leave staff. All these ideas need examination in the light of local restraints, but a bit of imagination may well resolve some problems (see chapter 14).

Learning Contracts

Learning contracts are seen as an appropriate tool for a student-centred, adult style of education. They allow highly individualised learning needs to be clearly identified for student and teacher/manager (Keyzer, 1986). They clarify for the student and teacher/manager their responsibilities in meeting these needs. The potential for learning contracts with students is somewhat limited as continuous assessment of a standardised nature is being widely implemented (UKCC, 1983). However, all programmes include individual learning needs as well and this can be explored with students.

For qualified staff the learning contract is a useful way of harnessing what is potentially a diverse range of needs.

THE ROLE OF THE STUDENT IN A PRIMARY NURSING SETTING

Student nurses can and indeed should fulfil the role of associate nurse within a primary nursing environment (Burns, 1988). For them to achieve the competencies as laid down by statute (UKCC, 1983), they should experience assessing, planning, implementing and evaluating nursing care in a variety of nursing environments. However, as mentioned earlier, their relative lack of knowledge and nursing expertise in these various nursing environments indicates that they should be supervised in role to ensure patient safety.

The students need to be aware of their part in managing their learning, and they need to know what learning opportunities are available. Often clear guidelines need to be given, as self-initiated learning may be new to them. Early questioning from students must be encouraged and responded to promptly. Students are generally enquiring and interested in the practice and with minimal encouragement do ask questions. Students also need guidance on how to use their mentor – sometimes they expect mentors to be constantly available and able to answer all questions. Students need to recognise that they need to initiate some of the teaching and with current off-duty commitments search out their mentors. In a primary nursing setting students have the opportunity to follow patients from admission to discharge and give care to their patients continuously when on duty. They should also be encouraged to follow patients out of the ward to observe investigations and operations whenever possible. This allows the student to gain an overall picture and deeper understanding of patients' perceptions of treatments. It is also of benefit to patients as they are escorted by a known person and so may feel reassured by the familiar company. Exciting programmes facilitating students following patients after discharge home or elsewhere in the community are ideas that may become more feasible in practice.

THE ROLE OF MENTOR IN A PRIMARY NURSE SETTING

The mentor role is crucial to the successful outcome of learning for students. Mentors need to be prepared well for the role. Qualified nurses should not be expected to take on this role for at least six months following appointment and registration. The mentor must feel confident of her clinical skills in a particular environment. Research (Lathlean et al., 1986) indicates that newly qualified nurses undergo major change in role during this time and it is inappropriate to expect them to encompass mentoring as well.

As experience is gained in mentoring, qualified staff need feedback on their effectiveness in the role. Within a primary nursing unit peer evaluation is fostered at all levels and this includes the mentor role. Mentors also need free access to the senior nurse so that potential problems can be thought through carefully. This sharing of problems allows mentors to learn from situations and develop further their skills, for example, in counselling a poor performer.

THE ROLE OF WARD SISTER/NURSE TEACHER

The two roles of ward sister and nurse teacher have been linked together to highlight that the division is false. The two roles are already to a greater or lesser extent invested in one person. Pembrey's (1980) research study indicated that sisters perceived an education role within their job. Further developments recently of joint appointments (Wright, 1985b) and lecturer practitioner posts (Vaughan, 1986) would seem to bear this out. The main aim of the role is, however, to foster throughout the qualified staff the learning of the students. Time and effort spent developing trained staff, identifying their learning needs and facilitating the achievement of learning goals will be repaid as they in turn work with the students. The ward sister fosters with her team the atmosphere of trust and permission to take risks – acceptable risks though, in terms of potential patient outcomes. One of the most important people in the team is the link teacher from the school of nursing. The link teacher needs to ensure that the nursing team knows the content and approach taken within the basic curriculum so that they too can work within it and therefore give congruent support to students.

In a primary nursing setting the opportunities for nurse teachers to have clinical responsibility are much greater. The fragmentary care normally available when nurse teachers work with students clinically can be avoided. It is possible with careful planning that the teacher can take an associate nurse role and with more determination and organisation a temporary primary nurse role. It is helpful if nurse teachers can clear a few days each year for uninterrupted clinical work. This reaffirms for the nurse teacher the quality of her clinical skills and has great impact on the nursing team.

From this sound basis from which to work, role modelling of expert care in the primary or associate nurse role is a very potent learning strategy. It helps reduce the criticism levelled at nurse teachers commented on earlier that it is difficult to achieve clinical accountability. Acting as primary nurse to one patient does not necessarily need persistent ward presence. The teacher can negotiate with her patient when she will be on the ward/unit, identifying times during the day for direct care giving. The opportunities for interaction with other members of the health team are also useful, namely the clinical nurse specialists, doctors and social workers. It may also help to remove the traditional sister tutor image of nurse teaching, often held by other health care professionals – an image we could do well to remove as we try to move towards *Project 2000* and higher education.

Conclusion

Primary nursing has implications for all nurses involved in education. The whole ethos of primary nursing should pervade educational approaches, placing emphasis on the value of the individual and recognising and addressing the individual's needs. The choice of theory to underpin these approaches must be that of the progressive school described earlier. The basis is then set for the provision of quality nursing care by confident, knowledgeable nurses who are still learning.

PART 4

Conclusion

17

Primary Nursing in Perspective

Steven Ersser and Elizabeth Tutton

This final chapter will both draw on the issues raised throughout the rest of the book and extend these to a consideration of primary nursing, present and future.

PRIMARY NURSING IN THE UNITED KINGDOM

It is difficult to pinpoint the current stage of development of primary nursing in the UK. There are uncertainties that nurses are referring to the same entity when they use the term 'primary nursing'. Little is known about the actual extent of the uptake of the approach and how this is taking place. The ward level organisation of nursing may adopt various hybrid forms rather than the 'ideal types' commonly described (see chapter 1). Hybrid forms may arise for various reasons: the transition from one system of organisation to another; significant daily variation in skill mix; and a lack of understanding of the concepts that distinguish primary nursing from other systems.

Some crude indication of the degree of interest in primary nursing can be derived from the database of the King's Fund Primary Nursing Network. The Network is a communication and support forum comprising units in the UK claiming to practise primary nursing or choosing to work towards its introduction (described in detail later). In May 1989 there were over 189 units involved, with numbers growing weekly. To obtain a clearer picture of what is happening nationally, a survey of all member clinical units has been planned for early 1990.

The Department of Health has given its support for primary nursing. In January 1989 Jennifer Hunt, a Nursing Officer at the Department, gave her encouragement at the inaugural meeting of Primary Nursing Network. The document *A Strategy for Nursing* (Department of Health, 1989b: 32) said: 'The development of primary nursing should be encouraged'. In April 1989 the University of Surrey advertised in *Nursing Times* for a government funded Project Leader stating that the project leader will 'seek to characterise the nature of primary nursing'.

It is evident that the nurses described in Part 2 often faced similar difficulties in establishing primary nursing in diverse clinical settings. Primary nursing was seen to be largely a planned development, but one often requiring some degree of adaptation of the 'ideal types' described previously (see chapter 1).

Adaptation of Theory to Practice

Primary nursing, like other major clinical nursing developments over the last decade, has involved attempts to transform theoretical ideas into practice. Within the nursing literature, nursing developments have appeared to follow a particular pattern. This is illustrated by the case of the nursing process. The chronological pattern of the literature reflects a move from speculative and theoretical ideas, such as in Yura and Walsh (1978), toward a more pragmatic approach, such as McFarlane and Castledine (1982). The literature that followed was more evaluative and critical in nature (e.g. Hardy and Engel, 1987). A similar pattern was also seen with nursing models. For example, Riehl and Roy's (1980) book, *Conceptual Models for Nursing Practice*, is largely theoretical. This was followed by Pearson and Vaughan's (1986) *Nursing Models for Practice* and Wright's (1986) *Building and Using a Model of Nursing*, which attempted to clarify these ideas and aid clinical application. Also in 1986 Webb combined both practical illustrations with critical comment in her book *Woman's Health*. Within the primary nursing literature the distinction between theory and practice has been less evident. Writing by Manthey (1980) and Hegyvary (1982) and to some degree Pearson (1988a) tends to be a combination of argument for primary nursing and a consideration of practical issues involved in the change. Little detailed reference is made, however, to the realities of undergoing a major change in the organisation of nursing nor to criticisms of the system.

Part 2 illustrates the difficulties of working towards any change in the organisation of nursing and the frequent need for some degree of modification of practice. This modification may be around the central principles upon which the justification of the change is based. Adaptation is required for many reasons: the rate of change; the number and skill mix of staff; the average rate of patient turnover; the rate at which the patients' conditions change; the degree to which medical authority dominates nursing activity; the degree to which staff understand the concepts underlying the development; the attitudes of other team members and the level of managerial and educational support provided.

Several key adaptations of primary nursing were described in the practice chapters. There was the high degree of flexibility in the arrangements made to cover the primary nurse's absence and changes in the patient's condition requiring a review of the plan. Accountability for decision making about nursing care for a patient group is made possible by the primary nurse forward planning and having the capacity to change the plan on return. The units described have tended not to opt for the primary nurse being contacted in her absence. Instead, the associate nurse typically makes the decision (perhaps in conjunction with others), but this is within the overall direction of care set by the primary nurse. Manthey (1970) has described such practice, with the primary nurse retaining responsibility, at the very least, for all fundamental changes in the design of the plan.

The Ward Co-ordinator

The development of a co-ordinator's role was a common adaptation. Wards that claimed to be particularly busy, such as the general medical wards described (chapters 6 and 11) and the surgical ward (chapter 5) with a high patient turnover, required the development of a nurse co-ordinator role to supplement the established primary nursing roles. These are not to be confused with the ward co-ordinator role as described by Pearson (1988a), which refers to an extended ward clerk role. The co-ordinator's responsibilities are held temporarily by an individual nurse. These include directing information between nurses and multidisciplinary team members, monitoring the bed state and attending doctors' rounds, putting the primary nurses' points forward and relaying points back. The allocation of newly admitted patients to nurses and the provision of support on a daily basis have also been mentioned (chapter 6).

The co-ordinator may also be required to direct events in the event of a cardiac arrest or a fire. In the unit for people with AIDS it was found not to be necessary to have a co-ordinator owing to the small size of the unit (chapter 9). The co-ordinator does not relate hierarchically to the nurses on the ward.

The development of the co-ordinator's role in the acute units may suggest that direct person-to-person communication is more difficult to achieve effectively in such units. However, the co-ordinators do not hold detailed information about patients and so, with the primary nurses continuing to forge key discussions with all those involved in a patient's care, the principle could be said to be retained in practice. It is interesting that little reference is made to the co-ordinator's role in the literature, particularly that from the USA.

The literature describes the staged introduction of primary nursing by firstly moving towards team nursing (Malby, 1988). In both this situation and another (Watson, 1977b), the authors explain the progression towards an approach which allowed an increasing degree of continuity to be provided through assigning a smaller number of nurses to the same patient and establishing a team leader. Again, this may be represented theoretically as movement along the continua described in chapter 1.

Difficulties Faced

The practice chapters also reveal the difficulties faced by units developing primary nursing. The numbers and skill mix of nurses have been important factors influencing the way nursing is organised, as seen in chapter 1 and in current practices (Part 2). Various questions had to be considered: What is the optimal and realistic case load for each primary nurse? How many nurses in the ward team have the attitude and competence to practise as primary nurses? How should the off-duty rota be organised? How does primary nursing operate on night duty?

Manpower Issues

It is evident in Part 2 that primary nursing may not necessarily require more staff but that it needs a particular skill mix which perhaps involves a greater proportion of qualified staff relative to unqualified staff in the ward establishment. The issue of skill mix in primary nursing is also described elsewhere in the literature (Binnie, 1984) and has been said to be both logical and clinically desirable (Pembrey, 1984). A shift in skill mix towards a higher proportion of qualified staff is compatible with primary nursing. However, the question of how the projected numbers and skill mix of nurses and lay carers available in the future will correspond with primary nursing needs further exploration.

The manpower crisis facing nursing has been said to be imminent (Dean, 1987), although there are strong indications that it is already here, with some health authorities reporting as much as 25% below establishment (Glendill, 1987). Traditionally, nursing is a female occupation, 90% of nurses are women and the average length of stay in nursing is 3 or 4 years (RCN, 1986). To provide a continual supply of nurses, the occupation is therefore dependent on a regular source of recruits. It is this supply which is currently diminishing. Demographic projections demonstrate a large drop in the number of 18-year-olds who will be available for service. Figures produced by Price Waterhouse show that currently more than 40% of nursing recruits are 18 years old, with between 5 O levels and 2 A levels. If the same proportion of the market is retained, this will lead to a gap between supply and demand that will be at its greatest in 1995 with an approximate shortage of 3000 entrants (UKCC, 1987a).

The situation is likely to be compounded by the *Project 2000* proposals for educational reform, which argue for students to have supernumerary status (UKCC, 1986). It is recognised that this would greatly exacerbate the manpower problem. *Project 2000* raised the issue about the degree to which learners contribute towards the nursing service. At present learners constitute less than 20% of the nursing workforce, a figure that has significantly diminished over the last 10 years (Bendall, 1986). Price Waterhouse suggest that the potential shortfall of nurses would be reduced by a student contribution of 20%. Clarke (1989) proposes a contribution of 1000 hours of rostered service over 3 years. The demand for nurses is also increased by the high degree of student wastage and a 10% wastage rate of qualified nurses per annum. Proposals to reduce the shortfall include reducing these rates, increasing the number of nurses returning to work, and widening the entry gate to training (UKCC, 1987a). If these measures are to succeed, Pearce (1988) suggests that radical advances in recruitment and retention practices need to be made.

Primary Nursing at Night

Part 2 also illustrated the potential difficulties with the organisation of staff on night duty. For some the issue is whether the number of staff on duty dictates whether primary nursing can be practised. However, irrespective of what system is being used, there will be the same ratio of staff to patients. Therefore the issue in fact becomes: how are the nursing staff most effectively deployed at night? Assuming the staff are associate nurses, the nursing that they provide will be in accordance with the overall direction of nursing planned by each of the different primary nurses on the ward. Furthermore, staff will be organised to work in such a way that continuity of contact with specific patients is maintained through the role of associate nurses. Obviously, because of limited numbers of qualified nurses on night duty, the consistency of patient assignment cannot be as great as that in the day. As with any other system the most senior or perhaps the only nurse on duty will supervise unqualified staff, including learners, and intervene accordingly. If a primary nurse is on duty, she can act as such for her patients and as associate nurse for some of those who are not. This again indicates the need for flexible practices which revolve around agreed principles.

The internal rotation of day staff onto night duty has been found to create problems such as the difficulty the primary nurse may have in making appropriate decisions about a patient's changing nursing needs within the day. One approach has been for either the ward sister or an associate nurse who has worked closely with a primary nurse to liaise with her when she is on night duty to ensure that the overall direction of care is appropriate and to deputise for her on nights off, when her absence will be prolonged. Chapter 8 describes the caretaker role assumed by the ward sister. In one setting (chapter 5) all night nurses worked as associate nurses; it was planned that the primary nurse would wind down her case load as night duty approached. Longer stay patients were handed over to other primary nurses. Before leaving the issue of manpower it is important to discuss the implications of primary nursing for Enrolled nurses and view this important group in relation to the manpower issue.

Primary Nursing and the Second-Level Nurse

Since the second-level or Enrolled nurse constitutes one-third of all qualified staff (RCN, 1986), their role in relation to primary nursing is important to clarify in order to prevent an exacerbation of the problem of misuse faced by these nurses (RCN, 1981; UKCC, 1986). These nurses have been used interchangeably with first-level nurses, for example RGNs and RMNs (Storey, 1988). An argument will be made for the suitability of the Enrolled nurse for the associate nurse's role, offering a means to employ both levels of qualified nurse appropriately, particularly with the growing shortage of skilled nurses.

Firstly, the skills and knowledge necessary to fulfil the responsibilities of a primary nurse will be described. These will then be looked at in relation to the Enrolled nurse's capacity to fulfil these requirements. A primary nurse will need to have the ability to:

1. Make decisions and plans about the nursing needs of those patients under her care and have the ability and knowledge to account for them when necessary. This requires knowledge and skill in:
    ● conducting an assessment of nursing needs upon which to plan a patient's nursing care;
    ● finding and making use of relevant information upon which to formulate an appropriate plan;
    ● providing nursing care, applying theory to practice;
    ● judging the value of the nursing decisions made and revising the plan in the light of this evaluation.

2. Communicate this plan, and the information necessary to devise it, between all
    those involved in the care of the patient.

Before discussing the second-level nurse it is important to emphasise that many
first-level nurses may not possess sufficient competence in these areas through lack
of experience, skill, knowledge or motivation, or may not be able to exercise it
because of having to work part-time hours. As such they would not be suitable to
adopt the role of primary nurse, although they could fulfil the associate nurse's
role. Also, a number of nurses may possess these skills on any single ward, and so a
decision would have to be made by the leader of that ward as to which nurses are
most appropriate to practise as primary nurses. From the foregoing comment the
question of whether an Enrolled nurse can assume the role of a primary nurse will
now be addressed.

Reference has been made to the need to allow Enrolled nurses the scope to
become primary nurses (Stroud, 1989). Although some second-level nurses may be
far more capable than RGNs in exercising the skills to act as a primary nurse it is a
fact that they remain in a very vulnerable position because of the nature of their
training. The risk of falling short of the acceptable level of competence is inevitably
far higher for these nurses because the set of abilities described above is more likely
to be the product of a first-level education programme. In this respect rule 18 of the
UKCC (1983) *Nurses, Midwives and Health Visitors Rules* (number 873) may
actually restrict Enrolled nurses in acting as primary nurses. It is accepted that
these rules relate to the nurse's competence at the point of qualification and
therefore it is perhaps unreasonable to assume no development of skill and
knowledge. Nevertheless, although this is a frustrating situation for those Enrolled
nurses capable of becoming primary nurses, such nurses would run the risks
referred to by Johnston and Ross (1988) and may be liable to professional
disciplinary action. Disquiet has already been expressed about the number of
Enrolled nurses coming before the professional conduct committee of the UKCC
(Vousden, 1987). A policy concerned with those nursing grades which could
potentially fill specific nursing roles, such as that of primary nurse has to be
directed towards selecting the grade most appropriate for the majority of nurses at
that level, for the sake of both staff and patient welfare. Zander (1985: 20),
referring to the nurse grade in the USA comparable to Enrolled nurses (Licensed
practical nurses), argues that such nurses are not prepared to be held accountable
for the outcome of nursing of a patient throughout his stay. In the light of these
arguments we now examine the possibilities facing Enrolled nurses who may
practise in a primary nursing system.

One of the most significant changes currently facing nursing is the educational
reforms to create one level of nurse (UKCC, 1986, 1987a). The obvious route for
Enrolled nurses with the ability and motivation to become primary nurses is for
them to be permitted and enabled to go through a conversion course to gain
first-level registration. This will help diminish the vulnerability of Enrolled nurses
by building on their existing knowledge and skills as well as providing them with a
just financial reward (alongside other registered nurses) for assuming this additional degree of responsibility.

The practical dilemmas facing many Enrolled nurses at present considering a conversion course include: the shortage of places on existing courses (Storey, 1988); their intensity (52 weeks); and their inaccessibility geographically and educationally. There is some hope that the present situation will be improved in that the ENB (1988: 67) have proposed a more flexible system of access by recognising previous learning to enable those nurses capable of converting to do so.

We have encountered many nurses working on wards where the skill mix is such that primary nursing would be difficult to operate effectively with so few first-level nurses. Two possible approaches could be adopted. Firstly, team nursing could perhaps be more suitable because the planning and delivery of nursing depend less on the ability of any one nurse, as in primary nursing, but rely more on the capacity of a group of nurses to pool knowledge and skill in planning care than primary nursing. Secondly, there may be a case for gradually changing the skill mix of a ward as shown by Binnie (1987) on a surgical ward. Such a change, however, may not necessarily result in a diminishing number of second-level nurses. Stroud (1989) describes the deployment of Enrolled nurses who are carefully selected as primary nurses. This includes those with special knowledge, skill and experience in a specialty, which reflect proven competence, working in close conjunction with the ward sister or co-ordinators. These issues clearly create dilemmas and anxieties for nurses and their managers. However, with sensitivity and resourcefulness, and by valuing the contribution of those Enrolled nurses, many of whom still have numerous working years, changes can be made in the organisation of nursing to harness effectively the contribution of the Enrolled nurse.

The second-level nurse's preparation would seem to be highly compatible with the responsibilities of an associate nurse. A job description to serve as a guide for a suitable role for second-level nurses, operating within a primary nursing system, is provided in Appendix II. The associate nurse's role provides scope for the comments of the second-level nurse to be considered by the primary nurse who writes the nursing plan. Although the primary nurse remains ultimately accountable for the nursing plan, she would be wise to draw on the resources of the associate nurses with whom she works, and invite their comment. Furthermore, the associate nurse can make an important contribution towards helping the primary nurse to evaluate care because the primary nurse also has significant responsibilities for planning care.

Nursing will continue to face the difficulties created by having more than one level of nurse. Multiple levels of nurses perpetuate the dubious belief that nursing can be coherently and effectively provided on the basis of an oversimplistic notion of a hierarchy of nursing skill. Such a notion interprets technical nursing activity to be of a higher status relative to fundamental care activities such as compensating for self-care difficulties. The relationship to a particular belief in a hierarchy of skill and the organisation of nursing is evident in the historical analysis provided earlier (see chapter 1). A more appropriate structure for matching nursing skill to nursing need would seem to be that of nurse and support worker to assist with nursing, as proposed by the UKCC (1986). However, recent proposals for the training of such a worker by the National Council for Vocational Qualifications (FEU, 1988) has caused the ENB alarm (*Nursing Times*, 1989a). The FEU paper suggests that after 2 years of NCVQ training support workers could be entitled to a 1 year reduction in first-level training. The Chairman of the *Project 2000* Implementation Group argues that the minimum training requirements for entry to the Register have not been set and that the modular training of the support worker could extend over a number of years. However, such a proposal may threaten a return to two levels of nurse and therefore a perpetuation of the problems we now face. A *Nursing Times* editorial (1989b) warned of the danger of such ideas lingering on and becoming part of common parlance.

In conclusion it would seem that rather than adding to the manpower problems nursing now faces, primary nursing may offer many units a logical system for effectively and sensitively deploying the two existing levels of qualified staff.

Primary nursing not only requires staff of a particular level of experience but also those with a certain level of competence to fulfil the necessary responsibilities. However, will there be sufficient nurses who possess the attitudes, knowledge and skills to practise in the way that primary nursing demands? There is also the issue of whether primary nursing will place even greater strain on the nurses' own welfare. Both of these issues raise questions about the support structures available to underpin the development of primary nursing. The supportive framework for the development of primary nursing will now be examined further.

A FRAMEWORK FOR PRIMARY NURSING

No change in clinical practice which is as significant as primary nursing can take place effectively without careful consideration of the factors which will make the change possible and sustain it in the long term. Two important areas of preparation involve the development of some form of strategic plan and of structures to support the change. These structures include those in education and management, and effective leadership of practice must be established at various levels.

The Need for Strategic Planning

All the chapters convey the need to plan any change carefully. Some describe the value of ward staff clarifying what they believe nursing to be, and what they are working towards. This review of beliefs and values about nursing describes the development of a ward philosophy. A working philosophy has been said to be like a rudder to a ship, keeping it on course (Prophit, 1986). The need to involve closely those who will undergo the change in coming to a consensus about how this may be achieved has been emphasised. Chapter 2 described some of the change strategies nurses could use in clinical development. Despite arguments for their use (Wright, 1985a; Pearson, 1985b) few are known to have used them and few have examined their value critically.

Supporting Structures

The change to primary nursing requires the development of different types of support structures for nurses: personal, educational and clinical. The development of a strategic plan is likely to require the active support of managers and educational staff. The transition nurses undergo when changing to primary nursing is often one that requires a change in thinking about nursing itself. There is a need to review the broad aims of practice of the nursing team and to make decisions about which actions are desirable or not. The skills to facilitate discussion of these issues may not exist within the nursing team. Furthermore, staff may require help in identifying and acquiring the knowledge and skills needed to operate within the new roles. This was explored in chapter 3.

There may be a problem in meeting the need for adequate support from educational staff. Rogers and Lawrence's (1987) survey of the opportunities for continuing education for nurses identified a considerable gulf between the ex-pressed commitment of health authorities and higher education institutions to this area and the practical provisions. The numbers of staff engaged in such work was appallingly low in many areas. This may be exacerbated further by the lack of staff with experience in supporting staff changing practice on a relatively large scale. This echoes the earlier reference made to Dean (1989). It may be necessary to explore other forms of educational support such as open learning, which allows students to choose the time, place and pace of study. It may help nurses to develop the ability to take greater control over their learning with the right support (Robinson, 1989) as advocated in chapter 3.

Chapters 11 and 13 drew attention to the need to consider the welfare of the nurse when making major changes in working arrangements. Chapter 13 indicated that it cannot simply be assumed that primary nursing is inevitably more stressful than other approaches. Since many units will be in the early days of practising primary nursing, the stress of adjustment in the change of responsibilities and the development of new skills will make any comparison with their former situation difficult. Nevertheless, it has been emphasised that the issues of personal support for nurses needs closer attention whatever the system of organisation in use. Bowman (1989) is at present completing a study looking at nurses' stress levels with different methods or styles of work organisation.

An important feature of the supporting framework for primary nursing is the development of appropriate management practice and clinical leadership, particu-larly at unit level. From chapter 14 it will be seen that the manager, at whatever level in the hospital, may help to create the conditions to make primary nursing possible. The devolution of authority to the clinical level has been said to require a reorientation of managers from a supervisory position to one in which they work as facilitators, providing active support to nurses. Such changes are supported by Zander (1980) and Manthey (1980). Zander (1980: 3) believes that the nurse manager of primary nurses walks a fine line between:

● . . . providing structure without stifling creativity, allowing autonomy without abandoning, teaching without telling and fostering growth without undermin-ing confidence.

Senior nurses need to liaise closely with general managers to explain carefully the reasons for changing the organisation of nursing and the means by which this change is going to be achieved. This is all the more important as most general managers are not nurses (Buchan, 1987). Emphasis on the exercise of accountability by primary nurses could be said to be highly compatible with government thinking about management control in public sector services. The Griffiths Report (1983) proposed that the efficiency and effectiveness of the NHS could be improved by establishing clearer lines of managerial accountability. Bowers (1989: 16) suggests that at ward level primary nursing represents a 'miniature reflection of general management in the NHS'.

If the quality of nursing is to be maintained and improved during and after the introduction of primary nursing, nurses will have to press to create the necessary conditions. Persistent attempts need to be made at all levels to influence decisions that affect the quality of the nursing service. This needs to be emphasised in the light of Strong and Robinson's (1987) observation that, in the process of restructuring, nursing has lost many of its experienced senior nurses, who guaranteed a voice in policy decisions. There is a risk that by losing the senior ranks young sisters, particularly with underdeveloped roles, may not be able to defend the interests of nursing.

Attention has been drawn to the lack of leadership at a wider professional level within nursing (McFarlane, 1989). Dean (1989: 20) has also expressed concern about leadership in nursing, saying 'Nurse leaders with a knowledge of nursing are noticeable by their absence'. He highlights the difficulties which have arisen from the post-Salmon Report emphasis on the management role of senior nuses to the exclusion of the nursing role. He also argues that nursing expertise in management has diminished as repeated reorganisations have created a vast gulf between those who know about nursing and those who think they know. This will make it even harder to exert the nursing perspective in arguing for changes in health care policy. Attention is drawn to the fact that the management of nurses and the management of nursing are not the same activity. Dean (1989) also argues that there is a need for nurses who can lead the development of practice as a career opportunity, a suggestion made in the Department of Health Report (1988) *The Way Ahead*.

Leadership at Ward Level

One of the critical role changes involved in the change to primary nursing is that required of the ward sister. This is in terms of the degree to which her responsibilities may change and also her important role in leading her staff through the turbulent period of transition. Potentially the role adjustment of the ward sister is a weak link in the chain of transition on the ward because the sister is required to provide leadership in keeping the unit operational while undergoing a significant change in her own role. This has also been observed by Watson (1977b). Zander (1980) describes the clinical leadership role of the head nurse and her continuing responsibility for the overall management of care. This refers to the overall monitoring of the quality of care on a unit and her role as a resource person and teacher of staff. It is evident that the ward sister does not, in the traditional sense, act as the person in charge. Primary nurses need to retain their autonomy if it is they who are selected to manage the overall direction of nursing for a group of patients. Chapter 15 discusses the changes in the power and communication patterns that occur with primary nursing.

The ward sister has been described as a general manager in the real sense by Pembrey and Binnie (in Slack, 1986) and Dean (1989). There are few who would doubt the demands of the sister's role, whatever the method of organising care. However, these demands often reach an unacceptably high level because of the appalling lack of practical support available to the sister to allow her to work effectively for patient and staff welfare. This issue requires careful consideration (Ciske, 1974; Pembrey, 1987).

Some ward sisters will welcome the opportunities to stand back from the day-to-day responsibility for the care of a patient group and to provide support and leadership (see chapter 10). However, for others there is the understandable feeling of losing control of decision making as well as perhaps the traditional status vested in this role. Some of the accounts describe the difficulty of getting the balance right between the ward sister providing leadership and being able to stand back from becoming so involved that primary nursing is disrupted (e.g. chapter 9). The problem may be exacerbated by the managerial and clinical inexperience of the primary nurses. Many of the sisters practised as associate nurses in addition to their leadership role (chapters 8 and 10). This is a consequence of the fact that their responsibilities do not often allow them to work effectively as primary nurses.

CAREFUL STEPS FORWARD

The future of primary nursing is in part dependent on the opportunities nurses have for the exchange of information about it, the application of its principles to practice and its strengths and weaknesses to the system. Furthermore, it is hoped that the future of primary nursing will also be shaped by the development of research programmes to monitor its consequences for nurses and patients and the careful use of the research already available.

Establishing a Communication Network

Nurses require a forum in which they are able to ask questions and check their understanding of both the theory and the practice of clinical developments with those who have learnt by their mistakes. To create opportunities for nurses to meet in this way, discussions took place with Jane Salvage, Director of Nursing Developments at the King's Fund Centre for Health Service Development, London, to establish a grassroots communication network.

The Primary Nursing Network was launched in 1989. Its aim was to enable those practising or working towards primary nursing to exchange information and to provide a framework for mutual support on a UK scale (see chapter 1 and Appendix I). The Network has a rapidly growing membership. A regional structure has been created to meet local need. This covers most of the UK and operates through a regional link person and meetings. Information on all Network members is available on a database at the King's Fund for members to contact each other. Information is also exchanged through a newsletter and both national and regional meetings. The next step in the Network's development will be to open up the opportunities for learning and development that an exchange scheme will provide by creating a starting point for members to spend some time in each other's units, matching units by geographical and interest area. The Network will provide a forum for the systematic collection of survey data on primary nursing. The Network provided the opportunity to have the first national forum on primary nursing research at the King's Fund Centre, London, in November 1989. The government's current White paper on the health service reinforces the requirement on nurses to evaluate the consequences of such practices (Department of Health, 1989a: 5).

Primary nursing represents a major change in the organisation of hospital nursing. Despite the government's strident efforts to control NHS costs, the implications that primary nursing has for the effectiveness of the hospital nursing service must also of course come under professional scrutiny. This raises issues about the need for ardent debate and the need to review the value of current research studies on primary nursing and the direction of future research.

Primary Nursing Research Issues and Implications

A central theme throughout this book has been the attempt to adopt a critical look at primary nursing. The study of primary nursing is, however, a complex activity making it a difficult subject of study. Two interrelated research issues will be addressed:

● The operational definition of primary nursing.
● The evaluation of primary nursing (which encompasses the operational definition).

Finally, some suggestions are made for the further study of primary nursing arising from the issues described.

Operational Definition of Primary Nursing

Primary nursing constitutes a complex series of variables and as such is very difficult to measure. Any method of organising nursing work represents a whole set of nursing behaviours which can be difficult to isolate and describe as a discrete whole. The component features were illustrated in chapter 1. Giovannetti (1981: 520–521) highlighted this problem when attempting to study primary nursing. She said:

● . . . all modes of nursing organisation are lacking operational descriptors.

Later she concluded in her review of research on primary nursing:

● . . . without exception, no investigator provided an operational definition of primary nursing or any of the other organisational modes studied. This omission represents the single most pervasive problem characterising the research to date. (Giovannetti, 1986: 129)

A recent attempt, however, has been made to operationalise the principles of primary nursing to a form that would allow measurement of changes which had occurred in the organisation of nursing work. This would then allow the relationship between the practice of primary nursing and various patient outcomes to be explored (MacGuire, 1990a, b). Giovannetti (1986) describes how the concepts of authority, responsibility and accountability used repeatedly to describe primary nursing are not described in measurable terms.

MacGuires's quasi-experimental study has reached the stage of introducing and describing a whole series of organisational changes which reflect the introduction of primary nursing into an elderly care unit (MacGuire, 1989a, b). The association of primary nursing (the experimental variable) to the various outcome indicators (12 in total) such as the average daily dependency and pressure sore rate was explored. This study also reflects the complexity of conducting such research, which requires the use of multiple methods to measure both the changes involved in nursing practice and the consequences for patients.

It could be argued that those who attempt to study primary nursing face a paradox in trying to ensure the valid measurement of how nursing is being organised on a ward. The measurement of primary nursing requires the researcher, in effect, to atomise it into its component parts or features. For example, the researcher may seek to identify whether a particular pattern of accountability is exercised by nurses. However, depending on how this is conducted, the qualities of the approach that characterise it as primary nursing may be lost; it is in this sense that primary nursing may be seen as greater than the sum of its parts selected for measurement.

Evaluation of Primary Nursing

The literature on primary nursing is voluminous. MacGuire (1990) located 200 articles originating from the USA from 1984 and the UK from 1980. Young et al.'s (1981) review and critique of primary nursing literature revealed that almost 80% of that identified did not constitute research and demonstrated overt support for primary nursing. Furthermore, Giovannetti's (1986) paper describes a comprehensive review of empirical work published from 1970 to 1984 involving several hundred articles. Only 29 studies met her inclusion criteria for review. Most of the studies on primary nursing are directed towards demonstrating its effectiveness (see chapter 12). There are many complex issues involved in conducting such research; Giovannetti (1986) has looked closely at these; they include:

● The introduction of primary nursing to a clinical unit is often accompanied by renewed interest in concepts not exclusive to primary nursing such as nursing process, standards of care, discharge planning and patient involvement.
● It is unlikely that there is one ideal way of delivering nursing care given the high degree of variation in patients' sets of needs, levels of nurses and clinical setting.
● The theoretical foundations of primary nursing are not completely clear.
● Typically, the methods used to measure the outcome criterion lacked adequate assessment of reliability and validity.

The difficulties involved in assessing the rigour of patient outcome measures have been highlighted in chapter 12. Furthermore, the difficulty of controlling the influence of significant extraneous variables such as nurses' competence has been illustrated in the studies of Felton (1975) and Shukla (1981, 1983). Despite the strength of MacGuire's (1989) study in attempting to define the need to operationalise the principles of primary nursing, the problematic areas stated above also apply to her study. Other critical comments on this study include the inadequate control provided through the quasi-experimental design and the threat to validity of the researcher being involved in the change process within this design. Also, the validity and reliability of some of the patient outcome tools were either not referred to, such as the KTC dependency formula, or are thought by some to be questionable (see Brittle and Marsh's (1986) critique of Senior Monitor).

Obstacles to the study of primary nursing are considerable for the researcher attempting to describe and pinpoint a change to primary nursing and attempting to evaluate its consequences for patients and staff. However, the important work of Giovannetti (1986) and MacGuire (1990a, b) at least chart many of the inherent difficulties. Other researchers have provided comment on such difficulties and propose some strategies for overcoming them (see Exley et al., 1980).

The development of effective evaluation strategies will be dependent in the first instance on the understanding of what constitutes the introduction of primary nursing into a ward, and then on developing and testing an appropriate set of methods to measure it, assuming that this may be possible, which may not be so. It would seem appropriate at this early stage in the study of methods or approaches to organising nursing work that a series of broad research and theoretical questions be posed which may be worthy of further exploration. These are:

1. What are the essential features which in composite define the organisation of ward-based nursing as primary nursing and differentiate it from other organisational approaches?
2. To what extent are the methods of organising ward-based nursing demonstrably different terms of nurses' observable behaviour?
3. How do those qualified nurses who believe they practise primary nursing interpret the nature of their work and respond to changes in the organisation of their work? (This could be extended to other organisational approaches providing a broader basis for differentiation and comparison.)

Study of the interpretation of social change by the people involved would lend itself to use of a qualitative research design. Furthermore, such an approach would provide a basis for developing concepts and propositions on aspects of nursing on which we have little knowledge.

4. What is the pattern of verbal interaction between
   ● nurse and patient;
   ● nurse and nurse on hospital wards practising primary nursing and those which are not, and in what ways do these patterns compare? Such a study may focus on particular areas of nursing such as co-ordination of care/ discharge planning.

There is also a need for research studies that provide detailed descriptions of the change which clinical units undergo when attempting to develop the organisation of their work together. Descriptions of the social consequences of such changes are also necessary. Intensive systematic study of individual clinical units, in the form of case studies, may provide nurses with insights into the complexities of introducing changes into the social structure of the hospital ward. Case studies may complement the plethora of experimental studies which have been used to evaluate changes in the organisation of nursing.

CONSEQUENCES OF PRIMARY NURSING

Patient Welfare

One of the major areas covered in this book concerns the implications of primary nursing for patients and nurses. From chapter 12 it is apparent that there is difficulty in identifying whether this system would benefit patients; however, some ways in which this may occur were identified. Although few research studies help to clarify this area, an attempt was made to provide a rational review of the issue.

There appear to be many logical reasons to suggest that primary nursing may be of value to patients. This is perhaps most clearly understood when the concepts of primary nursing described in chapter 1 are considered. For example, the greater continuity of nursing that accompanies primary nursing should at the very least provide opportunities for the nurse to use effectively those methods which benefit from a consistent approach, such as patient teaching. Primary nursing may create the conditions for the nurse; however, it does not ensure her competence. In both a medical ward (chapter 6) and an acute psychiatric unit (chapter 10) the authors expressed belief in the potential therapeutic benefits arising from the relationship developed between nurses and patients enhanced through primary nursing.

The literature on patients' satisfaction with primary nursing is problematic. There is difficulty in designing patient satisfaction tools that provide a valid measure. It is also unclear whether satisfaction arises from primary nursing or other features of change; furthermore, it is assumed that the patient is able to compare his experiences of nursing.

From a different perspective, the section on humanising hospital care (chapter 1) looked at what changes in hospital care, within nurses' control, may benefit the patient through minimising the alienating features of hospital care.

Nurses' Welfare and Resource Issues

In addition to the need to provide a framework of emotional support for nurses, particularly when undergoing changes in the way they work, the issue of nurses' morale requires particular attention. Many of the changes within nursing during the 1980s have posed a threat to the morale of nurses. If this is so, it would seem that there are indications that a small but significant benefit could be gained from primary nursing by alleviating a few of the sources of low morale and improving job satisfaction. In addition, there are also manpower implications which may also have a bearing on the situation.

Nurses' Morale

Was there evidence of widespread low morale among nurses in the UK in the 1980s? In recent years nurses have undergone numerous upheavals due to frequent changes both within nursing itself and from the wider changes within the NHS as a whole. These include major reorganisation within the NHS structure in 1982 and the development of general management (DHSS, 1983). Nurses have also undergone a considerable rethink in nursing practices, with greater emphasis being placed on providing care for the individual patient. Issues of considerable concern have included the funding of the health service, staff shortages, declining standards and subsequent low morale (RCN, 1984). Disputes over pay have received national attention, including the bitter dispute of 1982 and more recently the widespread disparity between the spirit and reality of the Clinical Grading Review (Nursing and Midwifery Staffs Negotiating Council Staff Side, 1988; Ferriman, 1988; Timmins, 1988).

In the national press, Clay (1988) has stated that the nursing profession's grievances over the health service go much wider than pay, saying:

- At its simplest nurses are dismayed because the system they are working in does not allow them to do the job they were trained to do. At the end of a shift they go home frustrated, feeling they have failed their patients. Added to this, they believe the government do not value their contribution.

Nurses have had to make significant adjustments to the rapid developments in medical technology. There is also increasing pressure to shorten the length of patient stay in hospital, leaving a higher proportion of dependent patients (Dean, 1987). There is a continual pressure for greater efficiency and cost benefit, as evident in the recent government White Paper on the health service (Department of Health, 1989a).

At ward level there are numerous sources of dissatisfaction. Studies have highlighted the persistent and fundamental problems facing staff nurses. Few are adequately prepared in their new role and many receive little support once in the job (Lathlean et al., 1986). Their preparation is directed towards producing competent nurses, but the reality is that they are often frequently moved between ward management and the nursing of a group of patients, and often find it difficult to do either well, which creates strain and dissatisfaction (Binnie, 1988). Furthermore, the management position many of these newly qualified nurses find themselves in is not one they face with confidence (Vaughan, 1980).

Set against this climate it would be of no surprise to find a great many nurses demoralised. Many of the causes of the problem are to do with lack of resources or a just wage, with inadequate staffing levels and with change itself. All these factors are likely to have a bearing on the ability of the nurse to work effectively and to achieve satisfaction in her work. Clearly primary nursing is going to make little impact on the source of these problems. Furthermore, it could be said that changes in the organisation of nursing may potentially exacerbate the situation. However, it is worth exploring this particular change more closely because there are indications that it may help to improve job satisfaction and perhaps have a positive effect on the manpower difficulties we currently face.

Job Satisfaction and the Organisation of Nursing

Studies evaluating primary nursing often attempt to establish the extent of job satisfaction of primary nurses. A relationship has been said to exist between job satisfaction, staff turnover and productivity. (MacPhail, 1988). If this is so, job satisfaction may increase for nurses who practise with greater autonomy, with a corresponding reduction in staff turnover and sickness rate. However, as yet, the evidence to support this premise is sketchy. In comparison with team nursing, primary nursing has been found to offer greater job satisfaction (Roberts, 1980; Laforme, 1982; Sellick, 1983; Reed, 1986). Betz (1981) revealed a decline in job satisfaction after introducing primary nursing, while the levels for team nurses remained stable. Examining the association between staff satisfaction, and turn-over and sickness rates, Betz (1981) found a higher staff turnover among nurses practising primary nursing than among those in team nursing. In contrast, Laforme (1982) found primary nurses to have high morale, 29 fewer sick days and a turnover rate that dropped from 48 to 13%. Marram's (1976) study reported reduced sickness rates in primary nurses but did not look at satisfaction levels. A major criticism of many of the studies is the lack of reliability and validity testing of the research tools.

Binnie's (1988) study provides a different perspective by highlighting the experiences of staff nurses who experienced a feeling of alienation from their work. She suggests that primary nursing would provide many nurses with the control over their work that they seek. It is perhaps difficult for most staff nurses to be skilled managers and leaders of a ward and to practise as skilled, knowledgeable nurses providing direct care.

Monitoring and Controlling the Patient Case Load

Can the system of primary nursing place nurses in a position to argue more effectively for an improvement in the staff establishment on a ward? The case assignment system provides greater clarity about how many patients, of a particular dependency level, may be cared for by a qualified nurse. Such decisions have to be made continually with primary nursing, adjusting case load number and type as people with different degrees of need are admitted and discharged.

The nursing leader of a primary nursing unit may collect information on patient dependency and monitor the quality of care they receive. Furthermore it is simpler to identify what each nurse can be responsible for using the case system. This provides a strong rational basis for arguing for appropriate establishment levels.

Clearly, the typical number of patients a primary nurse can look after varies within the setting. Both medical wards (chapters 6 and 11) described case loads of six or seven patients. Very dependent patients, such as those in the AIDS hospice (chapter 9), required one primary nurse to care for three patients. In a young disabled person unit, each primary nurse had four in-patients plus some coming in for day care. In the acute psychiatric unit (chapter 10) qualified nurses acted as the primary nurse for two patients and associate nurse for three. These figures are referred to as illustrations rather than guides.

Primary Nursing: The Nurse and Unqualified Carer

Primary nursing may also contribute towards the creation of the conditions in which more qualified nurses are able to give direct nursing care. Clay (1987: 62) has said: 'Primary nursing – in a modified form, if necessary – is, I believe, the key to the achievement of a qualified nursing workforce.' This is likely to improve the quality of care and complement the proposed move to supernumerary status for students. The manpower consequences of primary nursing require a consideration of the role of unqualified carers whose role is required to change.

Nursing auxiliaries currently provide a range of services from domestic worker to providing direct care. This perhaps creates the overall impression of a flexible worker filling gaps when there are staff shortages. *Project 2000* (UKCC, 1986) made a clear statement about the need to create a new role of aides or helper, with the emphasis on assisting with nursing. Requests have been made by some senior nurses for the role of auxiliaries to be standardised and extended to take on more direct nursing care (Harrison, 1988). It is of concern if this belief is still widespread, particularly with emphasis being placed on a qualified nurses giving care.

Currently it is not uncommon for nursing to be provided by unqualified staff (Melia, 1987). *Project 2000* proposals (UKCC, 1986) will lead to the need to employ more qualified nurses to provide direct care, unless the support worker role is to be abused. One description of such change in skill mix, in which it was possible to remain within budget, has been described (Binnie, 1984).

Munson and Clinton (1979) said that with primary nursing auxiliaries are directed away from giving direct patient care to adopting a supporting role which includes attention to equipment and supplies. The *Project 2000* helper role, in theory at least, should be compatible with such a change. The introduction of primary nursing may make the transition of role from care giver to supporter a little easier when it accompanies a more extensive change in the organisation of nursing, along with other staff.

Experimentation with the role of unqualified carer has already begun. To ensure that nurses gave direct care and to maximise the amount of time they spent with patients, Pearson *et al.* (1988b) developed a combined helper–domestic role termed Ward Orderly. Their role encompassed helping nurses when two people were needed, and carrying out tasks that did not require the skill of a nurse, such as running baths and making most of the beds. Domestic duties included some cleaning and preparing breakfast. In practice the ward orderlies occasionally gave some aspects of direct care. However this took place under a specific set of circumstances and normally under the close supervision of a qualified nurse, in accordance with the care plan, when the patient was nearing discharge (and so they would be like a relative or a care assistant in a Part 3 home). Although not ideal, this situation was very carefully controlled; staff were specifically employed to work as ward orderlies; the ward philosophy about nursing was very clear to all that patients had the right to the care of nurses, that nursing is an activity requiring skill and knowledge; this was the aim at all times.

Binnie (1984: 4) advocates the use of auxiliaries for housekeeping duties and helping with clerical work, but she also suggests that an auxiliary's contribution to nursing may be that of a caring relative. However, she argues that deployment of auxiliaries may lead to fragmentation of care. It would seem that primary nursing is likely to foster the role developments proposed by the UKCC (1986) and contribute towards clarifying the distinction between the nature of lay and professional care in practice, which is long overdue.

Primary Nursing: Economic Considerations

Studies reviewing the cost of implementing primary nursing are often of limited use, and there are difficulties in making comparisons. Most include different items in the costings and are also located in the American health system. Marram (1976) found team nursing to be more expensive than primary nursing; however, much of the difference was spent on staff salaries because of the longer period in post for staff on the team nursing unit (who were therefore higher up the salary scale). She also claimed that primary nursing used 35% fewer nursing hours over a 4 month period, and absent days for sickness were fewer.

Giovannetti (1980) found primary nursing to be more expensive than team nursing. Primary nursing units also had a higher bed occupancy and used more nursing hours, yet patient dependency was not taken into account. Within the NHS the cost of primary nursing has not really been assessed; however, Pearson (1988a: 143) said that the Oxford Nursing Development Unit, which adopted primary nursing, had staffing costs which were 25% lower than the costs of any comparable wards in the health district. However, no further information has been given about how this figure was obtained. Roberts (1980) found that primary nursing could be introduced within existing budgets. It is not possible to generalise from the chapters in Part 2 about staffing costs.

Recruitment and Retention

It may also be that primary nursing is an effective attraction for recruitment if the premise that many qualified nurses want to nurse rather than 'run a ward' is true. Finally, it would seem that it has much to offer learners. If primary nursing does improve job satisfaction, offering the prospect of allowing nurses to nurse as they have been prepared to do, this may help to reduce the high learner wastage rates. There may also be greater opportunity to observe skilled nursing by working alongside a nurse and to see the progression from assessment to the planning of care and the possibilities for evaluation made possible through consistent patient contact. Aspects of patient management are probably learnt more quickly on a small patient group scale than by attempting to get to grips with ward management before any mastery in nursing patients has been achieved. Primary nursing provides a basis for staff to develop an effective student mentor system through developing their own clinical expertise and being in a position to monitor more closely the competence of learners.

Conclusion

In this book we have attempted to show the complexity and significant implications of making major changes to the organisation of nursing work. From a personal point of view we have had to consider our moral position in helping nurses to undergo such changes when the welfare of patients and nurses may be affected for better or worse. We believe that as a first step there was a need to make an attempt to place primary nursing in some sort of perspective which would provide nurses with a basis for further debate.

Appendix I

Primary Nursing

Network Information

King's Fund Centre for Health Services Development

The Primary Nursing Network aims to provide a national forum for sharing and spreading information on primary nursing in the UK. This will serve as a basis for assessing and facilitating its development and evaluating its use.

Primary nursing is a method of organising care which can potentially make nursing more humane and more effective. The relationship between patient and nurse is of paramount importance; each patient has a named registered nurse responsible for planning and delivering his/her care, and accountable for it 24 hours a day. This offers significant potential benefits, and is being adopted enthusiastically around the UK. Careful monitoring is needed of its direction, alongside ongoing critical reivew of the benefits, and any associated problems.

Anyone involved in introducing primary nursing in their work setting is eligible to join. The network is co-ordinated by Jane Salvage, director, nursing developments, King's Fund Centre; Steve Ersser, Institute of Nursing, Oxford; and Liz Tutton, Buckinghamshire College of Higher Education.

The network's activities include:

- *Setting up a database for information storage and exchange.* As well as providing an accessible and up-to-date list of network members, it records what is happening and where – providing the information needed to scrutinise the innovation and plan a strategy for its development.

- *Information exchange for network users.* This includes putting nurses in touch with others working in the same geographical area or speciality; and publishing a regular newsletter including short articles on developments, book reviews and journal abstracts, and listing of relevant events.

- *Study days and workshops.* These range from small workshops to explore specific issues, through to regional events, national conferences and research seminars.

- *Dissemination of information.* Joint conferences will be explored as a means of communicating with nurses who are interested in primary nursing but not yet using it. Collections of papers on work in progress and relevant issues will be published by the King's Fund.
- *Research.* The network and database offer a means of providing raw data and co-ordinating research on primary nursing.

Appendix II
Examples of
Job Description

PRIMARY NURSE

JOB TITLE   Primary Nurse
GRADE   F
HOURS   Full time
ACCOUNTABLE TO   Senior Sister
MONITORED BY   Senior Sister/Ward Sister

Minimum Requirements

1. 2 years post-registration experience.
2. 9–12 months nursing experience in relevant specialty.
3. Evidence of professional development (completed/in progress), e.g. degree, diploma, primary nursing module, research course, relevant ENB course, other evidence of continuing study.
4. Evidence of teaching qualification (completed/in progress), e.g. mentor's course, ENB 998, City & Guild's 730).

Purpose

● To be responsible and accountable for assessing, planning, implementing and evaluating the nursing care for a named group of patients.
● To develop and maintain high standards of nursing care, reflecting the beliefs about nursing practice outlined in the unit philosophy.
● To contribute to the continuing development of the unit.
● To provide unit cover in the absence of unit sisters.
● To manage a small team of associate nurses.

Key Result Areas

Patient Care Skills

- To be responsible and accountable for assessing, planning, implementing and evaluating the nursing care for a named group of patients.
- To maintain accurate and legible records of care.
- To act as associate nurse, as required, to a named group of patients.

Organisational Skills

- To lead a team of associate nurses, acknowledging their contribution to patient care and decision making.
- To promote effective communication, liaising with other members of the health care team.
- To act as co-ordinator, i.e. organiser of ward activity and communications, on a regular basis, in rotation with other registered nurses.
- To provide unit cover on a regular basis in the absence of the unit sisters.
- To accept responsibility for specific administratative tasks as delegated by the ward sister.
- To act as mentor to student nurses allocated to the unit.
- To be aware of budgetry implications when prescribing care.
- To assist in maintaining the safety of unit personnel, unit environment and unit equipment.
- To ensure that health authority policies are adhered to.
- To contribute to achieving and maintaining the clinical learning environment criteria.
- To assist the ward sister in developing and maintaining the job performance review programme.

Personal Development

- To demonstrate research-based care.
- To maintain own personal and professional growth.
- To contribute to the continuing development of the unit.

ASSOCIATE NURSE (E GRADE)

JOB TITLE	Associate Nurse
GRADE	E
HOURS	Full time/Part time
ACCOUNTABLE TO	Ward Sister*
MONITORED BY	Ward Sister

---

*This represents a stage in the development of primary nursing. The associate nurse is accountable to the primary nurse for carrying out the care planned to an acceptable standard. However, accountability for other aspects of her job come under the sister's sphere of responsibility.

Minimum Requirements

1. 1 year post-registration experience within the last 3 years.
2. Evidence of attendance on mentor's course (completed/in progress) or equivalent.

Purpose

- To assist the primary nurse in assessing, planning, implementing and evaluating the nursing care for a named group of patients.
- To develop high standards of nursing care, reflecting the beliefs about nursing practice outlined in the unit philosophy.
- To contribute to the continuing development of the unit.
- To provide unit cover in the absence of unit sisters, when necessary.

Key Result Areas

Patient Care Skills

- To be a member of a nursing team led by a primary nurse.
- To assist the primary nurse in assessing, planning, implementing and evaluating the care for a named group of patients.
- To contribute to the plan of care, as appropriate, in the absence of the primary nurse.
- To discuss with the primary nurse all matters concerning the named group of patients being cared for by the nursing team.
- To assist other primary and associate nurses in the ward team as necessary.
- To maintain accurate and legible records of care.
- To have access to and consult with senior nurses within the unit.

Organisational Skills

- To promote effective communication, liaising with other members of the health care team.
- To provide unit cover in the absence of the unit sisters when necessary.
- To act as mentor to student nurses.
- To contribute to maintaining the clinical learning environment criteria.
- To be prepared to regularly support and supervise junior staff.
- To act as co-ordinator, i.e. organiser of ward activity and communications, in rotation with other staff on a regular basis.
- To be aware of budgetry implications when prescribing care.
- To ensure that health authority policies are adhered to.
- To assist in maintaining the safety of unit personnel, unit environment and unit equipment.

Personal Development

- To maintain own personal and professional growth.
- To demonstrate research-based care.
- To contribute to the continuing development of the unit.

ASSOCIATE NURSE (D GRADE)

JOB TITLE   Associate Nurse
GRADE   D
HOURS   Full time/Part time
ACCOUNTABLE TO   Ward Sister*
MONITORED BY   Ward Sister

Minimum Requirements

1. RGN (newly qualified, return to nursing after a 3 year or more gap).
2. EN, with minimum of 1 year relevant post-enrolment experience and/or qualification.

Purpose

- To assist the primary nurse in assessing, planning, implementing and evaluating the nursing care for a named group of patients.
- To develop high standards of nursing care, reflecting the beliefs about nursing practice outlined in the unit philosophy.

Key Result Areas

Patient Care Skills

- To be a member of a nursing team led by a primary nurse.
- To assist the primary nurse in assessing, planning, implementing and evaluating the nursing care for a named group of patients.
- To discuss with the primary nurse all matters concerning the named group of patients being cared for by the nursing team.
- To maintain accurate and legible records of care.
- To identify, have access to and consult with senior nurses within the unit.
- To assist other primary and associate nurses in the ward team as necessary.

Organisational Skills

- To promote effective communication, liaising with other members of the health care team.

- To develop ability in acting as co-ordinator, i.e. organiser of ward activity and communication, for the duration of a shift.
- To be aware of budgetry implications when prescribing care.
- To assist in maintaining the safety of unit personnel, unit environment and unit equipment.
- To ensure that health authority policies are adhered to.

Personal Development

- To participate in the continuing development of the unit.
- To develop and maintain personal and professional growth.
- To demonstrate research-based care.
- To support new and student members of staff and offer feedback to mentors as appropriate.

WARD SISTER

JOB TITLE   Ward Sister
GRADE   G
DEPARTMENT   Nursing
ACCOUNTABLE TO   Director of Nursing Services
MONITORED BY   Senior Sister/Lecturer Practitioner

Purpose

1. To lead the nursing team in providing a professional nursing service.
2. To facilitate innovative and creative nursing practice through a staff development programme.

Key Result Areas

Patient Care

- To liaise with primary and associate nurses to ensure a democratic patient allocation.
- To practise alongside the nursing team regularly.
- To act as consultant to the nursing team as required.
- To promote research-based practice and support clinical research projects within the unit.
- To contribute to the development of clinical practice of the unit.
- To monitor the quality of nursing and to give regular feedback to the nursing team and hospital management.

Ward Management

- To select and appoint the nursing team.
- To identify the nursing policies of the ward and district and ensure that they are adhered to.
- To ensure safe and effective nurse cover on the ward at all times.
- To promote the nurses'/patients' interests via good communication with the health care team.
- To develop close working relationships with the other unit sister and act as senior nurse covering the unit as required.
- To represent the ward/unit within the hospital.
- To manage the ward budget (staff salary and equipment).

Staff Development

- To support the nursing team in developing their professional practice.
- To encourage and assist staff in taking opportunities for developing their own practice.
- To monitor staff performance using the unit's job performance review schedule.
- To achieve and maintain the clinical learning environment criteria.
- To assist in planning, give support, supervise and teach all learners allocated to the ward, working closely with the tutor linked to the ward.
- To contribute to the development of the nursing degree programme, disseminating information to the ward appropriately.
- To maintain own personal and professional development.

NURSING AUXILIARY

JOB TITLE	Nursing Auxiliary
GRADE	A
HOURS	Full time/Part time
ACCOUNTABLE TO	Ward Sister
MONITORED BY	Ward Sister

Purpose

1. To assist the nursing staff with the direct care of patients.
2. To keep the ward environment tidy and well maintained.
3. To provide support to the nursing team which will contribute to the efficiency and smooth running of the ward.

Key Result Areas

Patient Care

● To assist a nurse with the care of patients.
● To carry out aspects of patient care under the direction of a qualified nurse (see guidelines).
● To feed back information about patients to the nursing team.
● To assist with patients' meals and to make drinks and snacks as required to supplement regular meals and beverage rounds.
● To escort patients within the hospital area when no nursing needs are identified by the requesting nurse and when escort by the portering staff is inappropriate.

Ward Environment

● To keep ward storage areas clean, tidy and appropriately stocked.
● To keep patients' lockers and other furniture surfaces in the ward clean and tidy.
● To strip, clean and remake beds of discharged patients.
● To dispose of dead flowers in the ward, change flower water regularly and keep vases clean.

Support for the Nursing Team

● To answer the telephone and take messages when the ward clerk is not available.
● To organise storage and maintenance of ward equipment as directed by the ward sister and to collect and deliver ward equipment within the hospital as necessary.
● To contribute to maintaining a happy working atmosphere within the ward.

General

● To be aware of and comply with relevant health and safety and fire policies.

WARD CARE ASSISTANT

JOB TITLE   Ward Care Assistant
GRADE   Nursing Auxiliary
HOURS   Varied
RESPONSIBLE TO   Senior Nurse Practitioner
ACCOUNTABLE TO   Nurse Practitioner/Associate Nurse on duty

Overall Objective

1. To work as part of the ward team by supporting and assisting qualified nurses, as and when required, to help facilitate and enhance patient comfort and care.
2. Contributing, under the direction of the nurses, to the safe, efficient and smooth running of the ward environment; in particular, by being responsible for keeping the ward clean, tidy and well maintained and ensuring that the patient's food is well presented.

Housekeeping/Ward Environment Duties

1. The Ward Care Assistant will be responsible for ensuring that patients receive the food and beverages either of their choice or as laid down for them.
2. To be responsible for ensuring that the ward environment is maintained to a satisfactory level in terms of safety, tidiness and cleanliness.
3. Specific duties here will include some or all of the following items:
   - Issue menu slips to patients and assist if required in the completion of the form.
   - Collect menu slips and return to the Catering Department.
   - Plate meals for patients in accordance with the menu ordered; serve and give assistance to help them eat, as necessary and directed.
   - Prepare the trolley, make and serve beverages and/or special diet snacks to patients. Lay up trays, trolleys and tables for each meal as required, and clear away the same to the kitchen on completion of the meal. Ensure surfaces are clean and condiments are full. All dishes and cutlery to be washed, dried and stored appropriately.
   - Check dry goods, bread and dairy produce; order as required. Accept and check deliveries, put away and accept responsibility for the control and security of items delivered to the ward.
   - Ensure food in the fridge is fresh and dispose of any out-of-date items.
   - Clean water jugs and glasses in the kitchen, refill and redistribute as required.
   - Display and dispose of flowers, changing water daily and cleaning vases after use.
   - Keep patients' lockers and other associated furniture tidy. Ensure that wash bowls and lockers are cleaned thoroughly on patients' discharge.
   - Strip clean and remake beds of discharged patients and make up unoccupied beds.
   - Be responsible for the care and maintenance of ward clothing and ensure that dirty linen is disposed of appropriately. Collect and dispose of rubbish on the ward.
   - Keep ward storage areas and sluice clean and tidy, and appropriately stocked by ordering according to preset lists, checking and putting items received away.
   - To ensure the ward and associated rooms are kept clean and tidy, clean up any accidental spillages of blood, faeces or vomit if required to do so.
   - Answer and take telephone messages when the ward co-ordinator is not

available and run errands for nursing staff as requested.
- To set up equipment for nurses' procedures and clear away when finished with.

Nursing Support/Assistance Duties

The Ward Care Assistant may, if requested, be required to *assist* one of the nursing staff in one or more of the following duties:

- The bathing of patients in bed or in the bathroom, and the preparation of the bathroom.
- The turning or lifting of patients using mechanical and bed appliances where appropriate.
- The care of the patient's hair, nails or oral hygiene.
- The toileting of patients according to their individual needs (i.e. bed pans, commodes, urinals, or up to the toilet).
- The dressing of patients who need assistance.
- The care of clothing and personal property of patients who are being admitted, transferred or discharged.
- The escorting of patients to clinical departments, the shop or chapel, when required.
- The weighing of patients.

General Requirements

1. To meet the requirements of the Health and Safety at Work Act in attending regular fire and safety instruction. To have a broad knowledge of the policies of the Health Authority on this subject.
2. To take all possible measures to ensure the safety of patients, visitors and staff in the ward. To report all incidents/accidents to the nurse in charge and assist in the completion of the relevant forms if appropriate.
3. To help ensure that all non-medical equipment is used correctly and to report any unsafe equipment immediately to the nurse in charge of the shift.
4. To have knowledge of the fire regulations of the Health Authority.
   - To read displayed notices giving instructions as to what to do in case of fire.
   - Know siting and use of fire-fighting equipment and siting of exits on your ward – these to be kept clear at all times.
   - To know the procedure for calling for assistance in the case of fire.

While this job description is not meant to be exhaustive, there may also be duties contained within it that the Ward Care Assistants will not necessarily be required to undertake. The details of these duties are as per the Ward Care Assistant manual, which will be issued on appointment.

The postholder will be expected to adopt a flexible attitude towards these duties, which may have to be varied subject to the needs of the patient as determined by the nurse and of the service as a whole.

The contents of the job description will be reviewed with the postholder at regular intervals.

Cumulative Bibliography

Abel-Smith B (1964) *A History of the Nursing Profession*. London: Heinemann.

Abercrombie N, Hills S and Turner B (1980) *The Penguin Dictionary of Sociology*. Harmondsworth: Penguin.

Aggleton P and Chalmers H (1986) *Nursing Models and the Nursing Process*. Houndsmith: Macmillan Educational Ltd.

Akehurst C J and Fitzsimons D (1988) *AIDS Newsletter*. Bureau of Hygiene and Tropical Medicine, 3(9–1): 21 July.

Alderman C (1983) Burford: a model for nursing individual care in action. *Nursing Times* **79**(3): 15–17.

Alexander C, Weisman C and Chase G (1981) *Organisational Correlates and Consequences of Primary Nursing*. Unpublished. Conducted under grant NU00568 from the Division of Nursing, Bureau for Health Manpower Health Resources Administration.

Alexander M F (1983) *Learning to Nurse: Integrating Theory and Practice*. Edinburgh: Churchill Livingstone.

Altschul A (1972) *Patient–Nurse Interaction: a Study of Interaction Patterns in Acute Psychiatric Wards*. University of Edinburgh, Department of Nursing Studies. Monograph No. 3. Edinburgh: Churchill Livingstone.

Anderson M and Choi T (1980) Primary nursing in an organizational context. *Journal of Nursing Administration*, **10**: 26–31.

Argyris C (1957) *Personality and Organisation: the Conflict between the System and the Individual*. New York: Harper and Row.

Argyris C and Schon D (1974) *Theory in Practice: Increasing Professional Effectiveness*. California: Jossey-Bass.

Atherton J S (1986) *Professional supervision in group care: A contract based approach*. London: Tavistock.

Bailey J T and Claus K E (1975) *Decision Making in Nursing*. St. Louis: C V Mosby Co.

Balint M (1957) *The Doctor, his Patient and the Illness*. London: Pitman.

Baly M (1975) *Professional Responsibility*. Chichester: John Wiley.

Baly M E (1980) *Nursing and Social Change*. London: Heinemann.

Barret J *et al*. (1975) *The Head Nurse*. New York: Appleton Century Crofts.

Batey M V and Lewis F M (1982) Clarifying autonomy and accountability in nursing service. *Journal of Nursing Administration*, September; 13–18.

Beckhard R (1969) *Organisation Development: Strategies and Models*. Reading, Mass.: Addison–Wesley.

Bellaby P and Oribabor P (1980) The history of the present – contradiction and struggle in nursing. In: *Rewriting Nursing History*, Davis C (ed.). London: Croom Helm.

Bendall E (1975) *So You Passed Nurse*. London: Royal College of Nursing.

Bendall E (1986) The disappearing nurses. *Nursing Times*, July 16: 28–30.

Benner P (1984) *From Novice to Expert*. Reading, Mass.: Addison–Wesley.

Bennis W, Benne K and Chin R (1976) 3rd edn *The Planning of Change*. Holt, Rinehart and Winston.

Bergman R (1981) Accountability, definitions, dimensions. *International Nursing Review*, **28**(2): 53–59.

Berry A and Metcalf C (1986) Paradigms and practices: the organisation of the delivery of nursing care. *Journal of Advanced Nursing*, **11**: 589–597.

Betz M (1981) Some hidden costs of primary nursing. *Nursing and Health Care*, **2**: 151–154.

Bevis E O (1983) *Curriculum Building in Nursing – A Process*, 3rd edn. St. Louis: C V Mosby Co.

Beyer J E and Marshall J (1981) The interpersonal dimension of collegiality. *Nursing Outlook*, November: 662–665.

Binnie A (1984) *Towards Professional Nursing Practice in Oxford. Are current nursing staff establishments appropriate for the development of a professional style of nursing in Oxford?* Unpublished. Discussion paper, Oxford Regional Health Authority.

Binnie A (1987) Primary nursing – structural changes. *Nursing Times*, **83**(39): 36–37.

Binnie A (1988) *The Working Lives of Staff Nurses: a Sociological Perspective*. Unpublished MA thesis, University of Warwick.

Blackham H J (1968) *Humanism*. Harmondsworth: Penguin.

Blair-Fish H M (1954) The patient in the ward today. *Nursing Times*, **21**(8): 902–903.

Blanchard K and Johnson S (1983) *The One Minute Manager*. London: Fontana/Collins.

Bond M (1982) Do you care about your colleagues? *Nursing Mirror*, October 20: 42–44.

Bond M (1986) *Stress and Self-awareness: A Guide for Nurses*. London: Heinemann Nursing.

Bowers L (1989) The significance of primary nursing. *Journal of Advanced Nursing*, **14**: 13–19.

Bowman J (1989) *Nurses' Stress Associated with Different Work Methods: Primary Nursing vs Team Nursing*. Unpublished paper.

Brech E F L (ed.) (1975) *The Principles and Practice of Management*, 3rd edn. London: Longman.

Breu C and Dracup K (1976) Implementing nursing research in a critical care setting. *Journal of Nursing Administration*, **6**: 14–17.

Brierton N (1987) Managing change. *Nursing Management*, **18**(10): 70.

Briggs A (Chairman) (1972) *Report of the Committee on Nursing*. London: HMSO.

Brittle J and Marsh J (1986) Monitor: Definition or Measurement. *Nursing Times*, 5th November.

Brooking J (1986) *Patient and Family Participation in Nursing Care: the Development of a Nursing Process Measuring Scale*. Unpublished PhD thesis, Department of Nursing Studies, King's College, University of London.

Brown E L (1966) Nursing and patient care. In: *The Nursing Profession: 5 Sociological Essays*, Davis F (ed.). New York: John Wiley.

Bruner J S (1966) *Towards a Theory of Instruction*. Cambridge, Mass.: Belknap.

Buchan J (1987) Reporting on Griffiths. *Nursing Times*, **83**(29): 34–35.

Buckenham J and McGrath G (1983) *The Social Reality of Nursing*. Sydney: Adis.

Burns S (1988) The role of the associate nurse. *Professional Nurse*, **4**(1): 18–20.

Burns S, Fitzgerald M and Vaughan B (1988) *Curriculum for the Primary Nursing Module*. Unpublished paper, Oxford School of Nursing.

Burns T and Stalker G M (1966) *The Management of Innovation*. London: Tavistock Publications.

Calsune S (1951) *Executive Behaviour: A Study of the Workload and Working Methods of Managing Directors*. Stockholm: Strombergs.

Carey R (1979) Evaluation of a primary nursing unit. *American Journal of Nursing*, July: 1253–1255.

Carpenter M (1978) Managerialism and the division of labour in nursing. In: *Readings in the Sociology of Nursing*, Dingwall R and McIntosh J (eds). Edinburgh: Churchill Livingstone.

Carson D (1988) Taking risks with patients – your assessment strategy. *The Professional Nurse*, **3**(7): 247–250.

Carter S L (1983) Rehumanising the nursing role: a question of love. *Topics in Clinical*

Nursing, **3**(3): 11–17.

Cassidy v. *Ministry of Health* (1951) 2 KB 343.

Castledine G (1980) 'My nurse' and 'my patient'. *Nursing Mirror*, **151**(6): 14.

CDR 90/44, Statistics prepared from voluntary confidential reports by Clinicians to CDSC and CD (Scotland) Unit, 2 November, 1990.

Central Health Services Council (1958) *Annual Report, Ministry of Health*. London: HMSO.

Chapman C (1977a) Concepts of professionalism. *Journal of Advanced Nursing*, **2**: 51–55.

Chapman C M (1977b) The paradox of nursing. *Journal of Advanced Nursing*, **8**: 323–333.

Chapman C (1983) The Paradox of Nursing. *Journal of Advanced Nursing*, **8**: 269–272.

Chavasse J (1981) From task assignment to patient allocation: a change evaluation. *Journal of Advanced Nursing*, **6**: 137–145.

Chin R and Benne K D (1976) General strategies for effecting change in human systems. In: *The Planning of Change*, Bennis W G *et al.* (eds). New York: Holt, Rinehart and Winston.

Ciske K (1974) Primary nursing evaluation. *American Journal of Nursing*, **74**(8): 1436–1438.

Ciske K (1980) Introduction of seminar and clarification of accountability in primary nursing. In: 'Primary Nursing' issue of *Nursing Dimensions*, Ciske K and Mayer G (eds), **II**(4): Winter.

Clark M (1978) Getting through the work. In: *Readings in the Sociology of Nursing*, Dingwall R and McIntosh J (eds). Edinburgh: Churchill Livingstone.

Clark P (1972) *Action Research and Organisational Change*. London: Harper & Row.

Clarke K (1989) Letter to Dame Audrey Emerton. United Kingdom Central Council for Nursing, Midwifery and Health Visiting.

Clarke M (1986) Action and reflection: practice and theory in nursing. *Journal of Advanced Nursing*, **11**: 3–11.

Claus K and Baily J (1977) *Power and Influence in Hospital Care*. St. Louis: Mosby.

Clay T (1987) *Nurses: Power and Politics*. London: Heinemann Nursing.

Clay T (1988) How to nurse the NHS back to health. *Daily Telegraph*, February 4.

Coates V (1985) *Are they being served? An investigation into the institutional care given by nurses to acute medical patients and the influence of ward organisational patterns on that care* London: RCN.

Cobbs P M (1975) The victim's perspective. In: *Humanising Health Care*, Howard J and Strauss A (eds). Berkley: University of California Press.

Cohen J Professor (Chairman) (1948) *Report of the Working Party on the Recruitment and Training of Nurses* (Cohen Report) Ministry of Health, Ministry of Labour and National Service. London: HMSO.

Coluccio M and Maguire P (1983) Collaborative practice: becoming a reality through primary nursing. *Nursing Administration Quarterly*, Summer: 59–62.

Crow J (1977a) The nursing process: theoretical background. *Nursing Times*, **75**(24): 342–346.

Crow J (1977b) Nursing care using a nursing care plan. *Nursing Times*, **73**(26): 938–940.

Crow R (1981) Research and the standards of nursing care: what is the relationship? *Journal of Advanced Nursing*, **6**: 491–496.

Culpepper R, Richie M, Sinclair V, Stephens N and Betz L (1986) The effect of primary nursing on nursing quality assurance. *Journal of Nursing Administration*, **16**(11): 24–31.

Cumberlege J (1987) Diary of nobody. *Nursing Times*, **83**(4): 28.

Daeffler R (1975) Patients' perceptions of care under team and primary nursing. *Journal of Nursing Administration*, March–April: 20–26.

Davies C and Francis A (1976) Perceptions of stress in NHS hospitals, In: *The Sociology of the NHS*, Stacey M (ed.). Sociological Monograph 22, University of Keele.

Davis C (1976) Experience of dependency in work: the case for nurses. *Journal of Advanced Nursing*, **1**(4): 273–282.

Davis C (1977) Continuities in the development of hospital nursing in Britain. *Journal of Advanced Nursing*, **2**: 479–493.

Davis C (1980) *Rewriting Nursing History*. London: Croom Helm.

Davis F (1966) *The Nursing Profession: Sociological Essays*. New York: John Wiley.

Davis L E and Trust E (1974) Improving the quality of working life. In: *Work and the Quality of Life*, O'Toole T (ed.). Cambridge, Mass.: MIT.

De la Cuesta C (1983) The nursing process: from development to implementation. *Journal of Advanced Nursing*, **8**: 365–371.

Dean D (1987) *Manpower Solutions*. London: Royal College of Nursing.

Dean D (1989) Managing a future. *Nursing Times*, **85**(13): 20.

Deirman P A, Noble E and Russell M E (1984) Achieving a professional practice model. *Journal of Nursing Administration*, July/August: 17.

Delamothe, T (1990) *British Medical Journal*, **301**, 27 October.

Delbecq A, Van der Ven A M and Gustafson D A (1975) *Group Techniques for Program Planning: a Guide to Nominal Group and Delphi Processes*. Glenvieur, Illinois: Scott Foreman.

Demers P M (1981) Developing a primary nurse. *Nursing Management*, **12**(12): 28–30.

Department of Health (1988) *The Way Ahead: Career Pathways for Midwives and Health Visitors: A Report of the NHS Management Board DH Nursing Division Career Development Project Group*. London: HMSO.

Department of Health (1989a) *Working for Patients*. London: HMSO.

Department of Health (1989b) *A Strategy for Nursing: A Report of the Steering Committee of the DH Nursing Division*, London: HMSO.

Dewey J (1933) *How we Think: A Restatement of the Relation of Reflective Thinking to the Educative Process*. Chicago: Henry Regnery.

DHSS (1973) *Report of the Committee on Hospital Complaints Procedure*. London: HMSO.

DHSS (1986) *Mix and Match: A Review of Nursing Skill Mix*. London: DHSS.

Dickinson S (1982) The nursing process and the professional status of nursing. *Nursing Times* Occasional paper, **78**(16): 61–64.

Dingwall R, Rafferty A and Webster C (1988) *An Introduction to the Social History of Nursing*. London: Routledge.

Donabedian A (1969) Quality of care: problems of measurement. Part II: Some issues of evaluating the quality of nursing care. *American Journal of Public Health*, **59**: 1833–1836.

Drucker P (1977) *People and Performance: The Best of P Drucker on Management*. London: Heinemann.

Duberley J (1977) How will the change strike you and me? *Nursing Times*, **73**(45): 1736–1738.

Eichhorn M and Frevert E I (1979) Evaluation of a primary nursing system using the quality patient care scale. *Journal of Nursing Administration*, **9**(10): 11–15.

ENB (1985) *Professional Training/Training Courses*. Consultation Paper. London: ENB.

ENB (1987) *Managing Change in Nursing Education. Pack One: Preparing for Change*. London: ENB.

ENB for Nursing, Midwifery and Health Visiting (1988) *Spectrum of Opportunities for Enrolled Nurses*. Paper 5. London: ENB.

Ersser S (1987) *Clinical Practice: Development Work, June–September*. Unpublished report, Didcot Hospital, Berkshire.

Ersser S J (1988) *An Ethnographic Study to Explore and Compare the Existence and Nature of Nurses' and Patients' Views about the Therapeutic Effect of Nursing. First Stage Fieldwork*. Unpublished report, Institute of Nursing, Oxford.

Ersser S J (1990) A search for the therapeutic dimensions of nurse–patient interaction. In: *Nursing as Therapy*, Pearson A and McMahon R (eds). London: Chapman and Hall.

Exley E, Barstow R, Ventura M, Hegedus K S and McCormick K (1980) Questions and answers, *Western Journal of Nursing Research*, **2**(3): 609–621.

Fagin C and Diers D (1983) Nursing on a metaphor. *New England Journal of Medicine*, **309**: 116–117.

Faulkner A (1988) The need for education. *Nursing*, **28**: 3rd series, April: 1014–1018.

Faulkner A and McGuire P (1988) The need for support. *Nursing*, **28**: 3rd series, April: 1010–1012.

Fein R (1975) A request for precision. In: *Humanising Health Care*, Howard J and Strauss A (eds). New York: John Wiley.

Felder L A (1983) Direct patient care and independent practice. In: *The Clinical Nurse Specialist in Theory and Practice*, Hamric A B and Spross J (eds). Florida: Grune and Stratton.

Felton G (1975) Increasing the quality of nursing care by introducing the concept of primary nursing: a model project. *Nursing Research*, **24**(1): 27–32.

Ferriman A (1988) Nurses to go on strike as protest grows. *The Observer*, November 27.

Filkins J (1986) Introducing change. *Nursing Times*, **82**(7): 26, 29–30.

Flint C (1986) *Sensitive Midwifery*. London: Heinemann.

Fowler F and Fowler H W (1969) *The Pocket Oxford Dictionary*. Oxford: Oxford University Press.

Fox R and Ventura M (1984) Internal psychometric characteristics of the quality patient care scale. *Nursing Research*, **33**(2): 112–117.

Friedson E (1970) *Professional Dominance: the Social Structure of Medical Care*. Chicago: Aldine Publishing Co.

Friedson E (1975) *The Profession of Medicine*. New York: Dodds, Mead.

Further Education Unit (FEU) (1988) *National Council for Vocational Qualifications and its Implications* 1988. Paper No. 1. London: FEU.

Gamarnikow E (1978) Sexual division of labour; the case of nursing. In: *Feminism and Materialism*, Kuhn A and Wolfe A (eds). London: Routledge and Kegan Paul.

General Nursing Council (1977) *General Nursing Council for England and Wales, 1977. Training Syllabus for Register of Nurses (General Nurses)*. London: General Nursing Council.

Gieger J (1975) Causes of dehumanisation in health care and prospects for humanisation. In: *Humanising Health Care*, Howard J and Strauss A (eds). New York: John Wiley.

Giovannetti P (1980) A comparison of team and primary nursing care systems. *Nursing Dimensions*, **7**(4): 96–100.

Giovannetti P (1981) *Primary Nursing – Is it the Answer?* Proceedings RCN Research Society Conference: Canterbury.

Giovannetti P (1986) Evaluation of primary nursing. In: *Annual Review of Nursing Research*, Weilty H H, Fitzpatrick J J and Tauton R L (eds). New York: Springer.

Girouard S (1983) Theory based practice: functions, obstacles and solutions. In: *The Clinical Nurse Specialist in Theory and Practice*, Hamric A B and Spross J (eds). Florida: Grune and Stratton.

Glendill R (1987) Nursing shortage 'is at crisis level'. *The Times*, September 21.

Goddard H A (1953) *The Work of Nurses in Hospital Wards* (Goddard Report). London: Nuffield Provincial Hospitals Trust.

Goldstone L A, Ball J A and Collier M M (1983) *Monitor*. Newcastle: Newcastle upon Tyne Polytechnics Products Ltd.

Graham H (1986) *The Humanistic Psychology in its Historical, Social and Cultural Context*. Milton Keynes: Open University Press.

Griffiths R (1983) *NHS Management Inquiry*. London: DHSS.

Hall L (1963) A center for nursing. *Nursing Outlook*, **11**: 805.

Hall, L (1964) *Project Report: The Solomon and Betty Loeb Center at the Montefiore Hospital*. New York: The Center.

Hall L E (1969) The Loeb Center for Nursing and Rehabilitation, Montefiore Hospital and Medical Center, Bronx, New York. *International Journal of Nursing Studies*, **6**: 81–97.

Hall L, Alfons G, Rifkin E and Levine H (1975) *Final Report: Longitudinal Effects of an Experimental Nursing Process*. Unpublished report. New York: Loeb Center for Nursing.

Hardy L and Engel J (1987) The search for professionalism. *Nursing Times*, April 15: 37–39.

Harrison D (1988) Nursing auxiliaries – an asset not to be wasted. *Senior Nurse*, **8**(3): 29–31.

Harrison E (1981) Activation of patients with strokes in clinical nursing care: effects on patients and staff. *Abstracts of Uppsala Dissertations*. Faculty of Medicine 407, University Hospital, Uppsala, Sweden.

Haussmann R K B, Hegyvary S T and Newman J F (1976) *Monitoring Quality of Nursing Care Part II: Assessment and Study of Correlates* (HRA Report no. 76–7). Bethesda, MD: Dept. of Health Education and Welfare.

Hays R and di Matteo M R (1984) Toward a more therapeutic physician–patient relationship. In: *Personal Relationships 5: Repairing Personal Relationships*, Duck S W (ed.). London and New York: Academic Press.

Hayward J (1986) *Report of the Nursing Process Evaluation Working Group*. London: King's College, University of London NERU.

Hegyvary S (1977) Foundations of primary nursing. *Nursing Clinics of North America*, **12**(2): 187–196.

Hegyvary S T (1982) *The Change to Primary Nursing: A Cross-Cultural View of Professional Practice*. St. Louis: C V Mosby Co.

Hegyvary S T and Hausmann R K D (1981) *The Process of Change to Primary Nursing*. Boston: C V Mosby Co.

Heller R (1972) *The Naked Manager*. London: Barrie and Jenkins.

Henderson V (1980) Prescribing the essence of nursing in a technological age. *Journal of Advanced Nursing*, **5**(3): 245–260.

Hersey P and Blanchard K H (1977) *Management of Organisational Behaviour*. Englewood Cliffs, New Jersey: Prentice Hall.

Herzberg F (1968) One more time: how do you motivate employees? *Harvard Business Review*, **46**(1): 53–62.

Heslop A and Bagnall P (1988) A study to evaluate the intervention of a nurse visiting patients with disabling chest disease in the community. *Journal of Advanced Nursing*, **13**(1): 71–77.

Hochschild A R (1983) *The Managed Heart: The Commercialisation of Human Feeling*. Berkley: University of California Press.

Hockey L (1984) Conclusion. In: *Communication*. Recent Advances in Nursing series. Edinburgh: Churchill Livingstone.

Holmes S W (1987) Managing the stress of primary nursing. *Nursing Management*, **18**(3): 62–66.

Horder Lord (Chairman), Royal College of Nursing, Nursing Reconstruction Committee (1942) *The Assistant Nurse, Section I*. London: Royal College of Nursing.

Horder Lord (Chairman), Royal College of Nursing, Nursing Reconstruction Committee (1943) *Education and Training, Section II*. London: Royal College of Nursing.

Horder Lord (Chairman), Royal College of Nursing, Nursing Reconstruction Committee (1943) *Recruitment, Section III*. London: Royal College of Nursing.

Horder Lord (Chairman), Royal College of Nursing, Nursing Reconstruction Committee (1944) *The Social and Economic Conditions of the Nurse, Section IV*. London: Royal College of Nursing.

Horn B and Parker J (1975) *Reorganisation of Nursing Resources in Hospitals*. Ann Arbor, School of Public Health, University of Michigan. Unpublished manuscript, cited in Munson and Clinton (1979).

Howard J (1975) Humanisation and dehumanisation of health care: a conceptual view. In: *Humanizing Health Care*, Howard J and Strauss A (eds). New York: John Wiley.

Hunt M (1987) The process of translating research findings into nursing practice. *Journal of Advanced Nursing*, **12**: 101–110.

Illich I (1976) *Limits to Medicine, Medical Nemesis: The Exploration of Health*. Harmondsworth: Penguin.

Inman U (1975) *Towards a Theory of Nursing Care: An Account of the RCN and DHSS Research Project*. London: Royal College of Nursing.

International Council of Nurses (1973) *Code of Nursing Ethics*. Geneva: ICN.

Jacquerye A (1984) Choosing an appropriate method of quality assurance. In: *Measuring the Quality of Care*, Willis L and Linwood M (eds). Edinburgh: Churchill Livingstone.

Jarvis P (1983) *Professional Education*. Worcester: Croom Helm.

Jarivs P (1986) Contract learning. *Journal of District Nursing*, November: 13–14.

Jarvis P (1987) Lifelong education and its relevance to nursing. *Nurse Education today*, **7**: 49–55.

Jenkinson V M (1953) Group or team nursing? *Nursing Times*, January 17 & 24.

Johns C C (1988) *Individual Performance Review Tool*. Unpublished document, Brackley

Cottage Hospital, Northants.

Johns C C (1989) Developing a philosophy. *Journal of Nursing Practice* (Nursing Standard Supplement), **3**(1): 2–4.

Johns C C (1990a) Developing a philosophy for practice: Part 2. *Nursing Practice*, **3.2**, 2–5.

Johns C C (1990b) Antonomy of primary nurses; the need to both facilitate and limit antonomy in practice. *Journal of Advanced Nursing*, **15**, 886–894.

Johns C C (1990c) *Becoming a primary nurse*. BNDU research publication, Burford, Oxon.

Johns C C (1991 forthcoming) *Developing clinical practice*. Harrow: Scutari Press.

Johns C C and Kingston S (1989) *Holbech Action Research Project*, **2**, Stage 1 report. BNDU Publications, Burford, Oxon.

Johnson T J (1972) *Professions and Power*. London: Macmillan.

Johnston M and Ross M (1988) *The Way Forward. Clinical Development for Enrolled Nurses: a Guide for Managers*. Oxford, OHA.

Jones D C (1975a) *Food For Thought*. London: Royal College of Nursing.

Jones K (1975b) Study documents: effect of primary nursing on renal transplant patients. *Hospitals, Journal of the American Hospital Association*, **49**: 85–89.

Jones W L (1977) Management by crisis or by objectives? *Nursing Times*, 10 & 17 March (10 & 11): 342–343, 388–390.

Jourard S M (1971) *The Transparent Self*. New York: D Van Nostrand.

Kagan C M (1985) *Interpersonal Skills in Nursing: Research and Applications*. London: Croom Helm.

Kemmis S (1982) *The Action Research Planner*. Deakin University, Victoria, Australia.

Keyzer D (1986) Using learning contracts to support change in nursing organisation. *Nurse Education Today*, **6**: 103–106.

Kirovac S and Fortin F (1976) A randomised control trial of preoperative patient education. *International Journal of Nursing Studies*, **13**: 11–24.

Kitson A (1984) *Steps toward the Identification and Development of Nursing Therapeutic Functions in the Care of Hospitalised Elderly*. Unpublished PhD thesis, University of Ulster, Coleraine.

Kitson A (1986) Indicators of quality in nursing care – an alternative approach. *Journal of Advanced Nursing*, **11**: 133–134.

Klein D C (1968) *Community Dynamics and Mental Health*. New York: John Wiley.

Knowles M S (1970) *The Modern Practice of Adult Education: from Pedagogy to Andragogy*. Cambridge: Cambridge Book Co.

Körner E (DHSS) (1982) *A Report on the Collection and Use of Information about Hospital Clinical Activity in the NHS* (Steering group of Health Services Information). London: HMSO.

Kramer H E (1974) The philosophical foundation of management rediscovered. *Management International Review*, **15**: 2–3.

Kratz C (1979a) *The Nursing Process*. London: Baillière Tindall.

Kratz C R (1979b) Primary nursing: letter from Australia – 2. *Nursing Times*, **75**(42): 1790–1791

Kron T (1971) *The Management of Patient Care: Putting Leadership Skills to Work*, 3rd edn. London: W B Saunders.

Laforme S (1982) Primary nursing: does good care cost more? *The Canadian Nurse*, April: 42–49.

Lancaster J (1982) Change theory: an essential aspect of nursing practice. In: *The Nurse as a Change Agent*, Lancaster J and Lancaster W (eds). St. Louis: C V Mosby Co.

Lanceley A (1985) Use of controlling language in the rehabilitation of the elderly. *Journal of Advanced Nursing*, **10**: 125–135.

Langrish J (1977) Technological determination. In: *Humanising the Workplace: New Proposals and Perspectives*, Ottaway R N (ed.). London: Croom Helm.

Lathlean J (1987) *Job Sharing a Ward Sister's Post*. A report of an evaluation commissioned by the Riverside Health Authority, London.

Lathlean J, Smith G and Bradley S (1986) *Post-Registration Development Schemes Evaluation*. Nursing Education Research Unit Report No. 4, King's College, London.

Lee M E (1979) Towards better care: primary nursing. *Nursing Times* occasional paper, **75** (33): 133–135.

Lelean S (1973) *Ready for Report, Nurse?* London: Royal College of Nursing.

Lembright M F (1983) Why nursing is not a profession. Free enquiry. *Creative Sociology*, **11**(1): 59–60, 64.

Leininger M (ed.) (1976) *Transcultural Nursing: Theories, Concepts and Practices*, New York: John Wiley.

Levanthal H (1975) The consequences of depersonalisation during illness and treatment. In: *Humanising Health Care*, Howard J and Strauss A (eds). New York: John Wiley.

Lewin K (1951) *Field Theory in Social Science*. New York: Harper and Row.

Lewin K (1958) Group decision and social change. In: *Readings in Social Psychology*, Maccoby E (ed.). New York: Holt, Rinehart and Winston.

Lewis F and Batey M (1982) Clarifying autonomy and accountability in the nursing service, Part 2. *Journal of Nursing Administration*, October: 10–15.

Ling M W O (1986) Critical analysis of literature on the nursing process. *The Hong Kong Nursing Journal*, **40**: 29–35.

Lippitt G L (1973) *Visualising Change: Model Building and the Change Process*. La Jolla, California: University Associates.

MacGuire J M (1980) *The Expanded role of the Nurse*. London: King's Fund.

MacGuire J (1989a) An approach to evaluating the introduction of primary nursing in an acute medical unit for the elderly. Part 1: Principles and practice. *International Journal of Nursing Studies*, **26**(3): 243–251.

MacGuire J (1989b) An approach to evaluating the introduction of primary nursing in an acute medical unit for the elderly. Part 2: Operationalising the principles. *International Journal of Nursing Studies*, **26**(3): 253–260.

Macleod-Clarke J (1984) Verbal communications in nursing. In: *Recent Advances in Nursing. 7: Communication*, Faulkner A (ed.). Edinburgh: Churchill Livingstone.

MacPhail J (1988) Job satisfaction in the nursing profession. In: *Recent Advances in Nursing*. Hudson: Longman.

McDonald M (1988) Primary nursing: is it worth it? *Journal of Advanced Nursing*, **13**: 797–806.

McFarlane J K (1982) *A Guide to the Practice of Using the Nursing Process*. London: C V Mosby Co.

McFarlane J K (1989) Profession is in disorder and disarray. Olive Anstey International Conference, Australia. *Nursing Times*, **84**(50): 6.

McFarlane J K and Castledine G (1982) *A Guide to the Practice of Nursing Using the Nursing Process*. London: C V Mosby Co.

McIntosh E (1951) *The Concise Oxford Dictionary*. Oxford: The Clarendon Press.

McMahon R A (1987) *An Analysis of Power and Collegial Relations among Nurses on Wards Implementing Hierarchical and Lateral Management Structures*. Unpublished MA dissertation, University of Warwick.

McMahon R (1988) Primary Nursing in Practice In: *Primary Nursing: Nursing in BONDU's*, Pearson A (ed.). London: Croom Helm.

McMahon R A (1989) Primary nursing: one to one. *Nursing Times*, **85**(2): 39–40.

McMahon R (1990) Collegiality is the key. *Nursing Times*, **86**, 42, 66–67.

Maggs C (1983) *The Origins of General Nursing*. London: Croom Helm.

Maggs C (1987) *Nursing History: the State of the Art*. London: Croom Helm.

Main T F (1957) The ailment. *British Journal of Medical Psychology*, **XXX**(3): 129–145.

Malby R (1988) All you need is thought. *Nursing Times*, **84**(51): 46–48.

Manfredi C (1986) Reliability and validity of the Phaneuf nursing audit. *Western Journal of Nursing Research*, **8**(2): 168–180.

Manthey M (1970) The history and development of primary nursing. *Nursing Forum*, **IX**(4): 359.

Manthey M (1973) Primary nursing is alive and well in the hospital. *American Journal of Nursing*, **73**(1): 83–87.

Manthey M (1980) *The Practice of Primary Nursing*. Boston: Blackwell Scientific.

Manthey M (1988) Can primary nursing survive? *American Journal of Medicine*, May: 644–647.

Manthey M and Kramer M (1970) The history and development of primary nursing. *Nursing Forum*, **IX**(4): 356–379.

Manthey M, Ciske K, Robertson P and Harris I (1970) Primary nursing: a return to the concept of 'my nurse' and 'my patient'. *Nursing Forum*, **IX**(1): 65–83.

Marcuse H (1964) *One Dimensional Man: Studies in the Ideology of Advanced Industrial Society*. Boston: Beacon Press.

Marram G (1976) The comparative costs of operating a team and primary nursing unit. *Journal of Nursing Administration*, **6**: 21–24.

Marram G D, Schlegel M N and Bevis E O (1974) *Primary Nursing: a Model for Individualised Care*. St. Louis: C V Mosby Co.

Marram G, Flynn K, Abaravich W and Carey S (1976) *Cost Effectiveness of Primary and Team Nursing*. Wakefield, Mass.: Contemporary Publishing.

Marram van Servellen G (1980) Evaluating the impact of primary nursing: outcomes. *Nursing Dimensions*, Winter: 48–50.

Marram van Servellen G (1982) The concept of individualised care in nursing. *Nursing and Health Care*, November: 482–485.

Marris P (1978) *Loss and Change*. London: Routledge and Kegan Paul.

Martin J P (1984) *Hospitals in Trouble*. Oxford: Blackwell.

Martin P and Stewart A (1983) Primary and non-primary nursing – evaluation by process criteria. *The Australian Journal of Advanced Nursing*, **1**(1): 31–37.

Maslow A H (1954) *Motivation and Personality*. New York: Harper and Row.

Matthews A (1975) Patient allocation – a review. *Nursing Times* occasional papers, **71** (1–4): 28, 29–31, 65–79.

Mauksch I G and Miller M H (1981) *Implementing Change in Nursing*. St. Louis: C V Mosby Co.

Mayer G (1982) The relationship between patient satisfaction with nursing care and the ability to identify the primary nurse. *Nursing and Health Care*, May: 254–257.

Meleis A I (1985) *Theoretical Nursing: Development and Progress*. Philadelphia: J G Lippincott.

Melia K M (1987) *Learning and Working: The Occupational Socialization of Nurses*. London: Tavistock.

Mellow J (1966) Nursing therapy as a treatment and clinical investigative approach to emotional illness. *Nursing Forum*, **5**(3): 64–73.

Menzies I E P (1960a) A case study in the functioning of social systems as a defence against anxiety. *Human Relations*, **13**: 95–120.

Menzies I E P (1960b) *The Functioning of Social Systems as a Defence against Anxiety*. London: Tavistock.

Menzies I E P (1960c) Nurses under stress: a social system functioning as a defence against anxiety. *International Nursing Review*, **7**(6): 9–16.

Menzies I E P (1960d) *A Case Study in the Functioning of Social Systems as a Defence against Anxiety: A Report of a Study of the Nursing Service in a General Hospital*. Tavistock Pamphlet No. 3, London: Tavistock Institute of Human Relations.

Merchant J (1985) Why task allocation? *Nursing Practice*, **1**(2): 67–71.

Mileur G (1987) Primary nursing revised. *Nursing Management*, **18**(10): 67.

Miller A (1985a) The relationship between nursing theory and nursing practice. *Journal of Advanced Nursing*, **10**: 417–424.

Miller A (1985b) Nurse/patient dependency – is it iatrogenic? *Journal of Advanced Nursing*, **10**: 63–69.

Miller A (1985c) A study of the dependency of elderly patients in wards using different methods of nursing care. *Age and Ageing*, **14**: 132–138.

Miller A E (1979) Nurses' attitudes towards their patients. *Nursing Times*, November 8: 1929–1933.

Millerson G (1964) *The Qualifying Association: A Study in Professionalization*. London: Routledge and Kegan Paul.

Mitchell R G (1988) The emotional cost of nursing. *Nursing*, 3rd series, **28**: 1021–1025.

Moores B and Thompson A G H (1986) What 1357 hospital inpatients thought about aspects of their stay in British acute hospitals. *Journal of Advanced Nursing*, **11**: 87–102.

Moos R (1974) *Evaluating Treatment Environments: A Social Ecological Approach*. New York: John Wiley.

Moritz D A (1979) Primary nursing: implications for curriculum development. *Journal of Nurse Education*, **18**(3): 33–37.

Mountain G (1984) *The Planning of Nursing Care for the Individual about to be Discharged from Hospital to Home; a Study at the Descriptive Level*. Unpublished BSc (Hons) project, Polytechnic of the South Bank, London.

Muetzel P A (1988) Therapeutic nursing. In: *Primary Nursing: Nursing in BONDU's*, Pearson A (ed.). London: Croom Helm.

Munson F and Clinton J (1979) Defining nursing assignment patterns. *Nursing Research*, **28**(4): 243–249.

Murray R and Zettner J (1974) *Nursing Concepts for Health Promotion*. Englewood Cliffs, NJ: Prentice Hall.

Naisbitt J (1982) *Megatrends: Ten New Directions Transforming our Lives*. London: Futura, Macdonald.

Nelson M L (1988) Advocacy in nursing. *Nursing Outlook*, **36**(3): 136–141.

Nightingale F (1859) *Notes on Nursing*, 1980 edn. Edinburgh: Churchill Livingstone.

Northedge A (1981) *Studying at University. Social Sciences: a Foundation Course*. Milton Keynes: Open University Press.

Nursing and Midwifery Staffs Negotiating Council Staff Side (1988) *A Guide to the Clinical Grading Structure*.

Nursing Standard (1988) *Understanding Clinical Grading, A Nurse's Guide to the New Pay Structure*. Harrow: Scutari Projects.

Nursing Times (1953a) Royal College of Nursing conferences discusses the College Working Party's comments on the Job Analysis Report. *Nursing Times*, December 5: 1238–1240.

Nursing Times (1953b) Concluding the Royal College of Nursing conference which has been discussing the College working party's comments on the Job Analysis Report. *Nursing Times*, December 12: 1273–1275.

Nursing Times (editorial) (1958) The ward sister's exacting task. *Nursing Times*, February 7: 143–144.

Nursing Times Support Worker training plans condemned (News Item) *Nursing Times* **85**(4): 5.

Oakley A (1981) *Subject Women*. London: Fontana Press.

O'Brien D, Clinto M and Cruddace H (1985) Managing and mismanaging change – the case of the nursing process. *Proceedings of the RCN Research Society Annual Conference*, Hawthorn P (ed.). London: Royal College of Nursing.

Ogier M E (1980) *The Effect of the Ward Sister's Management Style upon Nurse Learners*. PhD thesis, Birkbeck College, University of London.

Olson E M (1979) Strategies and techniques for the nurse change agent. *Nursing Clinics of North America*, **14**: 323–336.

Orem D (1985) *Nursing: Concepts of Practice*. 3rd Edn New York: McGraw-Hill.

Orlando I J (1961) *The Dynamic Nurse–Patient Relationship: Function, Principles and Process*. New York: G P Putnam and Sons.

Orton H D (1981) *Ward Learning Climate*. London: Royal College of Nursing.

Ottaway R M (1976) A change strategy to implement new norms, new style and new environment in the work organisation. *Personnel Review*, Winter, January 5: 13–18.

Otttaway R M (1982) Defining the change agent. In: *Changing Design*, Evans B, Powell J A and Talbot F (eds). Chichester: John Wiley.

Parsons T (1957) *The Social System*. London: Routledge and Kegan Paul.

Pearce C (1988) The nursing workforce. *Senior Nurse*, **8**(3): 25–27.

Pearson A (1974) *Quality Patient Care Scale in Wessex Regional Health Authority*. Report on proceedings of senior staff seminar on quality assurance, Wessex.

Pearson A (1983) *The Clinical Nursing Unit*. London: Heinemann.

Pearson A (1985a) *The Effects of Introducing New Norms in a Nursing Unit and an Analysis of the Process of Change.* Unpublished PhD thesis, Goldsmiths College, London.

Pearson A (1985b) Nursing as change agents and a strategy for change. *Nursing Practice,* **1**(2): 80–84.

Pearson A (ed.) (1987) *Nursing Quality Measurement: Quality Assurance Methods for Peer Review.* Chichester: John Wiley.

Pearson A (1988a) Trends in clinical nursing. In: *Primary Nursing,* Pearson A (ed.). London: Croom Helm.

Pearson A (ed.) (1988b) *Primary Nursing: Nursing in the Burford and Oxford Nursing Development Units.* London: Croom Helm.

Pearson A and Vaughan B (1984) Introducing change into nursing practice. In: *Open University: A Systematic Approach to Nursing Care.* Milton Keynes: Open University Press.

Pearson A and Vaughan B (1986) *Nursing Models for Practice.* London: Heinemann.

Pearson A, Morris P and Whitehouse C (1985) Consumer oriented groups: a new approach to interdisciplinary teaching. *Journal of the Royal College of General Practitioners,* **35**: 381–383.

Pearson A, Durand I and Punter S (1988a) *Therapeutic Nursing: An Evaluation of an Experimental Nursing Unit in the British NHS.* Oxford: Burford and Oxford Nursing Development Units.

Pembrey S (1975) From work routines to patient assignment. *Nursing Times,* **71**(45): 1768–1772.

Pembrey S (1980) *The Ward Sister – Key to Nursing.* London: Royal College of Nursing.

Pembrey S (1984) Nursing care: profession progress. *Journal of Advanced Nursing,* **9**(9): 539–547.

Pembrey S (1987) *District Guidance on Professional Nursing Practice in Oxfordshire.* Unpublished paper, Oxfordshire Health Authority.

Pembrey S (1988) *The Associate Nurse Role.* A guidance paper to the nursing policies group. Unpublished paper, Oxfordshire Health Authority.

Peplau H (1952) *Interpersonal Relations in Nursing.* New York: G P Putnam.

Peplau H (1987) Interpersonal constructs for nursing practice. *Nurse Education Today,* **7**: 201–208.

Per Alderson B-Blyth v. *Birmingham Waterworks Co.* (1856) 11 Ex 781, 784.

Phaneuf M C (1976) *The Nursing Audit: Profile for Excellence.* New York: Appleton-Century-Crofts.

Phillips K (1988) Well managed? *Nursing Standard,* September 3: 22–24.

Pinker R (1966) *English Hospital Statistics: 1861–1938.* London: Heinemann.

Plume, Sister (1989) *Sister Plume's Notes on Nursing.* Basingstoke: Macmillan.

Porter S (1988) Siding with the system. *Nursing Times,* **84**(41): 30–31.

Pratt R J (1988) *AIDS – A Strategy for Nursing Care.* London: Edward Arnold.

Prophit P (1986) *Developing a Philosophy of Nursing: Academic Exercise or Practical Prerequisite for an Effective Nursing Service.* Unpublished seminar given at ONDU, Oxford, February 4.

Punton S (1985) Coping with primary nursing. *Nursing Times,* **81**(1): 50.

RCN (1956) *Observations and Objectives.* London: Royal College of Nursing.

RCN (1981) *A Structure for Nursing.* London: Royal College of Nursing.

RCN (1984) *Nurse Alert.* London: Royal College of Nursing.

RCN (1985) *Commission Nursing Education. The Education of Nurses: A New Dispensation* (Judge Report). London: Royal College of Nursing.

RCN (1986) *A Manifesto for Nursing and Health.* London: Royal College of Nursing.

RCN (1987) *In Pursuit of Excellence: A Position Statement on Nursing.* London: Royal College of Nursing.

Reed S (1986) *A Comparison of Nurse Related Behaviour, Philosophy of Care and Job Satisfaction in Team and Primary Nursing.* Unpublished MSc thesis, Wolverhampton Polytechnic.

Reed S E (1988) A comparison of nurse-related behaviour, philosophy of care and job satisfaction in team and primary nursing. *Journal of Advanced Nursing*, **13**(3): 383–395.

Reiter F (1966) The nurse clinician. *American Journal of Nursing*, February: **66**(2): 274–280.

Revans R W (1964) *Standards for Morale: Cause and Effect in Hospitals*. London: Nuffield Provincial Hospitals Trust.

Riehl J and Roy C (eds) (1980) *Conceptual Models for Nursing Practice*. Norwalk, Conneticut: Appleton-Century-Crofts.

Risser N (1975) Development of an instrument to measure patient satisfaction with nurses and nursing care in primary care settings. *Nursing Research*, **24**(1): 45–52.

Ritter S (1984) Does the team work? *Nursing Times*, **80**(6) 53–55.

Roberts L (1980) Primary nursing. Do patients like it, are nurses more satisfied, does it cost more? *The Canadian Nurse*, December: 20–23.

Roberts C S (1982) Identifying the real patient problems. *Nursing Clinics of North America*, **17**(3): 481–489.

Robinson J and Strong P (1987) *Professional Advice after Griffiths: an Interim Report*. Nursing Policy Studies Centre, University of Warwick.

Robinson K (1983) Talking with clients. In: *Community Health*, Clark J and Henderson J (eds). Edinburgh: Churchill Livingstone.

Robinson K (1989) Loneliness of the long distance runner? *Nursing Times*, **85**(19): 72–73.

Robinson K M (1988) *Primary Nursing: A Discussion Note prepared for the Clinical Practice Development Group*. Unpublished document, Oxford Health Authority, Oxford.

Rogers C R (1967) *On Becoming a Person*. London: Constable.

Rogers M (1970) *An Introduction to the Theoretical Basis of Nursing*. Philadelphia: Davis.

Rogers C (1983) *Freedom to Learn for the 80's*. Columbus, Ohio: Merrill Publishing Co.

Rogers E and Shoemaker F (1971) *Communication of Innovations: A Cross Cultural Approach*. New York: The Free Press of Glencoe.

Rogers J (1987) The future of continuing professional education. *Professional Nurse*, **2**(7): 196.

Rogers J and Lawrence J (1987) *Continuing Professional Education for Qualified Nurse Midwives and Health Visitors*. Peterborough: Ashdale Press.

Rogers R and Salvage J (1988) *Nurses at Risk: A Guide to Health and Safety at Work*. London: Heinemann.

Rosser R R, Denford J, Heslop A, Kinston W, Macklin D and Minty K (1983) Breathlessness and psychiatric morbidity in chronic bronchitis and emphysema: a study of psychotherapeutic management. *Psychological Medicine*, **13**(1): 93–110.

Roy C (1976) *An Introduction to Nursing: An Adaptation Model*. Englewood Cliffs, New Jersey: Prentice Hall.

Rowden R. (1989) Support worker helper or hindrance? *Nursing Times* **85**(8): 52.

Runciman P J (1983) *Ward Sister at Work*. Edinburgh: Churchill Livingstone.

Salmon B (Chairman), Ministry of Health and Scottish Home and Health Department (1966) *Report of the Committee on Senior Nursing Staff Structure*. London: HMSO.

Salvage J (1985) *The Politics of Nursing*. London: Heinemann.

Salvage J (1988a) Professionalization – or struggle for survival? A consideration of current proposals for the reform of nursing in the United Kingdom. *Journal of Advanced Nursing*, **13**(4): 515–519.

Salvage J (1988b) *Partnership in Care? An Exploration of the Theory and Practice of the New Nursing in the UK*. Unpublished MSc dissertation, Royal Holloway and Bedford New College, University of London.

Salvage J (1988c) In the ghetto. *Nursing Times*, **84**(32): 22.

Sandford N (1970) Whatever happened to action research? *Journal of Social Issues*, **26**(4): 3–23.

Schön D (1971) *Beyond the Stable State*. New York: Random House.

Schön D (1983) *The Reflective Practitioner: How Professionals Think in Action*. London: Temple Smith.

Schön D (1987) *Educating the Reflective Practitioner: Toward a New Design for Teaching and Learning in the Professions*. San Francisco: Jossey-Bass.

Schrock R (1987) Professionalism – a critical examination. *Recent Advances in Nursing*, **18**:

12–24.

Schweiger J L (1980) *The Nurse as a Manager*. New York: John Wiley.

Sellick K (1983) Primary nursing: an evaluation of its effects on patient perception of care and staff satisfaction. *International Journal of Nursing Studies*, **20**(4): 265–273.

Shukla R (1981) Structure *vs* people in primary nursing: an inquiry. *Nursing Research*, **30**(4): 236–241.

Shukla R K (1982) Primary or team nursing? Two conditions determine the choice. *Journal of Nursing Administration*, **11**: 12–15.

Shukla R (1983) All-RN model of nursing care delivery: a cost benefit evaluation. *Inquiry*, **XX**: 173–184.

Shukla R K and Turner W E (1984) Patient perception of care under primary and team nursing. *Research in Nursing and Health*, **7**(2): 93–99.

Sigsworth J and Heslop A (1988) Self assessment and the student nurse. *Senior Nurse*, **8**(5): 14–16.

Simms L (1967) *Creating an Educational Climate in Nursing Practice*. New York: National League of Nursing Service Education in Public Health Nursing.

Skeet M (1983) Continuity of care. In: *Community Health*, Clark J and Henderson J (eds). Edinburgh: Churchill Livingstone.

Slack P (1980) What future for the ward sister? *Nursing Times*, November 12: 28–30.

Smith P (1988) The emotional labour of nursing. *Nursing Times*, **84**(44): 50–51.

Smith V M and Bass T A (1982) *Communication for the Health Care Team*. Adapted for the UK by Faulkner A. Cambridge: Harper and Row.

Snee T (1988), Nursing Officer, DHSS (AIDS Unit). Keynote address, 5th International Oncology Conference, September, London.

Sparrow S (1986) Primary nursing. *Nursing Practice*, **1**: 142–148.

Stein L (1978) The doctor nurse game. In: *Readings in the Sociology of Nursing*, Dingwall R and McIntosh J (eds). Edinburgh: Churchill Livingstone.

Stenhouse L (1975) *An Introduction to Curriculum Research and Development*. London: Heinemann.

Stoney M. (1988) 'Stoney slams scandal on ENB Dead-End Jobs' *Nursing Times* (News item) **34**(50): 6.

Stroud R (1989) First-level care by second-level nurses. Nursing Times (letters) **85**(5): 12–13.

Styles M (1982) *On nursing: toward a new endowment*. St. Louis: Mosby & Co.

Swaffield L, Taylor C, Pembrey S and Fitzgerald M (1987) Ever ready . . . or burn out. *Nursing Times*, **83**(12): 24–28.

Timmins N (1988) Pressure is mounting for extra funds to be provided for the nurses. *The Independent*, October 13.

Tingle J H (1988) Patient advocacy: the importance of recognising legal implications (letters). *Nursing Times*, **84**(44): 14.

Travelbee J (1971) *Interpersonal Aspects of Nursing*, 2nd edn. Philadelphia: F A Davies Co.

Truax C B, Altmann H and Millis W A (1974) Therapeutic relationships provided by various professionals. *Journal of Community Psychology*, **2**(1): 33–36.

Tschudin V (1985a) Too much pressure. *Nursing Times*, **81**: 30–31.

Tschudin V (1985b) Warding off crisis. *Nursing Times*, **81**: 45–46.

Turner V W (1969) *The Ritual Process*. Harmondsworth: Penguin.

Tutton L (1986) What is primary nursing? *The Professional Nurse*, November 39–40.

UKCC (1983) *The Nurses, Midwives and Health Visitors Rules Approval Order*. London: UKCC.

UKCC (1984) *Code of Professional Conduct for the Nurse, Midwife and Health Visitor*, 2nd edn. London: UKCC.

UKCC (1986) *Project 2000. A New Preparation for Practice*. London: UKCC.

UKCC (1987a) *Project 2000. The Final Proposals*. Project paper 9. London: UKCC.

UKCC (1987b) Counting the cost. *Senior Nurse*, **7**(1): 25–30.

Urwick L F (1947) *The Elements of Administration*, 2nd edn. London: Pitman.

Vaughan B (1980) *The Newly Qualified Staff Nurse: Factors Affecting Transition*. Unpublished MSc thesis, University of Manchester.

Vaughan B (1986) Bridging the gap, teaching roles in nursing education. *Senior Nurse*, **6**(5): 31.

Ventura M, Fox R, Corley M and Mercurio S (1982) A patient satisfaction measure as a criterion to evaluate primary nursing. *Nursing Research*, **31**(4): 226–231.

Vousden M (1987) Conduct unbecoming. *Nursing Times*, **83**(8): 33–34.

Walters K (1985) Organising nursing care, team nursing. *Nursing Practice*, **1**(1): 7–15.

Wandelt M and Ager J (1974) *Quality Patient Care Scale*. New York: Appleton-Century-Crofts.

Wandelt M and Stewart D (1975) *The Slater Nursing Competencies Rating Scale*. New York: Appleton-Century-Crofts.

Watkin B (1958) Team nursing and professional leadership. *Nursing Times*, February 7: 151–152.

Watson J N (1977a) New management attitudes to the humanisation of work. In: *Humanising the Work Place: New Proposals and Perspectives*, Ottaway R N (ed.). London: Croom Helm.

Watson J (1977b) Primary nursing – nursing care can be patient centred. *The Australian Nurses Journal*, **7**(2): 35–39, 54.

Watson J (1985) *The Philosophy and Science of Caring*. Colorado: Colorado Associated University Press.

Watson T (1987) *Sociology of Work and Industry*. London: Routledge and Kegan Paul.

Watts V H (1980) Ten components of primary nursing. *Nursing Dimensions*, **7**(4): 90–95.

Webb C (1981) Classification and framing: a sociological analysis of task-centered nursing and the nursing process. *Journal of Advanced Nursing*, **6**: 369–376.

Webb C (1986) *Woman's Health: Midwifery and Gynaecological Nursing*. London: Hodder and Stoughton.

Webb C (1987a) Speaking up for advocacy. *Nursing Times*, **83**(34): 33–35.

Webb C (1987b) Professionalism revisited. *Nursing Times*, **83**(35): 39–41.

Weber M (1947) *The Theory of Social and Economic Organization*. New York: Free Press of Glencoe.

Webster C (1988) *The Problems of Health Care: The British NHS before 1957*. London: HMSO.

White R (1984) Altruism is not enough: barriers in the development of nursing as a profession. *Journal of Advanced Nursing*, **9**: 555–562.

White R (1985) *The Effects of the NHS on the Nursing Profession, 1948–1961*. London: King's Fund.

Whittaker E and Oleson V (1978) The faces of Florence Nightingale: functions of the heroine legend in an occupational sub-culture. In: *Readings in the Sociology of Nursing*, Dingwall R and McIntosh J (eds). Edinburgh: Churchill Livingstone.

Wiedenbach E (1964) *Clinical Nursing*. New York: Springer.

Wilensky H (1964) The professionalization of everyone? *The American Journal of Sociology*, LXX(2): 137–157.

Wiles A (1988) Quality of patient care scale. In: *Nursing Quality Measurement: Quality Assurance Methods for Peer Review*, Pearson A (ed.) Chichester: John Wiley.

Williams A (1981) Student learning: team *vs* primary nursing. *Nursing Management*, **12**(9): 48–51.

Wilson-Barnett J (1977) *Patients' Emotional Reactions to Hospitalisation*. PhD thesis, University of London.

Wilson-Barnett J (ed.) (1983) *Patient Teaching*. Recent Advances in Nursing series. Edinburgh: Churchill Livingstone.

Wilson-Barnett J (1984) *Key Functions in Nursing*. London: Royal College of Nursing.

Wilson-Barnett J (1988) Nursing values: exploring the clichés. *Journal of Advanced Nursing*, **13**: 790–796.

Wood, Sir Robert (Chairman) (1947) *Report of the Working Party on the Recruitment and Training of Nurses* (Wood Report), Ministry of Health, Department of Health for Scotland and Ministry of Labour and National Service. London: HMSO.

World Health Organisation (1989) *World Literature on Human Retroviruses and Acquired*

Immunodeficiency Syndrome. Oncology Information Service. 5 March. Leeds University Press.

World Health Organisation (1990) *Weekly Epidemiological Record*, **36**, 7 September

Wright S (1985a) Change in nursing: the application of change theory to practice. *Nursing Practice*, **1**(2): 85–91.

Wright S (1985b) Reflecting on joint appointments. *Senior Nurse*, **3**(6): 8–9.

Wright S (1986) *Building and Using a Model of Nursing*. London: Edward Arnold.

Young J P, Giovannetti P, Lewison D and Thoms M C (1981) *Factors affecting nurse staffing in acute care hospitals: A review and critique of the literature*. DHEW Publication No. HRP 0501801: Hyattsville, MD Dept of Health Education and Welfare.

Yura H and Walsh M (1978) *The Nursing Process*. New York: Appleton-Century-Crofts.

Zander K S (1977) Primary nursing won't work unless the head nurse lets it. *Journal of Nursing Administration*, October 19–23.

Zander K S (1980) *Primary Nursing Development and Management*. Maryland: Aspen Systems Co.

Zander K (1985) Second generation primary nursing: a new agenda. *Journal of Nursing Administration*, March: 18–24.

Zeichener K M (1981) Reflective teaching and field based experience in teacher education. *Interchange*, **12**(4): 1–22.

Index

Absence of primary nurse 7, 71–2, 242
accountability
  24-hour 7
  in absence of primary nurse 242
  assignment methods compared
    patient allocation 10–11
    primary nursing 6–8
    task assignment 12
    team nursing 9
  case example, respirology ward 158, 161
  definitions 61–2
  legal implications 65–7
  preconditions 62
action research project 32
advantages of primary nursing
  management view 213–5
  see also evaluation
advocacy role of nurses, *see* patient advocate
AIDS ward, experience of primary nursing
  in 127–39
alienating aspects of hospital care 22–5, 30
appraisal, staff, *see* staff appraisal
assertiveness of nurses 41–2, 86
assignment methods
  case method 230
  compared 3–5
  patient allocation 10–11
  primary nursing 6–9
  task assignment 12–13
  team nursing 9–10
associate nurse
  in absence of primary nurse 7, 71–2, 242
  accountability 7
  educational preparation 56
  job description 264–7
  liaison with primary nurse when on night
    duty 245
  role, case examples
    AIDS ward 136–7
    continuing care unit 121
    psychiatric unit 146
    respirology ward 159
    surgical unit 82–3
  stress 189–90, 205
authority 158
  assignment methods compared
    patient allocation 10–11

    primary nursing 7
    task assignment 12
    team nursing 9
  definition 61
  delegation 67–8
autonomy
  assignment methods compared
    patient allocation 10–11
    primary nursing 7
    task assignment 12
    team nursing 9
  definitions 61, 220
auxiliaries, *see* nursing auxiliaries

Benefits of primary nursing
  management view 213–5
  see also evaluation
Briggs Committee (1972) 18
bureaucracy as an alienating aspect 22–3

Care
  continuity, *see* continuity of care
  co-ordination 178–9
  giver, *see* care giver
  planning, *see* care planning
  plans, *see* care plans
  quality, *see* quality of care
  standards 214–5
care assistant
  job description 269–71
  role 72
care giver
  assignment methods compared
    patient allocation 11
    primary nursing 8
    task assignment 12–13
    team nursing 10
  unqualified 258–9
care planning
  assignment methods compared
    patient allocation 11
    primary nursing 8
    task assignment 12–13
    team nursing 10
  need for contact with patient 178
care plans
  accountability of the primary nurse 69

case examples
    continuing care unit 123
    medical ward 96–7
    psychiatric unit 145
  as means of communication 230–1
  disregard of 204
  and nursing process notes 55–6
case examples
    AIDS ward 127–39
    continuing care unit 117–25
    disabled unit 103–16
    medical ward 87–102
    psychiatric unit 141–51
    respirology ward 153–64
    surgical unit 77–86
case load
  case examples
    AIDS ward 133
    medical unit 90
    surgical unit 82
  monitoring and control 257
case method 230
change
  action plan 36–7
  action research project 32
  agents 33–5
  approach, bottom-up versus top-down 33–4
  and culture 40–1
  forces affecting 47
  introduction and management of 31–48
  norms 31–2, 42
  planning and preparation, case examples
    AIDS ward 132–3
    continuing care unit 117–20
    disabled unit 108–11
    medical unit 87, 94–6
    surgical unit 79–81
  resistance to 35–40, 45–7
  in responsibilities 67–71
  strategies 31–2, 32–3, 45–6
  subsequent training 43–5
  viewing change 39
charge nurse, see ward sister
checklists, patient perceptions 170
clients, see patients
clinical grading review 200–2
Code of Nursing Ethics 29
Code of Professional Conduct 29, 62–3, 72
communication
  assignment methods compared
    patient allocation 11
    primary nursing 9
    task assignment 13
    team nursing 10
  care plan as means of 230–1
  case examples
    AIDS ward 133–4
    continuing care unit 122–4
    disabled unit 113
    medical unit 95, 96–8
  collegial 225
  development of skills 55
  network, see Primary Nursing Network

notice boards 89, 98
nurse/medical staff, see medical staff
nurse/nurse 44, 223–4, 230–1
nurse/patient, see nurse/patient relationship
concepts of primary nursing 4–5
continuing care unit, experience of primary
  nursing in 117–25
continuity of care
  assignment methods compared
    patient allocation 11
    primary nursing 8
    task assignment 12
    team nursing 9–10
  case examples
    medical ward 97–8
    surgical unit 83, 85
contract learning 59, 234–5
contribution of primary nursing 30
co-ordination of care 178–9
co-ordinator
  case examples
    AIDS ward 134
    medical unit 90–2
    surgical unit 84–5
  job description 91–2
  role 44, 243
coping with stress 186, 194
cost of implementing primary nursing 259
courses, see education
culture and change 40–1

Decentralised management 159
decision making 144, 158–9, 231–2
definitions
  accountability 61–2
  authority 61
  autonomy 61, 220
  primary nursing 4, 252–3
  responsibility 61
dehumanisation of hospital care 21–30
delegation of authority 67–8
demographic changes 227
Department of Health, support for primary
  nursing 241
development
  of primary nursing 19–21, 218
  of staff, see education
Director of Nursing Services (DNS), view of
  primary nursing 207–15
disabled unit, experience of primary nursing
  in 103–16
disadvantages of primary nursing, see evaluation
DNS, see Director of Nursing Services
doctors, see medical staff

Economic considerations 259
  funding education 203, 234
education
  associate nurses 56–9
  case examples
    continuing care unit 121, 122
    disabled unit 107, 109
    medical unit 99

respirology ward 162–3
  surgical unit 81
after change 43–5
communication skills 55
content 54–6
contract learning 59, 234–5
conversion courses for second level
  nurses 246–7
counselling 231
funding 203, 234
independent learning 49–50
philosophy of 51–2
primary nursing module 56–9
research 228–9
resources 233–4
specialist knowledge 55
study leave 234
theory and methods 52–4, 232–3
see also learning
Enrolled nurse, see second level nurse
establishment, see staffing levels and structure
evaluation 47–8, 206–7
  case examples
    AIDS ward 138–9
    continuing care unit 124–5
    disabled unit 111–16
    medical ward 100–2
    psychiatric unit 150–1
    respirology ward 163–4
    surgical unit 85–6
  methods, see quality of care
  of primary nursing 253–5

Feedback of performance 43, 44
funding of education 203, 234

General manager 250
  attitude to primary nursing 213
  and available resources 214
Goddard Report (1953) 16

Handover, case examples
  medical unit 97
  respirology ward 159–60
health of nurses 185
history of hospital nursing 13–21
Horder Committee (1942–1949) 15
hospital care
  alienating aspects 22–5, 30
  history 13–21
  humanisation 21–30
humanisation of hospital care 21–5
  a nursing response 25–30
humanism 28
humanistic philosophy 51–2

'Ideal types' of nurse assignment methods 5–6
implications
  for education 227–37
  for management 197–215
  for the nurse 183–95
  for the patient 167–81

Job descriptions
  associate nurse 264–7
  auxiliary, nursing 268–9
  care assistant, ward 269–71
  co-ordinator 91–2
  nursing auxiliary 268–9
  primary nurse 263–4
  ward care assistant 269–71
  ward sister 267–8
job satisfaction 26, 257
job sharing 155
joint appointments 236

King's Fund Primary Nursing Network, see
  Primary Nursing Network

Layout of ward, see ward structure and layout
leadership 249, 250
learning 162
  contracts 59, 234–5
  environment 233–5
  theory 232–3
  see also education
lecturer practitioner 236
legal issues 62–73
link teacher 236
Loeb Centre 20

Management
  decentralised 159
  Director of Nursing Services' viewpoint
    207–15
  nurse manager's viewpoint 199–207
  principles of 197–8
  role of senior nurse 71
  structure and power 221–2
  ward management in a psychiatric unit 147–8
  work organisation 198–9
manpower, see staffing levels
medical staff
  involvement in change process 43, 119
  relationship with nursing staff 66–7, 81,
    212–3, 222–3
medical ward, experience of primary nursing
  in 87–102
medication, administration of 159
mentor 235–6
morale 256
multidisciplinary teams
  case examples
    AIDS ward 134
    community hospital 202
    continuing care unit 123–4
    disabled unit 110, 115–6
    psychiatric unit 146
    respirology ward 155, 160
    surgical unit 81
  management view 210–3, 214–5
  relationships within 222–3

Needs of nurses 183, 184–5
negligence 63–4, 66
network, see Primary Nursing Network

night duty 244–5
    case examples
        AIDS ward 132
        continuing care unit 121–2
        medical unit 97
        surgical unit 83
night sister, role 208
norms, changing work norms 31–2, 42
notice boards 89, 98
nurse assignment, *see* assignment methods
nurse–client relationship, *see* nurse–patient
    relationship
nurse manager, view of primary nursing 199–207
nurse–patient relationship
    case examples
        AIDS ward 135–6
        disabled unit 110–11
        psychiatric unit 143–5, 147
        respirology ward 160–2
        surgical unit 83–4
    contact 176–8
    emotional involvement 205
    negotiation 144
    separation 149–50
    social environment 179–80
    stress 135–6, 184
nurse teacher 236–7
Nursing Audit 172
nursing auxiliaries
    as carers 258–9
    job description 268–9
    role 72
    stress 190–1
nursing officer, role 208

Off-duty rota, case examples
    AIDS ward 138
    continuing care unit 121
    medical ward 92, 93–4
    respirology ward 156–7
    surgical unit 80–1
operational definition of primary nursing 252–3

Patient advocate 29, 30, 210
patient allocation 10–11
patient orientation 17–19, 77, 178–80
patients
    participation in own care 27
    perceptions 169–170
    satisfaction 168–70
    surveys 169, 170
    teaching 178–9
    welfare 255
    well-being 174–6
performance indicators 173–4
performance review, *see* staff appraisal
Phaneuf's Nursing Audit 172
pilot site, case for 45
planning
    care, *see* care planning; care plans
    change, *see under* change
power 217–26
primary nurse

absence of, *see* absence of primary nurse
accountability for care planning and
        implementation 68–9
    as care giver 8
    education of 56–9
    job description 263–4
    learning needs 50–1
    and nursing process notes 55–6
    relationship with medical and paramedical
        staff, *see* medical staff
    relationship with other nurses 44
    role, case examples
        AIDS ward 136
        medical unit 96
        psychiatric unit 142–3
        surgical unit 82
    skills required 245–6
    see also primary nurse, job description
    standards 47–8
    stress 187–9, 210
Primary Nursing Network 241, 251–2, 261
principles of primary nursing 3–9, 27–30
    applied to education 229–32
professional conduct, *see Code of Professional
    Conduct*
professionalisation 218–9
    as an alienating aspect 24–5
professionalism 28–9, 219
Project 2000 227–8, 244, 258
psychiatric unit, experience of primary nursing
    in 141–51

Quality of care
    attributes 4
    performance indicators 173–4
    Phaneuf's Nursing Audit 172
    Qualpacs (Quality of patient care scale) 171
    results of studies 172
    Rush/Medicus quality measuring
        methodology 171
    Slater nursing performance rating scale 171–2
Qualpacs (Quality of patient care scale) 171
questionnaire, patient satisfaction 169

Recruitment and retention 259
reflection (thought) 44–5, 58
research
    nursing education 228–9
    primary nursing 252–5
respirology ward, experience of primary nursing
    in 153–64
responsibility
    assignment methods compared
        patient allocation 10–11
        primary nursing 6–7
        task assignment 12
        team nursing 9
    definition 61
    devolved from management 209
    legal implications 67–9
Risser patient satisfaction scale 169–70
Rush/Medicus quality measuring
    methodology 171

Second level nurse
  Enrolled nurse 118, 121
  as primary nurse 246–7
  suitability for associate nurse role 245–8
senior nurse, responsibilities 69–71
shift co-ordinator, *see* co-ordinator
sister, *see* ward sister
Slater nursing performance rating scale 171–2
staff appraisal 207
  case examples
    continuing care unit 123
    surgical ward 86
staff development, *see* education
staff nurse, stress 191–3
staff support
  case examples
    AIDS ward 133, 136
    continuing care unit 120
    medical ward 99–100
    respirology ward 161
  groups 194
  management implications 203–6
  role of ward sister 192
  support structures 248–50
  systems and strategies 193–4
staffing levels and structure
  case examples
    AIDS ward 128–31, 132
    community hospital 200–2
    continuing care unit 117
    disabled unit 105–6
    medical ward 88–90
    psychiatric unit 148–9
    respirology ward 155, 158
    surgical unit 80
  recruitment and retention 259
  staff shortage 243–4
standards 47–8, 214–5
strategic planning 248
A Strategy for nursing 241–2
stress 161, 183–95, 210
  associate nurse 189–90, 205
  coping with 186, 194
  management of 203–6
  nurse-patient relationship 135–6, 184
  nursing auxiliaries 190–1
  peer relationships 204
  primary nurse 187–9, 210
  staff nurse 191–3
  student nurse 231
  ward sister 191–3
student nurses
  case examples
    medical unit 99
    psychiatric unit 143
    respirology ward 158, 159, 163
    surgical unit 83
  research 228–9
  role 235
  stress 231
  supernumerary status 228

study leave 234
support, *see* staff support
support services 203–4, 211–2
support worker 72, 247–8, 258–9
surgical unit, experience of primary nursing
  in 77–86
survey of patients 169, 170

Task assignment 12–13
task orientation 18–19, 179–80, 186, 213–4
team, multidisciplinary, *see* multidisciplinary team
team nursing 9–10
technology as an alienating aspect 24
theory adaptation to practice 242
therapeutic aspects of nursing 175–6, 179–80
training, *see* education

Unit Executive 211–2, 213

Vicarious liability 64–5, 66

Ward care assistant, *see* care assistant
ward co-ordinator, *see* co-ordinator
ward philosophy 79–80
ward sister
  educational resources, responsibility for 234
  job description 267–8
  job sharing 155
  as leader 208, 250–1
  liaison with primary nurse when on night
    duty 245
  as manager 65–6
  position of power 221
  relationship with medical staff 212–3
  role, case examples
    AIDS ward 137–8
    continuing care unit 120–1
    disabled unit 106–7
    medical ward 92
    psychiatric unit 147
    respirology ward 160
  and staff support 192
  stress 191–3
  as supervisor 70
  support from management 209–10
  as teacher 231–2, 236–7
  ward structure and layout, case examples
    AIDS ward 129–30
    continuing care unit 118
    disabled unit 103–4
    medical ward 88, 89
    respirology ward 153–5
    surgical unit 78–9
welfare
  of nurse 255
  of patient 255
Wood Report (1947) 15
work norms, changing 31–2, 42
work organisation
  effect on pattern of care 176–7
  and management 198–9